MW00861457

Early Vocal Contact and Preterm Infant Brain Development

Manuela Filippa • Pierre Kuhn • Björn Westrup
Editors

Early Vocal Contact and Preterm Infant Brain Development

Bridging the Gaps Between Research and Practice

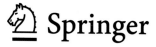 Springer

Editors
Manuela Filippa
Independent Researcher
Aosta, Italy

Björn Westrup
Karolinska Institute
Stockholm, Sweden

Pierre Kuhn
Médecine et Réanimation du
    Nouveau-né Hôpital de Hautepierre
CHU
Strasbourg, France

Laboratoire de Neurosciences
    Cognitives et Adaptatives
CNRS-Université de Strasbourg
Strasbourg, France

ISBN 978-3-319-65075-3   ISBN 978-3-319-65077-7   (eBook)
DOI 10.1007/978-3-319-65077-7

Library of Congress Control Number: 2017953386

© Springer International Publishing AG 2017
This work is subject to copyright. All rights are reserved by the Publisher, whether the whole or part of the material is concerned, specifically the rights of translation, reprinting, reuse of illustrations, recitation, broadcasting, reproduction on microfilms or in any other physical way, and transmission or information storage and retrieval, electronic adaptation, computer software, or by similar or dissimilar methodology now known or hereafter developed.
The use of general descriptive names, registered names, trademarks, service marks, etc. in this publication does not imply, even in the absence of a specific statement, that such names are exempt from the relevant protective laws and regulations and therefore free for general use.
The publisher, the authors and the editors are safe to assume that the advice and information in this book are believed to be true and accurate at the date of publication. Neither the publisher nor the authors or the editors give a warranty, express or implied, with respect to the material contained herein or for any errors or omissions that may have been made. The publisher remains neutral with regard to jurisdictional claims in published maps and institutional affiliations.

Printed on acid-free paper

This Springer imprint is published by Springer Nature
The registered company is Springer International Publishing AG
The registered company address is: Gewerbestrasse 11, 6330 Cham, Switzerland

Foreword

The newborn infant has generally been assumed to lack sensory awareness and consciousness and the word infant actually comes from the Latin for someone who cannot speak. In the past, parents were advised to leave their infants in a dark room and not to cuddle them and clinicians assumed that infants were not conscious of pain and did not require analgesia. The infant brain was assumed to be very immature, with relatively low activity, particularly in the cortex. Since then, several studies have demonstrated that infants are not only aware of pain, but also of different smells and auditory and visual impressions. They fulfill several criteria for being conscious, although this is at a minimal level (Lagercrantz, 2016; Zelazo, 2004). When infants are awake, they are aware of themselves and their environment and they can imitate facial and manual gestures (Meltzoff & Moore, 1977), feel emotions and express joy. They can also remember vowels and the language rhythms and music they heard before birth.

The infant brain is very active, and not a blank slate as earlier believed, with spontaneous resting state activity, particularly in the somatosensory, visual and auditory areas (Fransson, Aden, Blennow, Lagercrantz, 2011). The default mode network is starting to be formed (Doria et al., 2010). A newborn brain requires about 50% of the infant's blood sugar, compared to 20% in an adult. There is also very active synaptogenesis, which is of crucial importance for storing memories (Bourgeois, 2010).

But what about preterm infants, who are less awake and not as aware of their environment as infants born at term? They look at human faces longer than anything else and protect themselves with their hands if they feel threatened. They react to pain at a cortical level, indicating that they may be aware of it from at least 23 weeks of gestation (Garcia-Larrea & Jackson, 2016). From that week, the thalamocortical connections are established (Vanhatalo & Lauronen, 2006) and sensory impressions from the eyes, ears and the skin can be transmitted to the cerebral cortex. It is then important for the infant to be stimulated and to feel attached to their parents as they did to their mother in the womb.

Preterm infants who have been isolated in incubators with limited contact have been reported to display delayed language development (Pineda et al., 2014).

Therefore, it is so important to care for the infant by providing skin-to-skin contact and talking to them. Singing seems to be even more important, particularly calming the baby with lullabies. This interaction has probably happened since the beginning of human evolution.

These fundamental social interactions between the parents and their offspring may be disturbed by all the gadgets in the modern home, including the way that social media has replaced other forms of communication. This is even worse in the neonatal ward, where hi-tech equipment has replaced many human functions. Therefore, I welcome this book on the importance of early vocal contact for brain development, particularly of the preterm infant.

Although preterm infants cannot provide verbal feedback, it is possible to get some idea about their consciousness by studying their "the sucking, looking, touching, tracking, reaching and grasping", as pointed out by Colwyn Trevarthen in the first chapter of this book. Infants soon interact with their parents with proto-conversation and "share musical expressions…combining poetic narratives with actions of the body in universal human ways, which lead to learning of culture-specific habits".

Before it is even born, the infant has started to learn its mother's tongue, particularly the vowels and the metric of the language. American and Swedish newborn infants display different sucking patterns when they hear the vowels that are characteristic of their two languages (Chap. 2). Another indication that infants learn language in the womb is that French newborn infants cry with a rising pitch, while German newborn infants demonstrate a falling pitch, both of which correlate to the pitch of their native languages (Mampe, Friederici, Christophe, & Wermke, 2009).

Mothers talk to preverbal infants with a variable pitch and loudness and a greater sense of rhythm and warmer vocal tone than when they speak to adults. Infant-irected singing is more effective than infant-directed speech for stimulating emotions and arousal, according to Sandra Trehub (Chap. 3). Mothers sing to their infants in all cultures, which is why this process is probably driven by a biological instinct.

Intimacy and closeness between parents and very young infants form the basis of the protolinguistic system (Chap. 4) and the perception of emotion in their voice also seems to be important (Chap. 5).

The fetus perceives its environment as quiet, but complex. Once they are born, infants listen to speech longer than to artificial sounds, even if they display the same pitch contours. They recognize their mother's voice, which seems to be of particular importance, and prefer it to the voice of a stranger (Chap. 6). The loud, high frequency and artificial sounds in the neonatal intensive care unit (NICU) may disrupt their behavioral well-being (Chap. 7). Early live vocal contact is very important and essential for the foundation of bonding and attachment (Chap. 8). It also facilitates sleep and the organization of behavioral states.

There are several programs of ultra-early interventions described in this book: developmental care (Chap. 17), kangaroo or skin-to-skin care and family nurture intervention (Chap. 15). Most of the interventions are "cue-based" rather than "protocol-based". The first two will be quite familiar to readers. The third, family nurture intervention, emphasizes the vocal exchange of deep emotions and is based on the Pavlovian theory of co-conditioning and Tinbergen's four questions, which explore causation, ontogeny, function and evolution.

There is now biophysical evidence that the newborn infant is much more aware and conscious than we earlier believed. Nociceptive signals reach the somatosensory area and cingulus gyrus. There is also spontaneous brain activity, particularly in the somato-sensory, auditory and visual areas, although this is lower in the areas where we store our episodic memories for the future (Chap. 14).

A specific section of this book deals with empowering parents, so that they sing to their infants (Chap. 12), and music therapists discuss how to encourage parents to do this (Chap. 13).

Caring routines, including talking and singing to the infant, may have biological effects, based on epigenetic mechanisms. Animal experiments have shown that suboptimal caring increases methylation, which silences the gene and leads to the increased expression of glucocorticoid receptors and higher stress reactivity (Meaney & Szyf, 2005). The serotonin transporter gene is another key epigenetic regulator that is affected by early adverse experiences. Thus, good infant care that involves a lot of talking and singing may have a protective on DNA and even reverse it (Chap. 16).

This is a unique book that describes the phenomena and mechanisms of vocal interaction with infants, particularly preterm infants, and their practical and clinical implications. It reviews a number of studies that show the importance that exposing infants to talking and singing during early life has on brain development. It also presents practical guidelines on how to encourage parents to talk and sing to their baby. This seems to be more important than ever these days, when many parents communicate more frequently by using social media than by direct personal interaction. This comprehensive book is a real tour-de-force and should be read by all professionals working with infants. It will also be of great interest to new parents, particularly if their infant is born premature.

Hugo Lagercrantz, MD, PhD, Senior Professor
Karolinska Institute and
Astrid Lindgren Children's Hospital,
Solna, Sweden

References

Bourgeois, J.-P. (2010). The neonatal synaptic big bang. In H. Lagercrantz, M. Hanson, L. R. Ment, & D. Peebles (Eds.), *The newborn brain* (2nd ed., pp. 71–84). Cambridge, UK: Cambridge University Press.

Doria, V., Beckmann, C. F., Arichi, T., Merchant, N., Groppo, M., Turkheimer, F. E., et al. (2010). Emergence of resting state networks in the preterm human brain. *Proceedings of the National Academy of Sciences of the United States of America, 107*(46), 20015–20020.

Fransson, P., Aden, U., Blennow, M., & Lagercrantz, H. (2011). The functional architecture of the infant brain as revealed by resting-state fMRI. *Cerebral Cortex, 21*(1), 145–154.

Garcia-Larrea, L., & Jackson, P. (Eds.). (2016). *Pain and the conscious brain. Pain and the Conscious Brain*. Philadelphia, PA: IASP Press/Wolters Kluwer Health.

Lagercrantz, H. (2016). *Infant brain development*. Springer Nature: Cham.

Mampe, B., Friederici, A. D., Christophe, A., & Wermke, K. (2009). Newborns' cry melody is shaped by their native language. *Current Biology, 19*(23), 1994–1997.

Meaney, M. J., & Szyf, M. (2005). Maternal care as a model for experience-dependent chromatin plasticity? *Trends in Neurosciences, 28*, 456–463.

Meltzoff, A. N., & Moore, M. K. (1977). Imitation of facial and manual gestures by human neonates. *Science, 198*(4312), 75–78.

Pineda, R. G., Neil, J., Dierker, D., et al. (2014). Alterations in brain structure and neurodevelopmental outcomes in preterm infants hospitalized in different neonatal intensive care unit environments. *The Journal of Pediatrics, 164*, 52–60.

Vanhatalo, S., & Lauronen, L. (2006). Neonatal SEP – Back to bedside with basic science. *Seminars in Fetal & Neonatal Medicine, 11*(6), 464–470.

Zelazo, P. (2004). The development of conscious control in childhood. *Trends in Cognitive Sciences, 8*, 12–17.

Preface

The dramatic and continuous increase of survival of infants prematurely born over the last decade is very much due to the development of medical care and technological equipment that "inadvertently" led to separation of infants from their mothers. Despite this improvement in medical outcomes, vulnerable preterm infants remain at risk of altered neurodevelopment and it appears now essential to promote early, prolonged and as continuous as possible, contact between the infant and his/her parents. There is a growing consensus that the outcome of neonatal intensive care can be enhanced even further by not only perform needed tasks *upon* the infant but to do them in a collaborative manner *together* with infants and parents – moving from primarily task-oriented care to relationship based care. Subsequently, there is an increasing acceptance to invite parents to the nurseries and involve them in the caregiving and decision-making – empowering parents. It promotes continuity in the practical handling of the infant and, more importantly, it ensures the benefits of deep emotional contact with the infant that only parents can provide. This includes of course, skin-to-skin contact, breastfeeding and, early vocal contact to which this book is dedicated.

The main goal of this manual is to enlighten knowledge gained in the last decades on early vocal interactions with preterm babies. It aims first to clarify the multiple biological processes underlying the effects of early vocal contact in the normal development of fetuses, newborns, and in infants prematurely born. Second, it addresses the question of the efficiency of this intervention in preterm infants - in the Neonatal Intensive Care environment and according to preterm infants auditory, social and communicative development.

This book has to be considered in the broad context of developmentally supportive and family centered care. It is on maternal voice. However, with some exceptions, readers can substitute maternal voice, or maternal vocal contact, with parental voice, or vocal contact. The exceptions are linked to the specific role that the maternal voice has for fetuses during gestation. The father's and other caregiver's voice, in fact, are much less present that the mother's voice during pregnancy and gradually increase their role during infant development. However, the progressive increase in paternal presence can ensure the fundamental role of both parents.

This book is a multidisciplinary work with crossed views form different horizons. It navigates from theoretical perspectives to careful evaluation of specific implementations of early interventions, from neuroscientific data on cortical integration to behavioral analyses of social communication and interaction. This collaborative approach is a source of enrichment which lead also to constructive discussions and maybe partial controversies on some aspects between chapters. However, taken together all the chapters share a humane approach supporting close contact between infants and parents.

Obviously, the future health and development of prematurely born infants are depending both on sophisticated medical/technical care and also on parental involvement in the caregiving. As editors, we would like to draw the attention of the readers to one important point to keep in mind when considering the collaboration between professionals and parents to support early vocal contact. This intervention should be tailored to the physiological maturation and development of the infant, the infant's current medical condition as well as to the mental state of the parents. There is an enormous difference between a two-week-old infant born after 32 weeks of gestation without any technical support and a four-day-old infant born after 23 weeks on mechanical ventilation. Most of the reports in this book are based on studies of the more mature and stable infants. Hence, to guarantee the safety of the infant, parental vocalization in the NICU, as all interventions, must be adjusted to the need of the individual infant and family. This can only be ensured if the nursery can provide care according to infant-and family-centered developmentally supportive care principles, e.g., having staff trained in and providing guidelines based on Newborn Individualized Care and Assessment Program.

As editors, it has been very rewarding to reflect and interact with all authors. However, we should also bear in mind the other specialists, whose expertise in the field would have placed them as legitimate authors, but for different reasons were not able to contribute to the book. We hope that also the readers will enjoy reading about the various topics of the chapters, gaining new insights and that the book will contribute to support the future preterm infant's brain development and the strength and resilience of their families.

Aosta, Italy	Manuela Filippa
Strasbourg, France	Pierre Kuhn
Stockholm, Sweden	Björn Westrup

Contents

Contributors

Natascia Bertoncelli Neonatal Intensive Care Unit, Department of Medical and Surgical Sciences of Mothers, Children and Adults, University of Modena & Reggio Emilia, Modena, Italy

Joy V. Browne University of Colorado, School of Medicine, Center for Family & Infant Interaction, Aurora, CO, USA

Fielding Graduate University Santa Barbara, Santa Barbara, CA, USA

Emmanuel Devouche Laboratoire de Psychopathologie et Processus de Santé (LPPS), Institut de Psychologie - Université Paris Descartes, Paris, France

André Dufour Laboratoire de Neurosciences Cognitives et Adaptatives, CNRS-Université de Strasbourg, Strasbourg, France

Fabrizio Ferrari Neonatal Intensive Care Unit, Department of Medical and Surgical Sciences of Mothers, Children and Adults, University of Modena & Reggio Emilia, Modena, Italy

Manuela Filippa Independent Researcher, Aosta, Italy

Didier Grandjean Department of Psychology and Educational Sciences and Swiss Center for Affective Sciences, University of Geneva, Geneva, Switzerland

Maya Gratier Laboratoire Ethologie, Cognition, Développement, Université Paris Nanterre, Nanterre, France

Friederike Haslbeck Clinic of Neonatology at University Hospital Zurich and University Hospital Bern, Bern, Switzerland

Pernilla Hugoson University of Jyväskylä, Finland and Karolinska Institute, Solna, Sweden

Pierre Kuhn Médecine et Réanimation du Nouveau-né Hôpital de Hautepierre, CHU, Strasbourg, France

Laboratoire de Neurosciences Cognitives et Adaptatives, CNRS-Université de Strasbourg, Strasbourg, France

Laura Lucaccioni Neonatal Intensive Care Unit, Department of Medical and Surgical Sciences of Mothers, Children and Adults, University of Modena & Reggio Emilia, Modena, Italy

Robert J. Ludwig Nurture Science Program, Department of Pediatrics, Columbia University Medical Center, New York, NY, USA

Christine Moon Pacific Lutheran University, Department of Psychology, Tacoma, WA, USA

Rosario Montirosso 0-3 Centre for the at-Risk Infant, Scientific Institute, IRCCS Eugenio Medea, Bosisio Parini, LC, Italy

Luca Ori Neonatal Intensive Care Unit, Department of Medical and Surgical Sciences of Mothers, Children and Adults, University of Modena & Reggio Emilia, Modena, Italy

M. Kathleen Philbin Independent Researcher, Moorestown, NJ, USA

Livio Provenzi 0-3 Centre for the at-Risk Infant, Scientific Institute, IRCCS Eugenio Medea, Bosisio Parini, LC, Italy

Stéphane Rioualen Université de Brest, LIEN (EA 4685), Brest, France; CHRU Brest, Pôle de la Femme de la Mère et de l'Enfant, Brest, France

Jean-Michel Roué Université de Brest, LIEN (EA 4685), Brest, France; CHRU Brest, Pôle de la Femme de la Mère et de l'Enfant, Brest, France

Helen Shoemark Temple University, Philadelphia, PA, USA

Jacques Sizun Université de Brest, LIEN (EA 4685), Brest, France; CHRU Brest, Pôle de la Femme de la Mère et de l'Enfant, Brest, France

James E. Swain Department of Psychiatry and Psychology, Stony Brook University Medical Center, Stony Brook, NY, USA

Giovanna Talucci Neonatal Intensive Care Unit, Department of Medical and Surgical Sciences of Mothers, Children and Adults, University of Modena & Reggio Emilia, Modena, Italy

Sandra E. Trehub University of Toronto, Mississauga, Mississauga, ON, Canada

Colwyn Trevarthen University of Edinburgh, Edinburgh, UK

Martha G. Welch Nurture Science Program, Department of Pediatrics, Columbia University Medical Center, New York, NY, USA

Claire Zores Médecine et Réanimation du Nouveau-né Hôpital de Hautepierre, CHU Strasbourg, Strasbourg, France

Laboratoire de Neurosciences Cognitives et Adaptatives, CNRS-Université de Strasbourg, Strasbourg, France

About the Editors

Manuela Filippa Ph.D., is an independent researcher. She collaborates with a number of Universities and Research Centers. Dr. Filippa has a rich and varied experience in the field of early musical interventions with infants and parents. Her research activity focuses mainly on bio-behavioral effects of singing on preterm and newborn infants, early vocal contact, non-verbal vocal communication abilities and ontogenesis of musical experiences.

Pierre Kuhn MD, Ph.D., is Professor of Pediatrics and Neonatology at the University of Strasbourg, head of the NICU at Hautepierre Hospital. He is also researcher at the Institut de Neurosciences Cellulaires et Intégratives, CNRS Strasbourg, France. Pr. Kuhn is interested in individualized developmental care implementation and research. He has conducted research in the field of sensory system development in preterm infants.

Björn Westrup MD, Ph.D., is Senior Consultant and Lecturer at the Karolinska Institute and Director of the Newborn Individualized Developmental Care and Assessment Programme at Astrid Lindgren Children's Hospital, Karolinska University Hospital in Stockholm, Sweden. Dr. Westrup's field of research focusses on medical and physiological aspects of developmentally supportive care, family-centered care, and iron metabolism. He has been director of the Karolinska NIDCAP Training Center since its founding in 1999.

Part I
The Maternal Voice: A Link Between Fetal and Neonatal Period

Chapter 1
Maternal Voice and Communicative Musicality: Sharing the Meaning of Life from Before Birth

Colwyn Trevarthen

"Let the child lead the way"

Maori proverb, New Zealand

Abstract A mother talking and playing with her infant a few weeks old shares delicate patterns of movement with her child, matching rhythms and expressions of emotion. The infant is an active, sensitive, and creative partner, often taking the lead. The dynamics and affections or emotions of their relating depend on innate adaptations for moving the human body rhythmically to sustain vitality and for communicating their regulations of an intelligent life by shared motives and feelings. Mothers' affectionate speech is "musical" in ways adapted to fit with and celebrate the expressive impulses and feelings of the baby seeking company. Applying methods of acoustics physics, a musician Stephen Malloch developed a microanalysis of the "communicative musicality" both mother and infant enjoy in their vocal play. He traced how parameters of sound he identified in their voices were represented in proto-conversations of the first 2 months after a full-term birth and then how the impulse to share musical expressions invents playful rituals combining poetic narratives with actions of the body in universal human ways, which lead to learning of culture-specific habits and a language. Innate motives for the discovery of meaning in companionship that appear in the first efforts of a human self to share life in movement with affectionate friends constitute an essential support for any sensitive therapeutic care or education that adults may offer for a

Trevarthen, C. (2017, in press) Maternal voice and communicative musicality: Sharing the meaning of life from before birth. For "Maternal Voice Intervention and Preterm Infant's Brain Development". Edited by Manuela Filippa, Pierre Kuhn and Björn Westrup. Springer, Chapter 1.

C. Trevarthen (✉)
University of Edinburgh, Edinburgh, UK
e-mail: c.trevarthen@ed.ac.uk

© Springer International Publishing AG 2017
M. Filippa et al. (eds.), *Early Vocal Contact and Preterm Infant Brain Development*, DOI 10.1007/978-3-319-65077-7_1

developing child, especially for a prematurely born baby (Trevarthen and Fresquez, Body, Movement and Dance in Psychotherapy, 2015; Trevarthen and Malloch, The Nordic Journal of Music Therapy 9(2), 3–17, 2000).

Introduction: Accepting Neonatal Human Nature for Enjoyment of Shared Life

This article presents a provocative message which I hope will encourage delight in the strengths of a prematurely born infant, even though there will be concern that the process of development may not follow a full normal course and expert medical advice will be important.

Medical interventions to give direct aid to vital functions of the child's body may be essential for their survival, but at the same time, there are already formed capacities for engaging with the infant's mind in emotional ways with shared purposes or hopes of playful communication. I cite the clear message of the philosopher Barbara Goodrich (2010) and the psychologist Marc Wittmann (2009) that brain science must give attention to the vital processes that generate and regulate movements in measures of purposeful time, and I have summarized the findings that just these functions are the first to develop in a fetus. Attention of a rational psychology restricted to the later maturing cognitive functions neglects this foundation and its powers for supporting development.

I have mentioned the evidence from Alissandra Piontelli (2002) and Umberto Castiello et al. (2010) that, in the last trimester, twins interact with sensitivity for each other's awareness and show personality differences that continue through their childhood and that the mother is aware of these developments in her growing child and is normally attracted to them with love and anticipation of joy in companionship.

Studies of fetal movements with four-dimensional ultrasound movies, reviewed by Reissland and Kisilevsky (2015), teach us that rich powers of emotional expression are developing in mid-gestation and these movement patterns have astonishing sensitivity for the mothers movements, her vocalizations, and her emotions. Of primary importance is the shared sense of emotion in time expressed in complex facial and oral movements that give the foundation for vocal musicality of communication, which, in turn, anticipates the rhythms of narratives uttered in speech. This means that the mother's voice speaking or singing to her baby, projecting the modulated and gracious feelings of her love for the child, a voice that the fetus came to know even before a birth at 26 weeks, offers a course of "treatment" that will recognize the wishes of a baby who has been born to the outside world too soon and who may thrive with affectionate care. As Daniel Stern made clear, shared dynamics of inborn vitality make possible "application of a narrative perspective to the nonverbal … useful to many psychotherapies that rely on the nonverbal"

(Stern, 2000, p. xiv). It is not that music is training for intelligence to develop in the brain. Communicative musicality is the expression of motor intelligence seeking company and able to reward it.

Seeking Companionship in Dialogue when Born Too Soon

For a baby born 3 months prematurely, the sound of a sympathetic human voice, particularly the mother's voice, carries a vital message of joy and well-being, to which the baby's spirit is highly receptive. This simple message can encourage the small and inexperienced person to share the benefits of intimate skin-to-skin contact in kangaroo care, which protects life of the body when breathing and feeding may need artificial support, and while vision and other senses for awareness of the outside world are undeveloped. The baby's body and brain are adapted for this intimate sharing of life (Trevarthen, 2001).

Born before 6 months of gestation, the child is unlikely to survive outside the mother's body without elaborate medical care or special "kangaroo care" in intimate skin-to-skin contact (see Fig. 1.2). In gestation the visceral or *autonomic* "self-regulating" functions of the fetus take aid from the mother's regulations of her vitality, through the placenta and by ingestion of amniotic fluid. By exchange of hormones and nutrients, they form a cooperative *amphoteronomic* system of "mutual regulation," with controlled passage of the vital media across the boundaries between their separate organisms. Their biologies are "ruling together" to create a two-way relationship or "containment" of well-being (Trevarthen, Aitken, Vandekerckhove, Delafield-Butt, & Nagy, 2006, p. 70). They support one another.

At this stage, from the second month of gestation, the body and brain of the late embryo or early fetus are also preparing their anatomies in unique human ways for more active engagements, by growing organs of the face and mouth, nose, eyes, ears, and hands that are adapted for sharing vitality in movement when their bodies will be separate. Sense organs to appreciate an out-of-body world that includes other persons are being readied for social communication by exchange of expressive movements in "proto-conversation," which normally becomes functional and very attractive for a parent through the early weeks of infancy after a full 9 months of gestation (Fig. 1.1). Among the anatomical details that are already different from those of any other primate are the eyes with white sclera that will show clearly the moving focus of the baby's visual interest; expressions of a very complex face that will signal subtle differences in impulses of curiosity, surprise, sadness, fear, joy, and love; and hands designed for delicate gestures that are adapted to display signs of interest and self-satisfaction to others, as well as intricate exploration and transport of objects for the self (Trevarthen, 2015).

In mid-gestation the human voice, with a uniquely elaborate organ of hearing adapted to detect it and its emotional qualities in a rich world of other noises, is being prepared as a vital bridge between the expectant "other awareness" growing

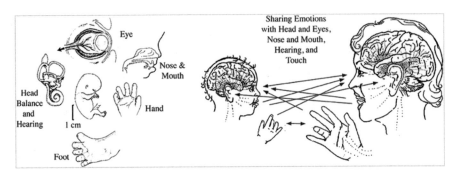

Fig. 1.1 *Left:* The organs for human communication begin to develop in the fetus and at 60 days are easily recognized. The senses and motor organs of are anatomically formed early in gestation, and they develop to serve awareness and production of signs for appreciation by touch, hearing, and sight. *Right:* The rhythm of behaviors in proto-conversation with a 2-month-old child uses all these organs for signaling interests and feelings. The baby's brain is smaller, with underdeveloped cerebral cortices, but has capacities to match the timing and emotional expressions of the adult and to coordinate senses and movements in a collaborative exchange

in a fetus and the conversational skills and playfulness that will be active in an infant with companions in the first 6 months after birth.

Study of the timing and melodious qualities of vocal play between infants and their parents has been guided by the neuroscience of animal emotions and their social functions in playful family life and cooperation in communities (Panksepp & Biven, 2011). But, special stories of companionship and cooperation in intelligent life grow in every human community by a unique richness of music-making, and a voice-making and voice-hearing brain and body with special talents of breathing and articulation of throat and mouth for exploring narratives of feeling are the principal organs for this (Malloch & Trevarthen, 2010; Porges, 2011; Trevarthen, 2001).

Readiness of a Premature Infant for Communication with the Rhythms of Speech

My appreciation of the inborn human sense of time in movement and its readiness for sharing in vocal communication with a parent was transformed when I saw a video made by a clinical psychologist Saskia van Rees and neonatal pediatrician Richard de Leeuw in an intensive care unit in Amsterdam (van Rees & de Leeuw, 1993). It recorded a vocal dialogue between a 2-month-premature girl, Naseera, and her father, who was kangarooing her skin-to-skin against his chest with affectionate care and pride (Fig. 1.2). Van Rees recorded both the gentle intimacy of the father's care and the loving response of his daughter expressed with gestures and face expressions and in an exchange of small "coos" which she created in precisely timed sequences with her father's imitations. They were sharing the pulse of

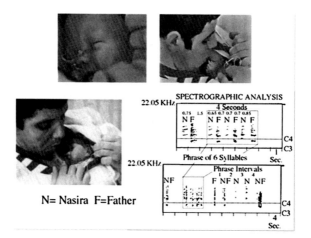

Fig. 1.2 Naseera (N), 2 months premature, with her father (F) who is holding her close to his body, "kangarooing," smiles, makes a gesture with her left hand, and then exchanges short "coo" sounds with her father's imitations. From a film by Saskia van Rees (van Rees & de Leeuw, 1993). Spectrographs produced by Stephen Malloch (1999). They share, with matching precision, the tempo and rhythm of syllables (0.3 s in duration and separated by 0.7 s) grouped in a phrase (of 4 s). In this phrase the interval between the last sound of Naseera and the response of the father is longer, 0.85 s, a good example of "final lengthening." Then they make a sequence of single sounds separated by the 4-second phrase-length intervals. For a short time, the father is not attending, and Naseera's second and third sounds vary in intensity or loudness in ways which express her wish for a response from him; then he responds to her fourth sound with a short utterance about "her little ear," which he is admiring

syllables and making an utterance that formed a phrase with final lengthening according to the universal human measures of vocal narration demonstrated by Lynch, Oller, Steffens, and Buder (1995) for infants 2–12 months after normal birth.

Naseera was born 3 months preterm in an intensive care unit where intimate body-to-body contact, "kangarooing," was used by the pediatrician Richard de Leeuw to aid the physical and mental development of every preterm babies and to support and encourage the confidence of their parents. Her mother began attending to Naseera, but soon had to be taken from her to have a surgical operation. Her father took over the kangarooing and with pleasure and pride accepted Naseera to his body under his clothes every day, cradling her against his skin and responding to her movements and expressions with gentle touching and speech. The development of their intimate relationship and Naseera's excellent progress were documented by videos made by a clinical psychologist Saskia van Rees.

As mentioned, Naseera's movements are made with the timing typical of adult conversational vocalizations. They demonstrate an innate human sense of time in movement or Intrinsic Motive Pulse (Trevarthen, 1999, 2016) and with signs of affection that correspond with normal adult intuitions for displaying actions with feeling (Trevarthen, 2009). They are combined in sequences with *narrative form* revealing that the vitality of experience passes through the measured phases identified by Malloch in the proto-conversation with Laura and also in baby songs in different languages (Delafield-Butt & Trevarthen, 2015; Trevarthen, 1999). They confirm the innate timing of vocal utterances with syllables and phrases that remains from infancy to mature adult speech (Lynch et al., 1995). They concord with observations made by filming behavior in utero (Reissland & Kisilevsky, 2015) that in the third trimester a fetus is ready to coordinate movements of the face, voice, and hands to express a pattern of expressions that seek to take part in consciousness of a delicately timed dialogue with a responsive adult (Trevarthen, 2016; Trevarthen & Delafield-Butt, 2017). They share "vitality dynamics" with "affective attunement" of "temporal feeling shapes" or "proto-narrative envelopes" described by Daniel Stern (Stern, 2010; Stern, Hofer, Haft, & Dore, 1985).

Developmental Neurobiology of the Human Sense of Lifetime and Vitality in Sympathetic Communication Before Birth

The development of the human body and brain before birth confirms the primary function of a core motivating system or self-representing mind of an intelligent individual and its formation for social cooperation with the motivations in minds of other selves. This mind is shaped to guide the body of a whole self in measures of time and space, enabling intentions to be directed to their goals, their consequences to be picked up in sensory stimulation, and objects to be perceived and evaluated with feelings that protect the well-being of the organism. The essential parts of the central nervous system for a psychology of embodied intentions and feelings are ancient and subcortical (Panksepp & Biven, 2011), as are those that have evolved from them to enable intimate communication with the intentions and feelings of other active human selves and to establish affectionate relations with those to be trusted (Porges, 2011).

The talents for communication we have described for newborn infants and the prematurely born Naseera were laid down as rudimentary organs of the affective mind many weeks before, while the fetus was sustained and nourished inside the vitality of mother's body. At first, as I explained earlier, they were entirely concerned with a shared autonomic or visceral existence, jointly regulated "amphotero-nomically," without engaging with experiences from an out-of-body world registered in a mind with functioning cerebral cortex.

The strategy of this developmental project is evident from the start. At 4 weeks the human body, a few millimeters long, is formed with trunk and limbs and has a head with rudiments of special sense organs – eyes, nose, ears, and mouth. The tissue for the central nervous system, the neurectoderm, is folded into a neural tube, and a brain forms. The interneuron systems of the autonomic nervous system – hypothalamus, reticular formation, basal ganglia, and limbic system – which will mediate intermodal sensory integration, the coordination of motor patterns, and direction of actions, appear between 30 and 40 days. They develop the foundations of the intrinsic motive formation (IMF) in the midbrain, before any cortical neurons are generated.

In the brain at 7 weeks, the core reticular system of neurons and cranial nerve nuclei, which are basic elements of the visceral brain that will take care of vital needs, is being transformed into the "polyvagal" emotional motor system that will communicate these (Porges, 2011). Cranial nerves develop for smelling and tasting, seeing, looking by rotating the eyes and focusing vision with lens movements, crying, making face expressions of emotion, feeling touch on the face, hearing, mouth movements of vocalizing, chewing, breathing, gasping, coughing, licking, sucking, expressions of voice, and speaking. All these brain stem sensorimotor organs also project nerve fibers into the forebrain hemispheres before the neurons of the cerebral cortex are differentiated, and this input influences neocortical growth and differentiation.

In the second month, the main lobes of the cerebral hemispheres are evident, and they are interconnected with the motor timing circuits of what will become a very large human cerebellum, which grows through childhood with developing motor skills for locomotion, manipulation, and communication (Llinás, 2001). The first generalized movements of the whole body of the fetus occur at this time, and the fetus swallows amniotic fluid at 11–12 weeks, "feeding" directly on maternal resources. By 8.5 weeks all the special senses of the head, face, hands, and feet are well formed and clearly human (Fig. 1.1). Core regulatory mechanisms of the central nervous system – the periaqueductal gray of the midbrain, the hypothalamus, reticular formation, basal ganglia, and limbic system – are laid down in the first trimester, but the systems of the cerebral cortex that will become cognitive of the resources of the world in infancy do not appear until the second trimester, after 13 weeks. The primary motivating and life-maintaining structures form a link between regulation of gene "instructions" for prenatal brain morphogenesis and the acquired adaptations or "information" taken up by the developing mind. Defects in this link are implicated in disorders of empathy and cognition, including autism and schizophrenia.

At 16 weeks the cerebral hemispheres and thalamus are swelling rapidly, but cortical cells are undeveloped. Brain stem monoaminergic neurons already penetrate the cortical plate at 13 weeks, and sensory thalamic axons arrive after that beginning the functions of body proprioception and touch sensing. Hemisphere development is accelerated with a surge of cell proliferation in the cortex at 10–20 weeks, toward the midpoint of gestation (Rakic, 1991), when the senses become functional and movements expressive of states of affect begin. For the sense of smell, the olfactory bulb has functional structure at 22 weeks and completes development in the following 3 months. At the same time, facial movements develop, including "cry face," "laughter face," and "pain-distress face." This improvement is a marker of healthy development.

Within the body of the fetus, proprioceptive and tactile senses for self-awareness, between moving body parts, grow. At 22 weeks self-touching movements are well directed and their forces sensitively controlled. These movements are part of a mental apparatus that is also other sensitive, capable of reacting to the rhythms and energy of the mother's life. Fetal expressions respond to and learn to recognize her voice, and they may imitate the sounds of adult speech with mouth movements (Reissland & Kisilevsky, 2015). Most astonishingly, the fetus's gestures can be influenced to show "sympathy" or an affective response to a mother's emotional state. Reissland and her colleagues have reported that a fetus in the last trimester can react to a mother's stress by self-comforting gesture to the face or head with the left hand. This introduces the phenomenon of cerebral asymmetry in sensorimotor functions and emotional states. Schore (1994) has shown the importance of the right hemisphere, activity of which is shown by expressions of the left hand, for emotional regulations of attachment in early childhood, when that hemisphere is growing more rapidly than the left (Trevarthen, 2001).

In the last trimester, the fetus develops many behaviors that will be essential for an intelligent and sympathetic human being. Beginning at 24 weeks, with developments in motor control, expressions of emotion are refined with awakening of awareness of the vitality and feelings of the mother. Facial movement patterns and general movement become more coordinated and complex with the maturation of elements of the motor control system in the brain stem and cerebellum. Respiratory movements and breathing appear several weeks before birth. Heart rate changes are integrated with phases of motor activity from 24 weeks indicating the formation of a prospective control of autonomic state coupled to readiness for muscular activity on the environment (Lagercrantz, 2016).

The Newborn Infant Is an Affectionate and Playful Human Person Seeking Meaning in Companionship

The pediatrician T. Berry Brazelton, supported by the educational reformer Jerome Bruner, changed medical care of newborns over 50 years ago by using careful observation of the baby's expressive behaviors and their sensitivity for engagement with an affectionate companion (Brazelton, 1961; Brazelton, Koslowski, & Main, 1974). He demonstrated the newborn's alertness to confirm parents' intuitions that their son or daughter is an intelligent human person, with intentions and feelings and wanting to share them. Bruner had, for decades, been supporting teachers to recognize a child as a creative learner, to accept that "human beings, uniquely among species, grow in a fashion that permits them to participate in human culture, to use its language, its kinship system, its technological way of organizing work" (Bruner, 1968/2015, p. 20). Brazelton, with the same belief in human nature, urged a new more sensitive approach to a newborn's awareness. "In performing the examination, we attempt to reproduce a mother's best efforts to communicate with her new baby as we elicit state changes and behavioral responses" (Brazelton, 1979, p. 81). He warned his medical colleagues that "to see the neonate as chaotic or insensitive provided us with the capacity to see ourselves as acting 'on' rather than 'with' him" (Brazelton, 1979, p. 79).

This ability to share "humanity in movement" is a special importance for care of prematurely born infants. New methods for filming the movements of fetuses in utero reveal that the unique human powers of expression are active from mid-gestation (Reissland & Kisilevsky, 2015). Before 20 weeks, midterm, hand movements explore the fetus's own body and surroundings with graceful intentionality proving a proprioceptive and tactile self-awareness, and the eyes turn in coordination with head movements as if directing selective sight to build awareness of the world. Twins adjust positions in the confined space, and gestures to touch one another are made "sympathetically" with slowed movements compared to self-directed actions (Castiello et al., 2010). There are "temperamental" differences in manner of moving between identical twin fetuses, which persist after birth (Piontelli, 2002). Fetuses hear from 20 weeks, developing special sensitivity for the pitch range of the human voice in the following 2 months, and babies recognize their mother's voice immediately after birth.

A pregnant woman feels the life of her fetus, and this prompts her to imagine the baby she will greet at birth, and sometimes she talks to the expected one. The baby's actions that anticipate her sympathy indicate that the talents for creating meaningful experiences by sensitive exchange of movements that Bruner and Brazelton described are developing in the first stages of growth of an active and aware human brain, before birth (Trevarthen & Reddy, 2016, in press). Research of the last 40 years has brought to light the primary impulses to share movement with rhythms and feelings of "musicality," and it has traced how these innate expressions of vitality lead a young baby to create with a playful companion artful meaning in movements that can tell an enjoyable story, share a game, or discover uses of an object (Malloch & Trevarthen, 2010; Trevarthen & Delafield-Butt, 2017).

Observing Babies as Intelligent Agents, Learning How to Discover the Human Meaning of Shared Life

In a project with Bruner and Brazelton in the Center for Cognitive Studies at Harvard, which Bruner had transformed by directing the research to developments before language, Martin Richards and I made films of mothers communicating with young babies, which showed how active and intelligent the babies were and how the expressive ways they moved with attention to another "person" were different from actions they directed to objects or "things" (Bruner, 1968/2015). Both ways of behavior showed intentions with prospective awareness and feelings, and they had the same rhythms and planned orientations in body-related space, but the tempo and feelings were presented quite differently to a person and obviously were expecting support from their responses.

In a spontaneous "conversation" between a 12-week-old boy and his mother, the infant, Jody, took a leading role (Fig. 1.3). His mother behaved like an interested and appreciative "audience" as he spoke his part, accepting his "story." This leading

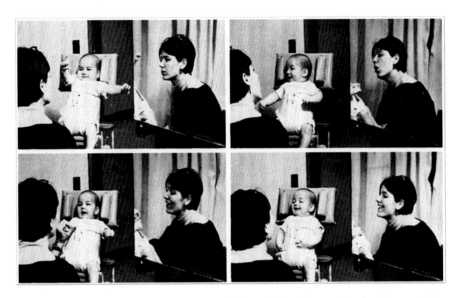

Fig. 1.3 Film record of a mother's communication with her interested and active son, Jody, 12 weeks old. The mother's imitations follow the infant's expressive movements by about one quarter of a second. She tends to imitate the emotional envelope, the calls and hand waving of the baby. Infants rarely reciprocate by imitating the mother (Trevarthen, 1974)

by the baby was confirmed by microanalysis of the body movements of this and other infants of the same age as recorded on film or television, when they were communicating face-to-face with their mothers or when they were tracking objects in motion that were offered to them in play. We made films week by week with five infants and their mothers from 2 to 6 months of age and compared how each infants behaved to the mother and to a suspended toy. The room was furnished as a quiet studio surrounded by heavy curtains, with carefully adjusted lighting. All films were taken with the infant propped up in the baby seat to be at eye level with the mother who was seated just in front of her baby and asked to just "chat." A camera was aimed to take a fullface view of the whole baby, and a front-surface mirror placed at an angle behind the baby gave a head and shoulders view of the mother. We made films at 16 frames/second when the mother and infant were left alone to have intimate communication without disturbance.

When I moved to Edinburgh University in 1971, I used these methods to make an intensive study of infant boys and girls through the first year, when they were communicating with their mothers or other people or using objects. A clear developmental plan was confirmed motivating the baby toward sharing of cultural meanings in progressively more elaborate ways before mastery of the advanced motor skills of speech. From the start the infants were using what the Scottish educational psychologist Margaret Donaldson (1978) called their "human sense" and learning to build cultural "common sense" (Donaldson, 1992) with their mother's companionship as a playmate.

The babies at 2 or 3 months after birth, mastering visual awareness for the first time, were making rich displays of feeling with face movements and hand gestures, including intricate sequences of "pre-speech" movements that could be matched to pictures of an adult articulating different syllables of language (Trevarthen, 1974, 1979). They made measured "utterances" or displays of face expressions, vocal sounds, and gestures that were cyclic. The mothers often responded as if the infant was making statements, telling a story, and they confirmed the infants' efforts with similar poetic or musical patterns of conversational engagement.

Discovery of Communicative Musicality with Its Innate Measures of Moving with Feeling for Composing Life Stories

In 1979 I recorded on film and with sound a short engagement between a 6-week-old girl Laura and her mother, and I used it to support a theory of infant semiotics or symbolic communication representing intuitive patterns of self-expression, which stimulate and guide the mother in her enthusiasm to share dialogic performances (Trevarthen, 1990). I concluded that the special melodic features of "infant directed speech," which Anne Fernald has described as "motherese" (Fernald, 1989), do not "teach" the infant to communicate interests and feelings, but they do give vital reward or confirmation for the infant's initiative.

In the same year, Mary Catherine Bateson reported her detailed study of films of an infant 7 and 14 months old with the mother. This is how she described the behaviors she discovered in "proto-conversation":

> The study of timing and sequencing showed that certainly the mother and probably the infant, in addition to conforming in general to a regular pattern, were acting to sustain it or to restore it when it faltered, waiting for the expected vocalization from the other and then after a pause resuming vocalization, as if to elicit a response that had not been forthcoming. These interactions were characterized by a sort of delighted, ritualized courtesy and more or less sustained attention and mutual gaze. (Bateson, 1979, p. 65.)

A trained linguist and anthropologist, Bateson described what she recorded as a "proto-conversation." She concluded that it constitutes a collaborative motivation based on "an innate, perhaps highly specific, ability to learn" (Bateson, 1979, p. 67). Her description of how a mother is attracted to support her infant's interest in a joint performance and the child's learning of actions to enrich it anticipates Bruner's (1983) proposal that any *language acquisition device* (LAD) in the infant's mind, such as Noam Chomsky had described, needs a *language acquisition support system* (LASS) from human companions.

Study of the expressive, prosodic features of mothers' talk to infants confirms a special mode of signing (Trevarthen & Marwick, 1986) – the affectionate and melodic discourse of Fernald's motherese (Fernald, 1989). Tests of the young infant's selective orientation to sounds of the human voice confirm that they are born with a preference for the higher range of the female voice and its affectionate modulations (Trehub, 2003). Infants a few weeks old make refined discriminations of pitch, harmony, and rhythm, and they prefer harmonious cords and melodic phrases to those that are dissonant and mechanical. Mechthild and Hanuš Papoušek (Papoušek & Papoušek, 1981) described the mother's "intuitive parenting" speech as showing "musicality." They concluded, with Bateson, that the intimate sharing of musical expressions guides the infant to learn language. This is confirmed by the timing of prelinguistic vocalizations of infants, which conform to universal patterns of syllables, utterances, and phrasing in adult speech (Lynch et al., 1995). The rhythmic impulses and playful rituals seeking company establish the baby as belonging to a family and set the basis for learning cultural habits and a language (Gratier & Trevarthen, 2008).

The story-making patterns of "musicality" are not confined to expressive actions of vocalization. They give temporal and energetic form to all body movements, especially those of postural attitude, head position and turning, eye movements with facial expressions, and the rich array of gestural movements of the hands, all of which accompany speech in any live conversation or shared occupation. The anthropologist Ray Birdwhistell (1970) studied the activities of "paraverbal" communication in different cultures and concluded that a large proportion of the meaning in the message of any human "dialogue" is actually "nonverbal." He established the principles of a science of "kinesics" to describe these behaviors.

Following work on the rhythms of adult vocal communication, William Condon, with the pediatrician Lou Sander, reported in 1974 that the gestures of a newborn may respond, in coordinated precision, to the prosodic rhythm of an adult voice (Condon & Sander, 1974). This phenomenon – along with the authors' claim that "inter-synchrony," the joint timing of expressions, is important for language acquisition – has been abundantly confirmed by subsequent studies. The pulse and modulation of the human-life-time in movement is infectious, adapted to make cultural narratives about a human-made world and its history in a community of minds (Donald, 2001). From birth, the rhythm of life and the stories of human vitality are shared to make life both enjoyable and meaningful, and to support well-being (Trevarthen & Delafield-Butt, 2015; Trevarthen, Delafield-Butt, & Schögler, 2011; Trevarthen & Fresquez, 2015; Trevarthen, Gratier, & Osborne, 2014; Trevarthen & Malloch, 2000).

In New York, Daniel Stern, a psychiatrist training in psychoanalysis, was inspired by Birdwhistell's "kinesics" and the work of Condon to study the natural dynamics of communication before language. He used microanalysis of film, which had been developed in the preceding decade as a method to reveal the natural rhythms of expression in dialogue (Jaffe & Felstein, 1970), to study playful communication of a mother with three-and-a-half-month-old twins and observed that the infants were actively directing their mother in exchanges of mutual attention by precisely timed engagement of expressive movements (Stern, 1971, 2004). This discovery led Stern away from conventional ideas of child psychiatry as a search for traumatic events in early life, to pathfinding studies of positive joy, which he reported in *The Interpersonal World of the Infant* (Stern, 2000) and richly demonstrated in accounts of further studies of normal mother-infant communication. He was attempting "to create a dialogue between the infant as revealed by the experimental approach and as clinically reconstructed, in the service of resolving the contradiction between theory and reality" (Stern, 1985, pp. viii–ix). And he built a new foundation for mutual emotional support in intimate communication, without resorting to the explicit verbal description of emotional "reactions" to distressing events of the past. With colleagues at Columbia University, he defined constructive dynamic principles of "affect attunement" (Stern et al., 1985) and later developed these in a practice of psychotherapy that sought to derive emotional benefit from intimate "moments of meeting," (Stern, 2004) using these as invitations to improved understanding in dialogues between therapist and patient as they explored their "implicit knowledge" of subjective experiences, both immediate and recalled (Boston Process Change Study Group, 2010).

With an interest in dance and choreography and after 40 years' experience expanding his awareness of the innate capacities of infants and their mothers for being in affective connection, Daniel Stern, in his latest book, *Forms of Vitality: Exploring Dynamic Experience in Psychology, the Arts, Psychotherapy and Development* (Stern, 2010), developed a comprehensive science of "vitality dynamics." Drawing on information from research on movements of fetuses, infants, and their mothers to the principles studied by performing artists, this concept of self-generated life in movement enriches our understanding of the nature of well-being and learning for human beings of all ages and of the appreciation of music as natural communication.

All our arts and sciences, our literature, and even much of creative invention in technology and industry draw inspiration from the expressive impulses of infancy explored in the work of Bruner, Brazelton, Stern and colleagues, Bateson, Condon and Sander, the Papoušeks, Lynch and colleagues, and Gratier. This work of the past 50 years established a new appreciation of the pulse, quality, and narrative of gestural and vocal meaning-making in concordant company, which Malloch defined as "communicative musicality" (Malloch & Trevarthen, 2010).

Rituals of Delight Performed with Pride in Action Games and Baby Songs

In studies to trace development of the dynamics of communication during the first year, my colleague Penelope Hubley charted how mothers respond to the infant's growing interest in the present environment at increasing distance from their selves, which draws the baby's interest away from the mother's familiar person. First mothers became more provocatively playful in the ways they addressed the babies, exaggerating the expressive dimensions of their attempts to play. Then they were led to bring objects that attract a baby's interest into the stories or games they invented together for fun (Hubley & Trevarthen, 1979; Trevarthen & Hubley, 1978). Their playful performances together develop the form of enjoyable rituals, with features that are remembered and recognized by the baby with pleasure at later times. For example, infants begin to imitate rhyming sounds in nursery songs and the pattern of movements in an action game, such as "Round and Round the Garden" or "Clappa-Clappa Handies." They display to their partner expressions of pride in making the response in the "conventional" way (Gratier & Trevarthen, 2008; Trevarthen, 2005; Trevarthen & Delafield-Butt, 2013; Trevarthen & Malloch, 2002).

The increasing playfulness signals a change in self-other awareness of the infants, which is presented as "self-consciousness" that reacts positively or negatively to being observed. Vasudevi Reddy has pioneered studies that reveal humorous avoiding or displaying behaviors that signal "coyness" and "showing off" of infants (Reddy, 1991, 2000). For example, if a mother holds a 3-month-old baby up to face a mirror, the baby shows first a curiosity for eye contact with the image then looks away with a timid smile of "embarrassment." The instantly reactive self-image, which returns a focused gaze, is felt to be intrusive. From this time babies also express stronger social awareness by becoming more "fun," enjoying and contributing to teasing with careful attention to timing as Hubley discovered. Numerous examples illustrating the developing richness of self-consciousness and both marking and remembering of playful performances of "joking, teasing, and mucking about" that excite and play with others' expectations are presented by Reddy in her book *How Infants Know Minds* (Reddy, 2008). These form the basis for feelings of trust and self-confidence parents and children feel in a particular culture with its habits of performance and explain the difficulties that arise for communication with young children when the family migrates (Gratier, 2003).

Measuring the Musical Motives for Human Companionship in Early Childhood

Twenty years after the recording of Laura and her mother Kay was made in Edinburgh, a *Special Issue* of the journal *Musicae Scientiae* edited by Irène Deliège for the European Society for the Cognitive Sciences of Music published the findings of detailed acoustic analysis of their vocal dialogue made by a musician and musical acoustics expert Stephen Malloch (Malloch, 1999). He used the evidence he obtained by computer-aided analysis of the sounds of the voices of mother and the infant in talking and singing to define the essential parameters of innate "communicative musicality."

In the *Special Issue*, which was entitled "Rhythm, Musical Narrative, and the Origins of Human Communication," a team that had been using Malloch's programs to portray sound trains of speech and song presented findings on many topics: how the rhythm and harmony of mother-infant vocal interaction is reduced when the mother has migrated to a different culture with a different language (Gratier, 1999), on the reduced emotional musicality of speech of a mother with postnatal depression to her baby (Robb, 1999), on the Intrinsic Motive Pulse that regulates the infant's sharing of talk and songs (Trevarthen, 1999), on coordination of timing in jazz duets (Schögler, 1999), on synchronous chorusing of vocal sounds to claim territory and form a community in insects and human primates (Merker, 1999), and on the time-keeping mechanisms of the brain for music perception and performance (Wittmann & Pöppel, 1999). These topics appear diverse, but they all confirm that an inborn sense of time and measures of energy and harmony in the movements of the voice, heard without and felt within, serves to link human, or animal, minds at all stages of development and this expression of the pulse and harmony of life force in sound is necessary for formation and sustaining of relationships and communities.

Ten years after the *Musicae Scientiae* publication, Malloch and I edited a book *Communicative Musicality: Exploring the Basis of Human Companionship* in which again Laura appeared as a star performer (Fig. 1.4). The description of her proto-conversation gave substance to the theory in many different applications and provided a common ground for 27 chapters by experts in brain science, human evolution, psychology, philosophy of art, education, therapy, and music performance. All considered "how speaking and moving in musical dance-like ways is the essential foundation for all forms of communication, even the most refined and technically elaborated, just as it is for parenting, good teaching, creative work in the arts and therapy to help disabled or emotionally distressed persons" (Malloch & Trevarthen, 2010, cover text).

The Infant's Innate Talents and Sympathy in Movement Support a Transformation of the Philosophy of Human Consciousness

The most significant finding of the work with infants is the demonstration that the sympathy for rhythmic agency expressing imagination for movement is already active and effective in a newborn baby. Contrary to firmly articulated beliefs of Sigmund Freud and Jean Piaget, a newborn baby may imitate expressions of another person's intention and feelings signaled by movements they see of the head, face, mouth, eyes, and hands, clearly discriminating different body movements deliberately presented as signs (Trevarthen, 2015) and passing them back to confirm a consensuality that will be necessary for the learning of a language and other cooperative social skills (Maturana, Mpodozis, & Carlos Letelier, 1995). The infant can synchronize movements of their hands with the rhythms of a person speaking, and they adjust posture and movements of their hands to being picked up and carried or to assist with breast feeding. The sequential pattern of movements in time that Malloch identified as "narrative" is already present and commensurate with the articulations of syllables, words, and phrases in speech (Delafield-Butt & Trevarthen, 2015). This hierarchy of rhythmic elements, which is also apparent in limb movements and hand gestures for different purposes, is developed further in the infants' participation in traditional baby songs in different languages (Trevarthen & Malloch, 2016, in press).

The question arises how does this ability to formulate movements with intention in time come about? Is it entirely innate, a product of the self-generation, or "autopoiesis" of a life activity of a human body with its brain, or does it require influence

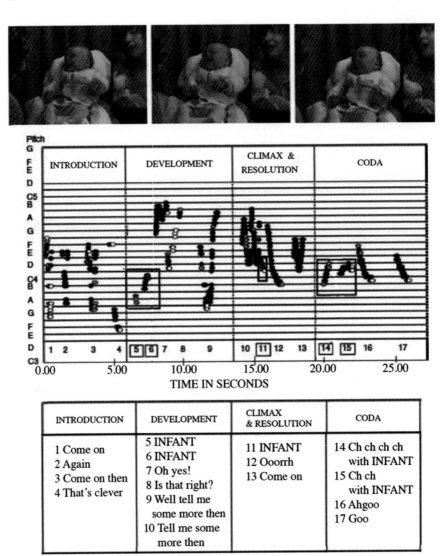

Fig. 1.4 Six-week-old girl, Laura, in proto-conversation with her mother. Malloch's pitch plot in quarter tones of their vocal exchange shows how their narrative developed with the aid of Laura's contributions. Each dot represents the pitch of the voice in 1.01 s. C4 indicates the pitch of Middle C. The infant's vocalizations are enclosed in rectangles (Malloch, 1999; Malloch & Trevarthen, 2010). Below is a transcript of the mother's speech and her nonverbal utterances, which harmonize with the infant's sounds

from outside from a more mature human being that offers "training" for nonmental developments in the child? Findings from the science of human brain development from embryo stages (Trevarthen, 2001), and new techniques for filming body movements of fetuses inside their mother's bodies (Reissland & Kisilevsky, 2015), give partial answers to these questions, and both strongly support the conclusion that the fetus has innate capacities for sharing a human kind of life in relationships. Most evident is the crucial role of a central intrinsic motive formation as an integrated core system of the brain-mind representing the potential forms of body movement and well-being (Trevarthen & Aitken, 1994; Trevarthen & Delafield-Butt, 2017) and as a neurochemical affective coordinator and regulator of movement and experience, animal and human (Panksepp & Biven, 2011).

This psychobiological endowment is evident both in the morphogenesis of brain systems that are essential for the coherent and imaginative sensorimotor intelligence of a freely active self (Llinás, 2001) and in the timing and emotional regulation of purposeful actions in beneficial engagements with elements of the outside world – physical, organic, animal, and human. There is a clear anticipation of human cultural life and how to appreciate it apparent in the life plan of a fetus. It is made for seeking and giving special value to cooperative company "in the relational manner of living that human language constitutes" (Maturana et al., 1995, p. 15) and its rhythms of musicality (Osborne, 2010; Panksepp & Trevarthen, 2010; Trevarthen, 2009).

Some philosophers have grasped the importance of the impulses for sharing life time and feelings and used this insight to oppose philosophies and psychologies that presume consciousness to be "self-reflective, passive, and timeless" (Goodrich, 2010, p. 331), rather than one founded on the regulation of deliberate and ambitious movement in time. Barbara Goodrich (2010), a veterinary care specialist and phenomenological philosopher, has made an eloquent account of the problem, welcoming the exceptional contributions of two neuroscientists Rodolfo Llinás and György Buszáki who recognize the creative timing of movements by the brain and its role in the pickup of information in consciousness, relating these to the phenomenological philosophies of Husserl and Merleau-Ponty.

One predecessor with a special appreciation of music as the expression of the human "innate sympathy," the natural feeling that guides an active aesthetic and moral life defined by his teacher Francis Hutcheson, was Adam Smith. He said:

> After the pleasures which arise from gratification of the bodily appetites, there seems to be none more natural to man than Music and Dancing. In the progress of art and improvement they are, perhaps, the first and earliest pleasures of his own invention. ... Without any imitation, instrumental Music can produce very considerable effects...: by the sweetness of its sounds it awakens agreeably, and calls upon the attention; by their connection and affinity it naturally detains that attention, which follows easily a series of agreeable sounds, which have all a certain relation both to a common, fundamental, or leading note, called the key note; and to a certain succession or combination of notes, called the song or composition. ... Time and measure are to instrumental Music what order and method are to discourse; they break it into proper parts and divisions, by which we are enabled both to remember better what has gone before, and frequently to foresee somewhat of what is to come after: .... the enjoyment of Music arises partly from memory and partly from foresight. (Smith, 1777/1982).

Observations of natural vocal communication between happy and affectionate mothers and their young infants and how they develop melodious games that become little rituals of a family culture prove that we are born to share precisely defined rhythms and expressive tones and to compose stories of vitality together.

Far beyond the singing of a blackbird, or a whale, or the imitations of parrot, telling of motives and feelings by the human voice has potentiality to become musical art or language with thousands of years of invention described in it. Thus human minds create meaning from infancy in stories of movement that will define a community and keep it alive through many generations and through many transformations of belief, rituals, and practice in art and technology.

References

Bateson, M. C. (1979). The epigenesis of conversational interaction: A personal account of research development. In M. Bullowa (Ed.), *Before speech: The beginning of human communication* (pp. 63–77). London, England: Cambridge University Press.

Birdwhistell, R. L. (1970). *Kinesics and context: Essays on body motion communication.* Philadelphia, PA: University of Pennsylvania Press.

Boston Process Change Study Group. (2010). *Change in psychotherapy: A unifying paradigm.* New York, NY: Norton.

Brazelton, T. B. (1961). Psychophysiologic reactions in the neonate. I: The value of observations of the neonate. *Journal of Pediatrics, 58,* 508–512.

Brazelton, T. B. (1979). Evidence of communication during neonatal behavioural assessment. In M. Bullowa (Ed.), *Before speech: The beginning of human communication* (pp. 79–88). London, England: Cambridge University Press.

Brazelton, T. B., Koslowski, B., & Main, M. (1974). The origins of reciprocity: The early mother-infant interaction. In M. Lewis & L. A. Rosenblum (Eds.), *The effect of the infant on its caregiver* (pp. 49–76). New York, NY/London, England: Wiley.

Bruner, J. S. (1968). *Processes of cognitive growth: Infancy.* (Heinz Werner Lectures, 1968) Worcester, MA: Clark University Press with Barri Publishers. (Republished in G. Marsico (Ed.). (2015). Jerome S. *Bruner beyond 100, cultural psychology of education* 2. Cham, Switzerland: Springer International Publishing. doi:10.1007/978-3-319-25536-1_2

Bruner, J. S. (1983). *Child's talk. Learning to use language.* New York, NY: Norton.

Castiello, U., Becchio, C., Zoia, S., Nelini, C., Sartori, L., Blason, L., … Gallese, V. (2010). Wired to be social: The ontogeny of human interaction. *PLoS One, 5*(10), e13199.

Condon, W. S., & Sander, L. S. (1974). Neonate movement is synchronized with adult speech: Interactional participation and language acquisition. *Science, 183,* 99–101.

Delafield-Butt, J. T., & Trevarthen, C. (2015). The ontogenesis of narrative: From movements to meaning. *Frontiers of Psychology, 6,* 1157. doi:10.3389/fpsyg.2015.01157

Donald, M. (2001). *A mind so rare: The evolution of human consciousness.* New York, NY/London, England: Norton.

Donaldson, M. (1978). *Children's minds.* Glasgow, Scotland: Fontana/Collins.

Donaldson, M. (1992). *Human minds: An exploration.* London, England: Allen Lane/Penguin Books.

Fernald, A. (1989). Intonation and communicative intent in mothers' speech to infants: Is the melody the message? *Child Development, 60,* 1497–1510.

Goodrich, B. G. (2010). We do, therefore we think: Time, motility, and consciousness. *Reviews in the Neurosciences, 21,* 331–361.

Gratier, M. (1999). Expressions of belonging: The effect of acculturation on the rhythm and harmony of mother-infant vocal interaction. In *Rhythms, musical narrative, and the origins of human communication. Musicae Scientiae, Special issue, 1999–2000* (pp. 93–122). Liège, Belgium: European Society for the Cognitive Sciences of Music.

Gratier, M. (2003). Expressive timing and interactional synchrony between mothers and infants: Cultural similarities, cultural differences, and the immigration experience. *Cognitive Development, 18*, 533–554.

Gratier, M., & Trevarthen, C. (2008). Musical narrative and motives for culture in mother-infant vocal interaction. *The Journal of Consciousness Studies, 15*(10–11), 122–158.

Hubley, P., & Trevarthen, C. (1979). Sharing a task in infancy. In I. Uzgiris (Ed.), *Social interaction during infancy: New directions for child development* (vol. 4, pp. 57–80). San Francisco, CA: Jossey-Bass.

Jaffe, J., & Felstein, S. (1970). *Rhythms of dialogue*. New York, NY: Academic.

Lagercrantz, H. (2016). *Infant brain development*. Cham, Switzerland: Springer Nature.

Llinás, R. (2001). *I of the vortex: From neurons to self*. Cambridge, MA: MIT Press.

Lynch, M. P., Oller, D. K., Steffens, M. L., & Buder, E. H. (1995). Phrasing in prelinguistic vocalisations. *Developmental Psychobiology, 28*, 3–25.

Malloch, S. (1999). Mother and infants and communicative musicality. In I. Deliège (Ed.), *Rhythms, musical narrative, and the origins of human communication. Musicae Scientiae, Special issue, 1999–2000* (pp. 29–57). Liège, Belgium: European Society for the Cognitive Sciences of Music.

Malloch, S., & Trevarthen, C. (Eds.). (2010). *Communicative musicality: Exploring the basis of human companionship*. Oxford: Oxford University Press.

Maturana, H., Mpodozis, J., & Carlos Letelier, J. (1995). Brain, language and the origin of human mental functions. *Biological Research, 28*(1), 15–26.

Merker, B. (1999). Synchronous chorusing and the origins of music. In I. Deliège (Ed.), *Rhythms, musical narrative, and the origins of human communication. Musicae Scientiae, Special issue, 1999–2000* (pp. 59–74). Liège, Belgium: European Society for the Cognitive Sciences of Music.

Osborne, N. (2010). Towards a chronobiology of musical rhythm. In S. Malloch & C. Trevarthen (Eds.), *Communicative musicality: Exploring the basis of human companionship* (pp. 545–564). Oxford: Oxford University Press.

Panksepp, J., & Biven, L. (2011). *Archaeology of mind: Neuroevolutionary origins of human emotions*. New York, NY: Norton.

Panksepp, J., & Trevarthen, C. (2010). The neuroscience of emotion in music. In S. Malloch & C. Trevarthen (Eds.), *Communicative musicality: Exploring the basis of human companionship* (pp. 105–146). Oxford: Oxford University Press.

Papoušek, M., & Papoušek, H. (1981). Musical elements in the infant's vocalization: Their significance for communication, cognition, and creativity. In L. P. Lipsitt & C. K. Rovee-Collier (Eds.), *Advances in infancy research* (vol. 1, pp. 163–224). Norwood, NJ: Ablex.

Piontelli, A. (2002). *Twins: From fetus to child*. London, England: Routledge.

Porges, S. W. (2011). *The polyvagal theory: Neurophysiological foundations of emotions, attachment, communication, and self-regulation*. New York, NY: WW Norton.

Rakic, P. (1991). Development of the primate cerebral cortex. In M. Lewis (Ed.), *Child and adolescent psychiatry: A comprehensive textbook* (pp. 11–28). Baltimore, MD: Williams and Wilkins.

Reddy, V. (1991). Playing with others' expectations; teasing and mucking about in the first year. In A. Whiten (Ed.), *Natural theories of mind: Evolution, development and simulation of everyday mindreading* (pp. 143–158). Oxford: Blackwell.

Reddy, V. (2000). Coyness in early infancy. *Developmental Science, 3*(2), 186–192.

Reddy, V. (2008). *How infants know minds*. Cambridge, MA: Harvard University Press.

Reissland, N., & Kisilevsky, B. (Eds.). (2015). *Fetal development: Research on brain and behavior, environmental influences, and emerging technologies*. London, England: Springer.

Robb, L. (1999). Emotional musicality in mother-infant vocal affect, and an acoustic study of postnatal depression. In *Rhythms, musical narrative, and the origins of human communication. Musicae Scientiae, Special issue, 1999–2000* (pp. 123–151). Liège, Belgium: European Society for the Cognitive Sciences of Music.

Schögler, B. W. (1999). Studying temporal co-ordination in jazz duets. In *Rhythms, musical narrative, and the origins of human communication. Musicae Scientiae, Special issue, 1999-2000* (pp. 75–92). Liège, Belgium: European Society for the Cognitive Sciences of Music.

Schore, A. N. (1994). *Affect regulation and the origin of the self: The neurobiology of emotional development*. Hillsdale, NJ: Erlbaum.

Smith, A. (1777/1982). Of the nature of that imitation which takes place in what are called the imitative arts. Republished in W. P. D. Wightman & J. C. Bryce (Eds.), 1982. *Essays on philosophical subjects* (pp. 176–213). Indianapolis, IN: Liberty Fund.

Stern, D. N. (1971). A micro-analysis of mother-infant interaction: Behaviors regulating social contact between a mother and her three-and-a-half-month-old twins. *Journal of the American Academy of Child Psychiatry, 10*, 501–517.

Stern, D. N. (2000). *The interpersonal world of the infant: A view from psychoanalysis and development psychology*. (Second Edition, with new Introduction. Originally published in 1985) New York, NY: Basic Books.

Stern, D. N. (2004). *The present moment: In psychotherapy and everyday life*. New York, NY: Norton.

Stern, D. N. (2010). *Forms of vitality: Exploring dynamic experience in psychology, the arts, psychotherapy and development*. Oxford: Oxford University Press.

Stern, D. N., Hofer, L., Haft, W., & Dore, J. (1985). Affect attunement: The sharing of feeling states between mother and infant by means of inter-modal fluency. In T. M. Field & N. A. Fox (Eds.), *Social perception in infants* (pp. 249–268). Norwood, NJ: Ablex.

Trehub, S. E. (2003). Musical predispositions in infancy: An update. In I. Peretz & R. Zatorre (Eds.), *The cognitive neuroscience of music* (pp. 3–20). New York: Oxford University Press.

Trevarthen, C. (1974). The psychobiology of speech development. In E. H. Lenneberg (Ed.), *Language and brain: Developmental aspects* (vol. 12, pp. 570–585). Boston, MA: Neurosciences Research Program Bulletin.

Trevarthen, C. (1979). Communication and cooperation in early infancy. A description of primary intersubjectivity. In M. Bullowa (Ed.), *Before speech: The beginning of human communication* (pp. 321–347). London, England: Cambridge University Press.

Trevarthen, C. (1990). Signs before speech. In T. A. Sebeok & J. Umiker-Sebeok (Eds.), *The semiotic web, 1989* (pp. 689–755). Berlin, Germany/New York, NY/Amsterdam, The Netherlands: Mouton de Gruyter.

Trevarthen, C. (1999). Musicality and the intrinsic motive pulse: Evidence from human psychobiology and infant communication. In I. Deliège (Ed.), *Rhythms, musical narrative, and the origins of human communication. Musicae Scientiae, Special issue, 1999–2000* (pp. 157–213). Liège, Belgium: European Society for the Cognitive Sciences of Music.

Trevarthen, C. (2001). The neurobiology of early communication: Intersubjective regulations in human brain development. In A. F. Kalverboer & A. Gramsbergen (Eds.), *Handbook on brain and behavior in human development* (pp. 841–882). Dordrecht, The Netherlands: Kluwer.

Trevarthen, C. (2005). Stepping away from the mirror: Pride and shame in adventures of companionship reflections on the nature and emotional needs of infant intersubjectivity. In C. S. Carter, L. Ahnert, K. E. Grossman, S. B. Hrdy, M. E. Lamb, S. W. Porges, & N. Sachser (Eds.), *Attachment and bonding: A new synthesis, Dahlem workshop report* (vol. 92, pp. 55–84). Cambridge, MA: The MIT Press.

Trevarthen, C. (2009). Human biochronology: On the source and functions of 'musicality', chap. 18. In R. Haas & V. Brandes (Eds.), *Music that works: Contributions of biology, neurophysiology, psychology, sociology, medicine and musicology* (pp. 221–266). Vienna, Austria/New York, NY: Springer.

Trevarthen, C. (2015). Infant semiosis: The psycho-biology of action and shared experience from birth. *Cognitive Development, 36C*, 130–141. doi:10.1016/j.cogdev.2015.09.008

Trevarthen, C. (2016). From the intrinsic motive pulse of infant actions, to the life time of cultural meanings. In B. Mölder, V. Arstila, & P. Øhrstrom (Eds.), *Philosophy and psychology of time, Springer studies in brain and mind* (vol. 9, pp. 225–265). Dordrecht, The Netherlands: Springer International. doi:10.1007/978-3-319-22195-3 ISBN 978-3-319-22195-3

Trevarthen, C., & Aitken, K. J. (1994). Brain development, infant communication, and empathy disorders: Intrinsic factors in child mental health. *Development and Psychopathology, 6,* 599–635.

Trevarthen, C., Aitken, K. J., Vandekerckhove, M., Delafield-Butt, J., & Nagy, E. (2006). Collaborative regulations of vitality in early childhood: Stress in intimate relationships and postnatal psychopathology. In D. Cicchetti & D. J. Cohen (Eds.), *Developmental psychopathology, volume 2, developmental neuroscience* (2nd ed.pp. 65–126). New York, NY: Wiley.

Trevarthen, C., & Delafield-Butt, J. (2015). The infant's creative vitality, in projects of self-discovery and shared meaning: How they anticipate school, and make it fruitful. In S. Robson & S. F. Quinn (Eds.), *The Routledge international handbook of young children's thinking and understanding* (pp. 3–18). Abingdon, Oxon/New York, NY: Routledge, Taylor & Francis Group.

Trevarthen, C., & Delafield-Butt, J. (2017). The development of consciousness. In B. Hopkins, E. Geangu, & S. Linkenauger (Eds.), *Cambridge encyclopedia of child development* (2nd ed.). Cambridge, UK/New York, NY: Cambridge University Press.

Trevarthen, C., Delafield-Butt, J., & Schögler, B. (2011). Psychobiology of musical gesture: Innate rhythm, harmony and melody in movements of narration. In A. Gritten & E. King (Eds.), *Music and gesture 2.* Aldershot, UK: Ashgate.

Trevarthen, C., & Delafield-Butt, J. T. (2013). Biology of shared experience and language development: Regulations for the inter-subjective life of narratives. In M. Legerstee, D. Haley, & M. Bornstein (Eds.), *The infant mind: Origins of the social brain* (pp. 167–199). New York, NY: Guildford Press.

Trevarthen, C., & Fresquez, C. (2015). Sharing human movement for wellbeing: Research on communication in infancy and applications in dance movement psychotherapy. *Body, Movement and Dance in Psychotherapy.* doi:10.1080/17432979.2015.1084948

Trevarthen, C., Gratier, M. and Osborne, N. (2014, March/April). The human nature of culture and education. Wiley Interdisciplinary Reviews: Cognitive Science, vol. 5, 173-192. doi:10.1002/wcs.1276.

Trevarthen, C., & Hubley, P. (1978). Secondary intersubjectivity: Confidence, confiding and acts of meaning in the first year. In A. Lock (Ed.), *Action, gesture and symbol: The emergence of language* (pp. 183–229). London, England/New York, NY/San Francisco, CA: Academic.

Trevarthen, C., & Malloch, S. (2000). The dance of wellbeing: Defining the musical therapeutic effect. *The Nordic Journal of Music Therapy, 9*(2), 3–17.

Trevarthen, C., & Malloch, S. (2002, September). Musicality and music before three: Human vitality and invention shared with pride. *Zero to Three, 23*(1), 10–18.

Trevarthen, C., & Marwick, H. (1986). Signs of motivation for speech in infants, and the nature of a mother's support for development of language. In B. Lindblom & R. Zetterstrom (Eds.), *Precursors of early speech* (pp. 279–308). Basingstoke, Hampshire: Macmillan.

Trevarthen, C. and Reddy, V. (2016, in press). Consciousness in infants. In, S. Schneider *and* M. Velmans (Eds.). Blackwell companion to consciousness, 2nd Edition. Oxford: Blackwells.

van Rees, S. and de Leeuw, R. (1993). *Born too early: The kangaroo method with premature babies.* Heythuysen, The Netherlands: Video by Stichting Lichaamstaal.

Wittmann, M. (2009). The inner experience of time. *Philosophical Transactions of the Royal Society of London, B Biological Science, 364,* 1955–1967.

Wittmann, M., & Pöppel, E. (1999). Temporal mechanisms of the brain as fundamentals of communication ì with special reference to music perception and performance. In I. Deliège (Ed.), *Rhythms, musical narrative, and the origins of human communication. Musicae Scientiae, Special issue, 1999–2000* (pp. 13–28). Liège, Belgium: European Society for the Cognitive Sciences of Music.

Chapter 2
Prenatal Experience with the Maternal Voice

Christine Moon

Abstract Research studies over the past 40 years have established that the maternal voice is a prominent feature of the prenatal environment, that the fetus responds to it, and that prenatal learning carries over into early postnatal life. The primary aim of the chapter is to describe what is known through research about prenatal exposure to the mother's voice, especially through audition. A second aim is to present a consideration of nonauditory experience such as the vestibular and, possibly, cutaneous sensations that are uniquely linked to auditory stimulation by the maternal voice. A third aim is to raise a question about the necessity of prenatal experience with the acoustic aspects of the maternal voice, given emerging data from deaf infants who receive cochlear implants many months after birth. The chapter concludes by considering implications for the care of hospitalized preterm infants who experience atypical experience with the mother's voice and other sounds. Chapter conclusions are (1) fetal auditory experience with the mother's voice begins around 24 weeks after conception, (2) the maternal voice is potentially a rich source of multimodal stimulation and information, and (3) for favorable postnatal development, the role that is played by very early exposure to the maternal voice is not yet understood.

> When Elizabeth heard Mary's greeting, the baby leaped in her womb, and Elizabeth was filled with the Holy Spirit. (Luke 1:41, Bible New International Version)

The scientific method has confirmed what has been passed down for at least two millennia. Research results converge to show that the fetus begins reacting to maternal and other acoustic signals before birth. Resourceful twentieth century investigators devised procedures to record what sounds could be generated within the womb or be transmitted from the outside. In addition, they learned how to measure both fetal and neonatal responses to particular sounds. Audio recordings in the womb show that a strong maternal voice signal is available to the fetus. Fetal cardiac and motor activity show a reaction to the mother's voice, and there is a good reason to believe that the sound of her voice is retained across the transition into postnatal life.

C. Moon (✉)
Pacific Lutheran University, Department of Psychology, Tacoma, WA, USA
e-mail: mooncm@plu.edu

© Springer International Publishing AG 2017
M. Filippa et al. (eds.), *Early Vocal Contact and Preterm Infant Brain Development*, DOI 10.1007/978-3-319-65077-7_2

For the fetus, this early experience is potentially a rich source of learning about the mother, language, and their contexts. The necessity of such prenatal auditory experience has not been established. Special cases such as children in the deaf community show us that there is considerable plasticity in early postnatal development.

Maternal Voice Is Available in the Womb

Recordings from inside the womb during labor show that the maternal voice is prominent among other sounds. Recordings exist of womb sounds because researchers have threaded a tiny microphone or hydrophone through the cervix after rupture of the amniotic sac with microphone placement next to the fetal head. In the most extensive study to date, five laboring women in a hospital in Roubaix, France, spoke both spontaneously and also under instruction ("live") while recordings were made both inside the womb and outside in the room (Querleu, Renard, Versyp, Paris-Delrue, & Crepin, 1988; Querleu, Renard, Versyp, Paris-Delrue, & Vervoort, 1988). Besides the live recordings, a loudspeaker in the room played comparable prerecorded male, female, and the maternal voices, and these stimuli were recorded both near the mother's belly in air and *in utero*. Analysis of the intrauterine recordings showed that the maternal live voice was more intense than other voices. Moreover, as the researchers pointed out, in everyday life a mother's voice is not only louder but is also normally more abundantly available than other voices. With every maternal utterance, sound waves from her vocal tract are both airborne and borne through her abdomen to the womb where they are likely to be delivered by soft tissue and liquid conduction to the cochlea (Adelman, Chordekar, Perez, & Sohmer, 2014; Perez, Adelman, & Sohmer, 2016). One would expect transmission through tissue and liquid to be more effective for lower frequencies, and the early recordings generally confirmed this. Frequencies above about 500 Hz showed overall attenuation. Interestingly, conduction transmission of sound waves to the fetal cochlea means that it probably isn't possible for the fetus to determine the location of sound sources. Sound localization requires time or intensity differences in the arrival of sound at the two ears. Nevertheless, neonates less than 2 h old have been reported to turn their heads in the direction of the mother's voice (Querleu et al., 1984). Thus, it appears that an ability that is not present in the womb is available immediately upon birth.

On the internal recordings, the Roubaix team discovered that the loudspeaker version of a male voice emerged and was more intense than a female non-maternal voice but was masked by internal low frequency sounds such as maternal vascular and digestive noises that are relatively intense. The non-maternal female voice, with its higher frequencies, although less intense, had less competition with other sounds. In comparison, the live maternal voice had both the advantage of greater intensity and less masking, and it was therefore the most prominent of the recorded voices. The intrauterine recordings also revealed the presence of sound emanating from the maternal cardiac and digestive systems.

In the Roubaix study, the research protocol included an intelligibility test of speech in the womb by using standard clinical speech-language lists of words and nonsense syllables. Blinded listeners then heard the intrauterine recordings and were asked to identify the vowels, consonants, and nonsense syllables or words. The frequency components in speech range from the fundamental frequency of the voice at around 200 Hz to about 8000 Hz. If the higher frequencies in speech are attenuated, one would expect difficulty for listeners identifying individual consonants and vowels that are information-rich in frequencies greater than about 150 Hz for men or 250 Hz for women. Identification of consonants was 14% for the recorded maternal voice but 30% for her live voice. For all voices together, intelligibility of the recorded speech hovered around 30%, individual phonemes, nonsense syllables, and words included. Similar intelligibility results have been reported in research on cochlear microphonics in fetal sheep (Smith, Gerhardt, Griffiths, Huang, & Abrams, 2003).

In contrast to the data suggesting that fetuses receive little exposure to frequencies greater than 1000 Hz, there are results suggesting that higher frequencies are available to the fetus. For the Roubaix study, the investigators used two microphones, one for lower and one for higher frequencies. The microphone *in utero* that was especially chosen for fidelity in recording frequencies greater than 1000 Hz showed that frequencies in a synthetic vowel emerged up to 10,000 Hz. In addition, the vowel /i/ (as in "feet"), requiring a second formant component of 2500 Hz for recognition, was one of the best recognized in intelligibility tests. Researchers have speculated that resonance patterns form among the sound waves inside the uterus, that attenuation of frequencies above 1000 Hz is not linear, and that, thus, higher frequencies are present. For a review and model, see Lecanuet et al. (1998).

If there is uncertainty about the extent of prenatal exposure to higher frequency sounds, there is no uncertainty about the lower frequency prosodic features of speech: rhythm, stress (relative loudness), and intonation (pitch). Prosody is well preserved on intrauterine recordings (D. Querleu, Renard, Boutteville, & Crepin, 1989). Prosody communicates emotion (Wiethoff et al., 2008) and intention (Hellbernd & Sammler, 2016) as well as grammatical function (e.g., for tone languages, or for English differentiation of questions and statements, and parts of speech like nouns and verbs).

Experiments show that the transmission of sound frequencies from outside into a specific location in the amniotic cavity depends on many factors: location of the sound source, how much tissue or fluid is present between the source and measurement site, whether the uterus is larger or smaller with thicker or thinner walls, and the acoustic structure of the outside environment (Gerhardt, 1989; Lecanuet et al., 1998; Turkewitz, 1988). The experience of the maternal voice is undoubtedly dynamic depending on the development of the fetal auditory system plus the external factors listed above. One conclusion has emerged from research over time: contrary to some earlier hypotheses (Fifer & Moon, 1988; Spence & DeCasper, 1987) the maternal voice can deliver more acoustic information to the developing fetus than lower frequency prosody. Individual sounds of speech (phonemes) seem to be available prenatally in addition to the prosody and unique characteristics of voices (Huotilainen, 2013; Moon, Lagercrantz, & Kuhl, 2013).

In addition to being richer in language information than previously thought, the maternal voice potentially delivers sensory information to other systems besides the auditory system. Sound transmission into the uterus is best described as multimodal (Moon & Fifer, 2000). For one thing, sound is transmitted in waves of compressed molecules that at high intensities and low frequencies can be felt as vibrations in the body. How the fetus experiences the non-cochlear components of sound delivery, particularly the mother's voice, has not been investigated. One question is the following: Are vibrations from the mother's voice available through the cutaneous senses when the fetus's skin is in direct contact with the uterus? This may be possible when a pregnant woman's voice is in the lower range as in the vocalist's "chest voice." If so, the experience of the maternal voice may be available earlier than the onset of hearing because the cutaneous senses are among the earliest sensory systems to develop (Hogg, 1941).

In addition to the cutaneous route, another nonauditory mode of transmission of the maternal voice is through the vestibular sense. For one thing, speaking requires movement of the mother's diaphragm and intercostal muscles in the chest in controlled expiration of air through the larynx. Respiratory inspiration motions are also synchronized with speech. These maternal motions are likely to cause at least small displacements of the fetus's body in space, depending on maternal effort and fetal size. Moreover, talking is accompanied by the speaker's motion of hands, arms, torso, and even legs, and this motion is very likely to affect the position of the fetus in space and be detected by the vestibular sense. Furthermore, as the fetus grows heavier over time, the nature of maternal body motion changes. For this type of motion, there is some research. In the late term fetus, passive motion of mother being propelled in a swing resulted in heart rate acceleration in the fetus when passive swinging was in an anterior-posterior direction but not side-to-side (Lecanuet & Jacquet, 2002). The study showed that fetuses are sensitive to motion of mother's body, but it doesn't address the conjugate prenatal stimulation by the maternal voice and motion that comes from her gestures and other body movements.

As a final point in the discussion of what the maternal voice may bring to the development of the fetus, there are circadian rhythms that bring together maternal voice and motion. When it is night and mother is lying in bed, for the most part she is not talking nor is anyone else. During the day when she is awake, upright, and actively moving, she is more likely to be speaking, and other voices are present.

Thus, there are at least three ways the maternal voice may be synchronized with nonauditory fetal sensation: vocal vibration, vestibular motion, and circadian cycles. Virtually nothing is known about how the relationship between maternal voice and motion affect prenatal and early postnatal development.

The Fetus Responds to Maternal Voice

The fetus is, of course, not readily accessible for observation of a response to a sound, and this poses a big research challenge. One potential source of information about fetal reaction to sound is the reports of pregnant women who feel startle-type responses to loud sounds. But maternal report of fetal movement in general is not a sensitive way to determine if a fetus has detected a particular sound. In one study, only 16% of fetal movement episodes detected by Doppler ultrasound were reported as such by mothers (Johnson, Jordan, & Paine, 1990). Researchers therefore use other methods. There are three targets of measurement for fetal detection of a particular sound: fetal brain activity, movement, and cardiac changes. The most frequently used methods have been (1) fetal motion detection through ultrasound visualization of the limbs or face, or detection of nonspecific motion through the use of Doppler ultrasound, and (2) measurement of fetal cardiac response to a sound through Doppler ultrasound. The method of Doppler ultrasound uses high frequency sound waves that penetrate through to the fetus and are affected by fetal motion, either of the heart or other parts of the body. The Doppler device receives the echo of the altered sound waves and provides data about them.

Doppler data on fetal motor activity has provided the most solid evidence thus far of the existence of fetal hearing at 24 weeks gestational age (GA). Forty-seven fetuses were tested with a rattle-like device (peak intensity 89 dB) 4 inches away from the maternal abdomen near the fetal head. Comparison of stimulation trials with sham trials showed a significant fetal motor, but not cardiac, response at 24 weeks. Fetuses at 36 weeks responded to the sound with both motor and cardiac changes (DiPietro et al., 2013). In a study conducted 20 years earlier, fetal movement to pulsed sound was reported for 20-week-olds (Shahidullah & Hepper, 1993). However, because 110 dB broadband sound (80–2000 Hz) was delivered through direct coupling with the maternal abdomen, it is possible that the fetal response was due to vibratory sensory characteristics of the sound and not cochlear reception. Acoustically complex, percussive sounds may be more effective at eliciting a response than pure tones, at least that seems to be the case for newborns (Clarkson & Berg, 1983). These experiments suggest that at 24 weeks, around the age of viability, the fetus is capable of detecting and responding to the acoustic features of the mother's voice. The conjoint features that accompany the maternal voice and that do not depend on a functioning fetal auditory system may be detected well before 24 weeks.

Very few studies have been published on fetal response to maternal voice per se. The studies that have been reported have used two types of stimulation, live speaking and recorded speech delivered by loudspeaker. These modes of delivery have different characteristics for the fetus. Live voice is the more familiar mode, is accompanied by synchronous auditory cardiovascular changes, and is multimodal. A recorded version of the mother's voice delivered from a loudspeaker is likely to be different in intensity and spectral properties compared to the live voice and is experienced during the audio recording process prior to loudspeaker testing as a live voice, and the voice is auditory only, not multimodal.

An older study with ten 36-week gestational age (GA) fetuses actually directly compared fetal motor responding to maternal live vs. recorded direct skin contact loudspeaker speech. Results showed differences in motor response to the two modes of stimulation (Hepper, Scott, & Shahidullah, 1993).

In a more recent Doppler ultrasound study of 74 fetuses at 36 weeks GA, only live speech was used in an effort to characterize the more typical circumstances of mother talking (Voegtline, Costigan, Pater, & DiPietro, 2013). In order to have some control over samples of talking, mothers read a passage aloud. This type of talking is arguably rare for fetuses. Fetuses showed a decrease in motor activity when the mother was speaking. Compared to a baseline period, fetal response to the voice was mediated by both the fetus's and the mother's prior state of arousal. The largest fetal motor and cardiac responses came from those who had been in a more quiescent state and whose mothers had previously been resting. But even the fetuses in a more active state of arousal responded with a heart rate-orienting response when their mother switched from conversation to reading aloud. In an even more recent study using ultrasound visual images, researchers coded five specific fetal movements of head, arms, and face in "awake" fetuses during live reading of one of two children's stories (Marx & Nagy, 2015). The fetuses were either in the second trimester ($N = 10$) or third ($N = 13$). Results showed no difference in the movements to voice compared to a control period with the exception of one of the six movements – yawning in third trimester fetuses (less frequent during speaking). The results should be considered preliminary due to the small N and low inter-rater reliability.

Taken together, these three studies, especially Voegtline et al. (2013), confirm that by the beginning of the third trimester, fetuses detect when their mother is talking, and they respond with changes in movement and heart rate. Fetal responses vary depending upon their own state of arousal and that of their mother when she begins to talk.

In an attempt to discern whether recognition of the mother's voice begins before birth, researchers have studied fetal response to audio recordings of mother vs. an unfamiliar female. In the studies, the two voices have been rendered equivalent by presenting them over a loudspeaker with the same words, equal duration, and equal intensity. One such study with ten fetuses showed no difference in fetal movement to the two voices (Hepper et al., 1993), whereas two studies from a different lab did find differences in heart rate response. In the first of these, at 38 weeks, fetuses responded with a sustained heart rate acceleration to a recording of a poem read by the mother, whereas the response to an unfamiliar female voice was a sustained deceleration (Kisilevsky et al., 2003). An important control for the within-subjects experimental design was that the maternal voice for each fetus served as the control voice for the subsequent one. In a later study, 104 fetuses of 33–41 weeks GA again showed a heart rate acceleration during a maternal voice recording compared to an unfamiliar female voice (Kisilevsky et al., 2009). The finding of heart rate acceleration to a recorded version of the mother's voice may reflect an increase in arousal because the recorded sound of her voice is unusual. This is supported by the 2003 study's deceleratory response to the novel voice. In neither the 2003 nor the 2009 research articles do the authors report fetal state of arousal prior to sound delivery. In other fetal perception studies, the stimuli are presented only when the fetus is in a state of low heart rate variability so that a small (usually deceleratory) orienting response to a moderately novel stimulus can be detected against background fetal heart rate fluctuations (Lecanuet, Granier-Deferre, & Jacquet, 1992).

To sum up the results from the few extant prenatal maternal voice studies, they provide a positive answer to the question of whether there is prenatal perception of the mother's voice and whether her voice is perceived as distinct from others.

Studies of fetal response to other types of sound stimuli are consistent with prenatal learning about the mother's voice, particularly exposure studies in which sounds, such as stories, are presented daily at home over time, and then the fetus is tested for evidence of having learned about them (DeCasper, Lecanuet, Busnel, Granier-Deferre, et al., 1994; Krueger, Holditch-Davis, Quint, & Decasper, 2004).

Postnatal Retention of Prenatal Experience

Newborn infants are much more accessible for observation than fetuses. Consequently there have been many more prenatal learning studies of babies than fetuses. The research strategy is based on the assumption that during the neonatal period, there has been so little opportunity to learn that infant responses reflect retained prenatal experience. Particularly informative have been studies that measure newborn "preference" for one sound compared to another. Preference has been inferred by exposing the infant in the laboratory to two alternatives, one presumably familiar and the other unfamiliar. Researchers measure the relative behavioral attraction to the two stimuli. For example, neonates make head turns in the delivery room toward live maternal voice more than toward an unfamiliar female voice (Querleu et al., 1984) or later after birth toward the maternal voice compared to turns toward the father's voice (Lee & Kisilevsky, 2014).

Most neonatal preference experiments do not rule out rapid postnatal learning, but there are a few that provide strong evidence of prenatal learning. One such experiment used infant-controlled presentation of sounds in headphones. Sound presentation was contingent on pacifier sucking, and the frequency and duration of production of one sound vs. another were assumed to reveal infant preference for the sound. Using this method, Spence and colleagues obtained results consistent with a preference for a synthesized prenatal version of the mother's voice, a sound not experienced postnatally (Spence & DeCasper, 1987; Spence & Freeman, 1996). In another study, DeCasper and Spence asked pregnant women to frequently read a story aloud, and then the neonates were tested for preference for the prenatal story vs. a novel one. The infants preferred the familiar prenatal story that they had not heard since being born (DeCasper & Spence, 1986).

Infant-controlled voice preference studies show that neonates alter sucking patterns to activate the sound of the mother's voice whether she was recorded reading a nursery story (DeCasper & Fifer, 1980) or conversing with another adult (Moon & Fifer, 1990). And they prefer a recording of the maternal language vs. a foreign one (Moon, Panneton Cooper, & Fifer, 1993) but show no preference for either of a bilingual mother's two languages (Byers-Heinlein, Burns, & Werker). The language recognition results were extended to show that neonates respond to a vowel from the maternal language as if it is familiar compared to a vowel from a foreign language. The number of hours of postnatal experience to the native language did not affect responding to the two languages, consistent with an effect of prenatal, and not postnatal, learning (Moon et al., 2013). The experiments comparing native and foreign languages show that frequencies above 1000 Hz are available in the womb because the vowels cannot be learned on the basis of lower frequencies alone (Huotilainen, 2013) and neither can most consonants. In a neonate brain imaging study on fetal exposure to a recorded pseudoword (not the mother's voice), response patterns to the familiar word were different compared to other stimuli, and the amount of pre-natal exposure was related to postnatal brain response strength (Partanen et al., 2013). In neonatal brain imaging studies, infants showed different brain evoked response patterns to a recording of their mother saying the word "baby" vs. an unfa-miliar female. Remarkably, they seemed to recognize the voice on the basis of less than a second of stimulus (Deregnier, Nelson, Thomas, Wewerka, & Georgieff, 2000). In contrast, results of a sucking behavior study using the single word "baby" showed no preference for mother vs. a stranger (Moon, Zernzach, & Kuhl, 2015). This seems to indicate that although voice recognition is present despite minimal information, it takes a richer sample of the maternal voice for newborns to mount a behavioral response and show a preference. Perhaps prosody is required. A study of 1-month-olds using the contingent sucking procedure showed no difference in responding to the voice of mother vs. a stranger when the recordings were monotone (Mehler, Bertoncini, Barriere, & Jassik-Gerschenfeld, 1978), and rhythm is an important feature of newborn language discrimination (Nazzi, Bertoncini, & Mehler, 1998). It is apparent from decades of research on prenatal experience with the maternal voice that the voice is a prominent feature of the intrauterine environment, that fetuses perceive it, and that they learn as a result of exposure. At the very least, they learn to recognize their mother's voice, and they learn about her language(s).

Prenatal Auditory Experience and Later Spoken Language Acquisition

Although experimental evidence converges on the existence of prenatal learning about voices and speech, hearing the mother's voice during the fetal period may not be necessary for acquisition of spoken language (Moon, 2011). Especially informa-tive are cases in which fetuses are exposed to little or no sound of maternal speech. One such example is the language acquisition of hearing children of deaf mothers who used little spoken speech during both the pre- and postnatal periods. Such chil-dren, KODAs (kids of deaf adults), are studied especially for their bilingual lan-guage acquisition. They learn both spoken and sign languages. Despite a relative paucity of experiencing spoken language compared to hearing children of hearing parents, KODAs meet acquisition milestones in their two languages at the same rate as hearing children of hearing parents (Brackenbury, Ryan, & Messenheimer, 2006; Petitto et al., 2001).

In contrast to the relatively rare research studies of KODAs, there is a large and growing research literature on language learning by children who were born deaf but were later able to perceive speech because of cochlear implants at the end of their first year at the earliest. Prior to being implanted, these children have had minimal experience with the sounds of speech, depending on their degree of deafness. Even after implantation, they do not have the full range of sound available because cochlear implants deliver only a portion of the audible frequencies to the auditory nerve. Nonetheless, under optimal conditions, children with cochlear implants (CI children) who had little to no prenatal auditory experience have been shown to score within the range of hearing children on standardized measures of language acquisition. In a recent prospective longitudinal sample of 60 CI children, predictors for language outcome at 10.5 years included implantation before 3 years of age, a high level of parent education and income, hearing aids prior to implantation, early professional speech and language intervention, and early mainstream classroom education. The participants' preschool speech/language ability predicted their ability at 10.5 years of age (Geers & Nicholas, 2013). This study is particularly informative because it shows that early intervention and nurturing conditions can alter a pre- and early postnatal developmental path that may seem fixed at birth.

This example speaks to early deprivation of acoustic stimulation and suggests plasticity in brain organization for speech perception and production at least up to the end of the second year of postnatal life (Kral & Sharma, 2012; Markman et al., 2011). In fact, it appears that there are multiple open windows for brain organization for different aspects of spoken language that close at different times in development (Markman et al., 2011). These results open many questions for both basic and applied research on aberrant early experience relevant to language acquisition. For basic research, what is the best way to describe the aspects of language that are under development at different times? What are the mechanisms that allow the development of one aspect of language before another? For applied research an important question is how to support language development both before and after intervening to make relatively typical auditory experience possible?

Preterm Infants

Deaf infants and preterm infants both experience unusual exposure to sound during very early development compared to hearing fetuses born at term. Without supportive intervention, both populations are at risk for delayed language development. An exception is deaf children of deaf mothers who use fluent sign language with them (Bornstein, Selmi, Haynes, Painter, & Marx, 1999). In contrast to hospitalized preterms at the same gestational ages, deaf fetuses experience the other forms of sensory stimulation that accompany maternal use of language, whether or not the mother uses spoken or signed language (Petitto, Holowka, Sergio, & Ostry, 2001). From CI infants, we can learn about the consequences of early auditory deprivation followed by intervention, and we can be optimistic about the plasticity of the auditory system and language acquisition in the first 2 years after birth if the right kind of support is provided. Hospitalized preterm infants are not comparable to deaf infants in that they do experience sounds during what would normally have been their fetal period, including speech sounds, but the acoustic characteristics are not the same as the ones they would have experienced at the same stage of development in utero. Research has yet to clearly specify the characteristics of those intrauterine sounds *as perceived by the fetus* at different points in development. If only we had a psychophysics of the fetus!

For the hospitalized preterm infant, the environment may provide a rich sound environment, perhaps even much richer compared to the womb – a broader range and different distribution of the sound frequency spectrum, machine sounds, and different voices but less maternal voice and no maternal digestive and cardiac sounds. This will vary, depending on the infant's circumstances. We have had research results for decades demonstrating that loud and unabated sound in the NICU is detrimental to hospitalized preterm infants (Graven, 2000). Compared to the womb, in the NICU there is most likely a relative paucity of sustained exposure to a particular voice, that of the mother. Furthermore, the impoverished experience with this one particular voice includes the lack of conjoint nonauditory sensory stimulation. The exception is when the mother is holding the baby, particularly with skin-to-skin contact as in kangaroo care (Feldman, Rosenthal, & Eidelman, 2014). We know next to nothing about the developmental role played by the absence of experience with one particular voice and with its conjoint multisensory stimulation.

In conclusion, many studies have been conducted on prenatal exposure and learning about the mother's voice. The studies confirm what many mothers and others have believed for millennia – that the developing child in the womb perceives the maternal voice, learns from it, and retains what was learned into early postnatal life. Much remains unknown about the prenatal effect of hearing the mother's voice, including even very basic information about the dynamic unfolding of the experience, what sensations are involved, and even whether the experience is necessary for favorable development.

Key Messages
- Fetal auditory experience with the mother's voice begins around 24 weeks after conception, and learning that occurred during prenatal life persists into early postnatal life.
- The maternal voice is potentially a rich source of multimodal stimulation that is comparatively absent for hospitalized preterm infants.
- Deaf infants with early cochlear implants appear to surmount early auditory deprivation and can be equivalent to hearing children in language acquisition. This suggests early human brain plasticity for language acquisition.
- The sound of the maternal voice and the complex of sensory experiences that accompany it are present for typically developing fetuses, but the necessity of the sound per se for favorable long term development has not been established, for either the fetus or the hospitalized preterm.

References

Adelman, C., Chordekar, S., Perez, R., & Sohmer, H. (2014). Investigation of the mechanism of soft tissue conduction explains several perplexing auditory phenomena. *Journal of Basic and Clinical Physiology and Pharmacology, 25*(3), 269–272. doi:10.1515/jbcpp-2014-0037

Bornstein, M. H., Selmi, A. M., Haynes, O. M., Painter, K. M., & Marx, E. S. (1999). Representational abilities and the hearing status of child/mother dyads. *Child Development, 70*(4), 833–852. doi:10.1111/1467-8624.00060

Brackenbury, T., Ryan, T., & Messenheimer, T. (2006). Incidental word learning in a hearing child of deaf adults. *Journal of Deaf Studies and Deaf Education, 11*(1), 76–93. doi:10.1093/deafed/enj018

Byers-Heinlein, K., Burns, T. C., & Werker, J. F. The roots of bilingualism in newborns. *Psychological Science, 21*(3), 343–348. doi:10.1177/0956797609360758

Clarkson, M. G., & Berg, W. K. (1983). Cardiac orienting and vowel discrimination in newborns: Crucial stimulus parameters. *Child Development, 54*, 162–171.

DeCasper, A. J., & Fifer, W. P. (1980). Of human bonding: Newborns prefer their mothers' voices. *Science, 208*(4448), 1174–1176.

DeCasper, A. J., Lecanuet, J.-P., Busnel, M.-C., Granier-Deferre, C., et al. (1994). Fetal reactions to recurrent maternal speech. *Infant Behavior & Development, 17*(2), 159–164.

DeCasper, A. J., & Spence, M. J. (1986). Prenatal maternal speech influences newborns' perception of speech sounds. *Infant Behavior & Development, 9*, 133–150.

Deregnier, R. A., Nelson, C. A., Thomas, K. M., Wewerka, S., & Georgieff, M. K. (2000). Neurophysiologic evaluation of auditory recognition memory in healthy newborn infants and infants of diabetic mothers. [Research Support, Non-U.S. Gov't Research Support, U.S. Gov't, P.H.S.] *Journal of Pediatrics, 137*(6), 777–784. doi:10.1067/mpd.2000.109149

DiPietro, J. A., Voegtline, K. M., Costigan, K. A., Aguirre, F., Kivlighan, K., & Chen, P. (2013). Physiological reactivity of pregnant women to evoked fetal startle. *Journal of Psychosomatic Research, 75*(4), 321–326. doi:10.1016/j.jpsychores.2013.07.008

Feldman, R., Rosenthal, Z., & Eidelman, A. I. (2014). Maternal-preterm skin-to-skin contact enhances child physiologic organization and cognitive control across the first 10 years of life. *Biological Psychiatry, 75*(1), 56–64. doi:10.1016/j.biopsych.2013.08.012

Fifer, W. P., & Moon, C. M. (1988). Auditory experience in the fetus. In W. P. Smotherman & S. R. Robinson (Eds.), *Behavior of the fetus*. Caldwell, NJ: Telford Press.

Geers, A. E., & Nicholas, J. G. (2013). Enduring advantages of early cochlear implantation for spoken language development. *Journal of Speech, Language, and Hearing Research, 56*(2), 643–653. doi:10.1044/1092-4388(2012/11-0347)

Gerhardt, K. J. (1989). Characteristics of the fetal sheep sound environment. *Seminars in Perinatology, 13*(5), 362–370.

Graven, S. N. (2000). Sound and the developing infant in the NICU: Conclusions and recommendations for care. *Journal of Perinatology, 20*, S88–S93.

Hellbernd, N., & Sammler, D. (2016). Prosody conveys speaker's intentions: Acoustic cues for speech act perception. *Journal of Memory and Language, 88*, 70–86. doi:10.1016/j.jml.2016.01.001

Hepper, P. G., Scott, D., & Shahidullah, S. (1993). Newborn and fetal response to maternal voice. *Journal of Reproductive and Infant Psychology, 11*(3), 147–153.

Hogg, I. D. (1941). Sensory nerves and associated structures in the skin of human fetuses of 8 to 14 weeks of menstrual age correlated with functional capability. *Journal of Comparative Neurology and Psychology, 75*, 371–410. doi:10.1002/cne.900750302

Huotilainen, M. (2013). A new dimension on foetal language learning. *Acta Paediatrica, 102*(2), 102–103. doi:10.1111/apa.12122

Johnson, T. R., Jordan, E. T., & Paine, L. L. (1990). Doppler recordings of fetal movement: II. Comparison with maternal perception. *Obstetrics and Gynecology, 76*(1), 42–43.

Kisilevsky, B. S., Hains, S. M. J., Brown, C. A., Lee, C. T., Cowperthwaite, B., Stutzman, S. S., … Wang, Z. (2009). Fetal sensitivity to properties of maternal speech and language. *Infant Behavior & Development*, *32*(1), 59–71. doi:10.1016/j.infbeh.2008.10.002

Kisilevsky, B. S., Hains, S. M. J., Lee, K., Xie, X., Huang, H., Ye, H. H., … Wang, Z. (2003). Effects of experience on fetal voice recognition. *Psychological Science*, *14*(3), 220–224.

Kral, A., & Sharma, A. (2012). Developmental neuroplasticity after cochlear implantation. *Trends in Neurosciences*, *35*(2), 111–122. doi:10.1016/j.tins.2011.09.004

Krueger, C., Holditch-Davis, D., Quint, S., & Decasper, A. (2004). Recurring auditory experience in the 28- to 34-week-old fetus. *Infant Behavior & Development*, *27*(4), 537–543.

Lecanuet, J.-P., Gautheron, B., Locatelli, A., Schaal, B., Jacquet, A.-Y., & Busnel, M.-C. (1998). What sounds reach fetuses: Biological and nonbiological modeling of the transmission of pure tones. *Developmental Psychobiology*, *33*(3), 203–219.

Lecanuet, J.-P., Granier-Deferre, C., & Jacquet, A. Y. (1992). Decelerative cardiac responsiveness to acoustical stimulation in the near term fetus. *The Quarterly Journal of Experimental Psychology*, *44B*(3/4), 279–303.

Lecanuet, J.-P., & Jacquet, A.-Y. (2002). Fetal responsiveness to maternal passive swinging in low heart rate variability state: Effects of stimulation direction and duration. *Developmental Psychobiology*, *40*(1), 57–67.

Lee, G. Y., & Kisilevsky, B. S. (2014). Fetuses respond to father's voice but prefer mother's voice after birth. Developmental Psychobiology, *56*(1), 1-11. doi: 10.1002/dev.21084.

Markman, T. M., Quittner, A. L., Eisenberg, L. S., Tobey, E. A., Thal, D., Niparko, J. K., & Wang, N.-Y. (2011). Language development after cochlear implantation: An epigenetic model. *Journal of Neurodevelopmental Disorders*, *3*(4), 388–404. doi:10.1007/s11689-011-9098-z

Marx, V., & Nagy, E. (2015). Fetal behavioural responses to maternal voice and touch. *PLoS One*, *10*(6).

Mehler, J., Bertoncini, J., Barriere, M., & Jassik-Gerschenfeld, D. (1978). Infant recognition of mother's voice. *Perception*, *7*(5), 491–497.

Moon, C. (2011). The role of early auditory development in attachment and communication. *Clinics in Perinatology*, *38*(4), 657–669. doi:10.1016/j.clp.2011.08.009

Moon, C., & Fifer, W. P. (1990). Syllables as signals for 2-day-old infants. *Infant Behavior & Development*, *13*(3), 377–390.

Moon, C., & Fifer, W. P. (2000). Evidence of transnatal auditory learning. *Journal of Perinatology*, *20*(8), S37–S44.

Moon, C., Lagercrantz, H., & Kuhl, P. K. (2013). Language experienced in utero affects vowel perception after birth: A two–country study. *Acta Paediatrica*, *102*(2), 156–160. doi:10.1111/apa.12098

Moon, C., Panneton Cooper, R., & Fifer, W. P. (1993). Two-day-olds prefer their native language. *Infant Behavior & Development*, *16*(4), 495–500.

Moon, C., Zernzach, R. C., & Kuhl, P. K. (2015). Mothers say 'baby' and their newborns do not choose to listen: A behavioral preference study to compare with ERP results. *Frontiers in Human Neuroscience*, *9*.

Nazzi, T., Bertoncini, A., & Mehler, J. (1998). Language discrimination by newborns: Toward an understanding of the role of rhythm. *Journal of Experimental Psychology: Human Perception and Performance*, *24*(3), 756–766.

Partanen, E., Kujala, T., Näätänen, R., Liitola, A., Sambeth, A., & Huotilainen, M. (2013). Learning-induced neural plasticity of speech processing before birth. *Proceedings of the National Academy of Sciences of the United States of America*, *110*(37), 15145–15150. doi:10.1073/pnas.1302159110

Perez, R., Adelman, C., & Sohmer, H. (2016). Fluid stimulation elicits hearing in the absence of air and bone conduction – An animal study. *Acta Oto-Laryngologica*, *136*(4), 351–353. doi:10.3109/00016489.2015.1113560

Petitto, L. A., Holowka, S., Sergio, L. E., & Ostry, D. (2001). Language rhythms in baby hand movements. *Nature*, *413*(6851), 35–36. doi:10.1038/35092613

Petitto, L. A., Katerelos, M., Levy, B. G., Gauna, K., Tétreault, K., & Ferraro, V. (2001). Bilingual signed and spoken language acquisition from birth: Implications for the mechanisms underlying early bilingual language acquisition. *Journal of Child Language, 28*(2), 453–496. doi:10.1017/s0305000901004718

Querleu, C., Lefebvre, C., Titran, M., Renard, X., Morillion, M., & Crepin, G. (1984). Reactivité du nouveau-né de moins de deux heures de vie à la voix maternelle. *Journal de Gynécologie Obstétrique et Biologie de la Réproduction, 13*, 125–135.

Querleu, D., Renard, X., Boutteville, C., & Crepin, G. (1989). Hearing by the human fetus? *Seminars in Perinatology, 13*(5), 409–420.

Querleu, D., Renard, X., Versyp, F., Paris-Delrue, L., & Crepin, G. (1988). Fetal hearing. *Journal de Gynécologie, Obstétrique et Biologie de la Reproduction, 28*(3), 191–212.

Querleu, D., Renard, X., Versyp, F., Paris-Delrue, L., & Vervoort, P. (1988). La transmission intra-amniotique des voix humaines. *Revue Française de Gynécologie et d'Obstétrique, 83*(1), 43–50.

Shahidullah, S., & Hepper, P. G. (1993). The developmental origins of fetal responsiveness to an acoustic stimulus. *Journal of Reproductive and Infant Psychology, 11*, 135–142.

Smith, S. L., Gerhardt, K. J., Griffiths, S. K., Huang, X., & Abrams, R. M. (2003). Intelligibility of sentences recorded from the uterus of a pregnant ewe and from the fetal inner ear. *Audiology and Neurotology, 8*(6), 347–353.

Spence, M. J., & DeCasper, A. J. (1987). Prenatal experience with low-frequency maternal-voice sounds influence neonatal perception of maternal voice samples. *Infant Behavior & Development, 10*, 133–142.

Spence, M. J., & Freeman, M. S. (1996). Newborn infants prefer the maternal low-pass filtered voice, but not the maternal whispered voice. *Infant Behavior & Development, 19*(2), 199–212.

Turkewitz, G. (1988). A prenatal source for the development of hemispheric specialization. In D. L. Molfese & S. J. Segalowitz (Eds.), *Brain Lateralizations in children: Developmental implications* (pp. 73–81). New York, NY: Guilford Press.

Voegtline, K. M., Costigan, K. A., Pater, H. A., & DiPietro, J. A. (2013). Near-term fetal response to maternal spoken voice. *Infant Behavior & Development, 36*(4), 526–533. doi:10.1016/j.infbeh.2013.05.002

Wiethoff, S., Wildgruber, D., Kreifelts, B., Becker, H., Herbert, C., Grodd, W., & Ethofer, T. (2008). Cerebral processing of emotional prosody – Influence of acoustic parameters and arousal. *NeuroImage, 39*(2), 885–893.

Chapter 3
The Maternal Voice as a Special Signal for Infants

Sandra E. Trehub

Abstract Mothers throughout the world vocalize to infants in the course of caregiving. This chapter describes (1) mothers' speech and singing to infants, including differences arising from cultural practices and individual circumstances, and (2) the impact of maternal speech and singing on infants. Vocalizations to infants are more expressive than vocalizations to others, and they are often accompanied by gestures in other modalities. Although infants are sensitive to voices in general, they are particularly sensitive to the expressive style of infant-directed vocalizations and to the familiarity of the maternal voice. Infant-directed vocalizations, whether speech or singing, are effective in capturing infant attention, but infant-directed singing is more effective than infant-directed speech for regulating infant emotion or arousal. The maternal voice seems to function as a source of security and stimulation for infants, enhancing mother-infant bonds and promoting infants' social, emotional, and cognitive development.

Human Vocalizations

Human vocalizations are biologically and socially significant for listeners of all ages. In the newborn period, infants listen longer to speech than to artificial sounds that mimic the pitch contours and timing of speech (Vouloumanos & Werker, 2007). A few weeks later, they smile socially to voices before they begin smiling to faces (Wolff, 1963). The unique timbre or sound quality of a natural voice activates voice-sensitive regions in infant and adult brains (Belin, Zatorre, & Ahad, 2002;

Preparation of this chapter was assisted by grants from the Natural Sciences and Engineering Council of Canada and by inspiration from AIRS (Advanced Interdisciplinary Research in Singing). Address correspondence to Sandra E. Trehub, University of Toronto Mississauga, Mississauga, Ontario, Canada L5L 1C6. Email: sandra.trehub@utoronto.ca

S.E. Trehub (✉)
University of Toronto, Mississauga, Mississauga, ON L5L 1C6, Canada
e-mail: sandra.trehub@utoronto.ca

© Springer International Publishing AG 2017
M. Filippa et al. (eds.), *Early Vocal Contact and Preterm Infant Brain Development*, DOI 10.1007/978-3-319-65077-7_3

Blasi et al., 2011; Grossmann, Oberecker, Koch, & Friederici, 2010), with the activation being more intense for emotional than for neutral vocalizations (Grossmann et al., 2010).

Familiar voices have more potent effects than unfamiliar voices, regardless of the age of the listener. For example, newborns recognize their mother's voice and prefer it to the voice of a stranger (DeCasper & Fifer, 1980), presumably on the basis of prenatal exposure. A number of factors facilitate the recognition of familiar voices, including timbre or voice quality, pitch patterning or intonation (Bergeson & Trehub, 2007), and timing (rhythm and speaking rate) (Vongpaisal, Trehub, Schellenberg, van Lieshout, & Papsin, 2010). Although familiar voices are a source of comfort and pleasure for infants, they also enhance speech perception in infancy (Barker & Newman, 2004), as in the preschool years (Ryalls & Pisoni, 1997) and beyond (Nygaard, Sommers, & Pisoni, 1994).

Infant Listening Skills for Speech and Music

Maternal vocal communication, which features the most familiar voice, has special significance for infants. For preverbal infants in particular, melodic patterns (i.e., combinations of pitch and rhythm) in maternal speech and song are highly salient (Fernald, 1992; Trehub, 2016; Trehub & Trainor, 1998). Before considering the nature of maternal speech and song, it is important to consider the perceptual skills that make those sounds accessible and potentially meaningful to infant listeners.

Infants detect subtle pitch changes (i.e., a semitone or less) in a melody (Trainor & Trehub, 1992; Trehub, Schellenberg, & Kamenetsky, 1999), but they are especially sensitive to pitch relations. For example, they perceive the similarity of a melody and its transpositions—absolute pitch differences but pitch relations preserved (Chang & Trehub, 1977a; Trehub, Thorpe, & Morrongiello, 1987). They exhibit long-term memory for the pitch relations of instrumental melodies but not their absolute pitch level (Plantinga & Trainor, 2005). For vocal melodies, however, infants exhibit long-term memory for their pitch level (Volkova, Trehub, & Schellenberg, 2006) and pitch relations (Mehr, Song, & Spelke, 2016).

In some circumstances, infants notice a single changed note in a melody, whether it alters the contour, or pattern of directional pitch changes (Trehub, Thorpe, & Morrongiello, 1985), or preserves the contour (Trainor & Trehub, 1993). In general, however, they focus on the pitch contours of melodies—their overall shape—while ignoring small interval changes (Trehub et al., 1987). Infants' focus on melodic shape rather than pitch accuracy should allay the concerns of mothers who consider themselves poor or middling singers.

Most research on infants' perception of pitch patterns has been conducted with awake, alert, and cooperative infants who are 5 months of age or older. Surprisingly, there are striking parallels in sleeping newborns (1–3 days of age), which have been documented with electrophysiological methods. Such studies have revealed that the neonatal brain is sensitive to changes in pitch direction—rising versus falling pitch (Carral et al., 2005)—and changes in interval size, large (seven semitones) versus small (two semitones) (Stefanics et al., 2009).

From 4 or 5 months of age, if not before, infants focus on the pitch contours of infant-directed speech (Fernald, 1989, 1992), which are often characterized as *speech melodies*. Note, however, that *speech melodies* have a loose correspondence to *musical melodies*. Pitch levels change much more rapidly in speech than in music, and intonation contours have larger and less precisely specified pitch excursions than melodic patterns in music (Zatorre & Baum, 2012). In any case, infants differentiate rising from falling pitch contours in speech (Frota, Butler, & Vigário, 2014; Soderstrom, Ko, & Nevzorova, 2011), but they do not link those differences to the speaker's intentions (e.g., questioning vs. stating). Infants also distinguish approving from disapproving/prohibition contours, which differ in the magnitude and smoothness of their pitch excursions (Fernald, 1993). Remarkably, the cries of French newborns are dominated by rising pitch, and those of German newborns are dominated by falling pitch, in line with the predominant pitch patterns of French and German speech (Mampe, Friederici, Christophe, & Wermke, 2009), a finding that implicates prenatal learning.

Infants are also sensitive to temporal aspects of music and speech. They detect changes in tempo (Pickens & Bahrick, 1995) and exhibit long-term memory for the tempo of familiar melodies (Trainor, Wu, & Tsang, 2004). They perceive temporal grouping or relative timing in music (Chang & Trehub, 1977b; Trehub & Thorpe, 1989) and the meter or pattern of strong and weak beats (Bergeson & Trehub, 2006; Hannon & Trehub, 2005). Temporal regularity is important for infant listeners, as evident by superior detection of pitch and timing changes in metrically regular music than in music with irregular timing (Trehub & Hannon, 2009). Even during sleep, newborn brains are sensitive to the beat of rhythmic music, as reflected in their responses to the omission of strong beats (Winkler, Háden, Ladinig, Sziller, & Honing, 2009).

Infants' perception of meter is influenced by movement experienced while listening to sound patterns. When 7-month-olds are bounced on every second beat to a drumming pattern with ambiguous meter (no accented beats), they perceive the pattern in duple meter; when bounced on every third beat, they perceive it in triple meter (Phillips-Silver & Trainor, 2005). Listening to rhythmic music also promotes rhythmic movement from about 5 months of age (Ilari, 2015; Zentner & Eerola, 2010), but such movement is not synchronized with the music. In fact, rhythmic movement does not become synchronized with music until about 4 years of age (McAuley, Jones, Holub, Johnston, & Miller, 2006). For younger children, greater synchronization is evident in social than in nonsocial contexts (Kirschner & Tomasello, 2009).

Synchronous movement to music has social as well as perceptual consequences. When 14-month-old infants are bounced to music and observe a synchronously or non-synchronously bouncing adult, they subsequently exhibit more prosocial behavior toward the adult who moved synchronously than to the other adult (Cirelli, Einarson,

& Trainor, 2014). Their prosocial behavior is selective rather than general, being directed to the synchronous bouncer and her friends but not to other adults (Cirelli, Wan, & Trainor, 2016). In the preschool period, synchronous singing and dancing promote prosocial behavior with peers (Kirschner & Tomasello, 2010).

Maternal Speech to Infants

As the most ubiquitous auditory signal for infants, it is not surprising that maternal vocal communication, speech in particular, has been the focus of extensive research. Mothers talk effusively to preverbal infants in a style that features higher pitch, more variable pitch and loudness, greater rhythmicity, slower rate, and warmer vocal tone relative to speech directed to adults (e.g., Fernald & Simon, 1984; Fernald et al., 1989; Narayan & McDermott, 2016). These various features contribute to the musical (Brandt, Gebrian, & Slevc, 2012; Fernald, 1989, 1992) and emotive (Trainor, Austin, & Desjardins, 2000) qualities of maternal speech. It is worth noting, however, that North American mothers' intonation patterns are more exaggerated than those produced by fathers and by mothers from other cultures (Fernald et al., 1989; Kitamura, Thanavisuth, Luksaneeyanawin, & Burnham, 2002). Moreover, individual differences within cultures are substantial (Narayan & McDermott, 2016).

Mothers intuitively adapt their speech to the age and needs of infants, which results in more comforting speech for 3-month-olds, more arousing speech for 6-month-olds, and more informing or directive speech for 9-month-olds (Kitamura & Burnham, 2003; Kitamura & Lam, 2009). The limited research on speech to newborns reveals predominantly soothing rather than stimulating vocal and nonvocal behaviors, reflecting caregivers' nurturing goals and concerns about overstimulation (Stern, Spieker, Barnett, & MacKain, 1983). In the case of congenitally deaf infants with cochlear implants (implants typically received at 12 months of age or later), mothers' use of approving and comforting speech is influenced by infant hearing experience (i.e., months of functional hearing) and age, and mothers' use of informing and directive speech is influenced by infant age or cognitive maturity (Kondaurova, Bergeson-Dana, Zu, & Kitamura, 2015).

In addition to the prosodic commonalities and variations that are evident within and across cultures (Fernald et al., 1989; Narayan & McDermott, 2016), there are unique or individually distinctive aspects of maternal speech. For example, each mother tends to use a limited set of unique interval sequences or *signature tunes* when speaking to her infant (Bergeson & Trehub, 2007), heightening the potency and memorability of her speech.

Mothers' vocal expressiveness or emotionality is also influenced by feedback from infants. When mothers interact face-to-face with infants, their speech is more emotive than it is in interactions at comparably close range but with infants obscured from view (Trehub, Plantinga, & Russo, 2016). The one-on-one, face-to-face context, which is typical of urban, middle-class interactions with infants from 2 or 3 months to at least 6 months of age, allows mothers to monitor infants' engagement and fine-tune their communicative behavior to the needs of infants.

Face-to-face contexts provide infants with distinctive visual as well as vocal input. For example, mothers produce facial expressions that convey nurturance, wonder, or joy (Chong, Werker, Russell, & Carroll, 2003). These and other visual cues vary across languages, enabling adults to distinguish one language from another on the basis of visual cues (Soto-Faraco et al., 2007). Infants as young as 4 months of age also differentiate a familiar language—the one usually heard in their environment—from an unfamiliar language solely on the basis of visual cues (Weikum et al., 2007). Other modalities are involved in typical mother-infant interactions. For example, mothers often touch infants while interacting face-to-face, but touch is more pervasive in the absence of face-to-face contact, as when holding or carrying infants. Maternal touch varies with infant age, being more affectionate (e.g., stroking, patting) for younger infants and more stimulating (e.g., tickling) for older infants (Ferber, Feldman, & Makhoul, 2008; Jean, Stack, & Fogel, 2009).

Maternal challenges—emotional, social, or economic—affect qualitative and quantitative aspects of their speech. For example, depressed mothers interact less, vocalize less, and exhibit less affectionate vocal and nonvocal behavior with infants than do non-depressed mothers (Field, Diego, & Hernandez-Reif, 2006; Herrera, Reissland, & Shepherd, 2004). Similarly, mothers from economically disadvantaged backgrounds typically have fewer one-on-one interactions with their young children than do mothers from more advantaged backgrounds (Hart & Risley, 1995). As a result, infants from disadvantaged families often experience less infant-directed speech than their middle-class counterparts (Weisleder & Fernald, 2013).

Effects of Maternal Speech

Newborns and older infants are more attentive to speech in the maternal style than to conventional adult-directed speech (Cooper & Aslin, 1990; Fernald, 1985; Werker & McLeod, 1989). The happy-sounding quality of such speech seems to underlie its attention-getting properties in the first year (Kitamura & Burnham, 1998; Singh, Morgan, & Best, 2002), with such effects continuing into the second year as well (Segal & Newman, 2015). Maternal visual signals also have important consequences, but most research has focused on auditory aspects of stimulation. When 3- and 5-month-old infants are presented with side-by-side displays of silent talking faces (videos) in infant- or adult-directed style, they look preferentially at the infant-directed faces regardless of whether they hear infant-directed speech, adult-directed speech, or silence (Kim & Johnson, 2014). Audiovisual renditions of infant-directed speech influence infant affect as well as attention (Werker & McLeod, 1989).

The visual gestures that accompany talking not only distinguish one language from another (Soto-Faraco et al., 2007; Weikum et al., 2007); they also distinguish one person from another. After hearing infant-directed speech or singing from an unfamiliar person, adults successfully judge which of the two successively presented silent videos corresponds to the person heard previously; 6- to 8-month-old infants look longer at the silent video of the previously heard person than at the video of a novel person (Trehub, Plantinga, Brcic, & Nowicki, 2013). These findings emphasize the unique, person-specific auditory and visual cues in speech and song.

In the early months of infancy, the mother's speech has wide-ranging social and emotional implications. Her sensitivity, which entails vocal and nonvocal behavior that is appropriate to the infant's age and needs, especially in the context of distress, is of particular importance (Leerkes et al., 2015). Nonvocal behavior such as holding and carrying, especially while moving (i.e., walking rather than sitting), is highly effective in calming crying infants (Esposito et al., 2013). Interestingly, maternal sensitivity in infancy has long-term emotional, social, and academic implications (Raby, Roisman, Fraley, & Simpson, 2015).

In later months, the quality and quantity of maternal speech have consequences for language development (Hoff, 2003; Hurtado, Marchman, & Fernald, 2007). By 18 months of age, notable differences in verbal processing and production are evident in children from economically disadvantaged backgrounds and those from more advantaged backgrounds (Fernald, Marchman, & Weisleder, 2013). The critical issue here is speech directed specifically to infants rather than speech that infants simply overhear. In fact, infants' exposure to one-on-one speech predicts language processing efficiency and vocabulary at 24 months of age (Weisleder & Fernald, 2013). Individual differences in attention also play an important role. For example, 12-month-olds' differential attention to speech and non-speech sounds is linked to expressive vocabulary at 24 months of age (Vouloumanos & Curtin, 2014).

Maternal Singing to Infants

Mothers across cultures sing to infants while providing care (Trehub & Gudmundsdottir, 2015; Trehub & Trainor, 1998). In societies where caregivers maintain almost constant physical contact with infants and value infant tranquility, lullabies are the songs of choice. In cultures that prioritize face-to-face contact and infant stimulation, play songs are more frequent, with lullabies reserved primarily for bedtime routines.

Analyses of caregivers' singing, which have focused largely on play songs, have revealed that mothers and fathers sing at a higher pitch level, slower tempo, and with warmer vocal tone when singing to infants than in other contexts (Trainor, Clark, Huntley, & Adams, 1997; Trehub, Unyk, & Trainor, 1993, Trehub et al., 1997). Infants' presence is necessary to elicit fully expressive performances, as indicated by parents' reduced expressiveness in infants' absence (Trehub et al., 1997). An infant audience in itself is insufficient; the infant must also be visible. For example, mothers sing less expressively when their infant is out of view—behind an opaque screen—rather than in view (Trehub et al., 2016), which indicates that visual feedback from infants maximizes maternal expressiveness. Bodily contact may also enhance maternal vocal expressiveness, but this issue has not been studied to date.

Fig. 3.1 Mean duration (in seconds) of maternal smiling while talking or singing to infants during a 60-second interaction when infants were in view or obscured from view (From Trehub et al. (2016))

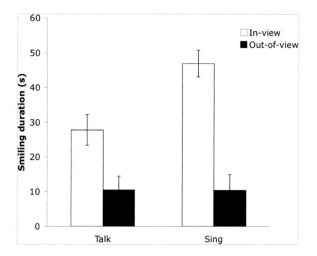

Although mothers produce distinctive facial expressions when talking to infants (Chong et al., 2003), they smile considerably more when singing than when talking (Trehub et al., 2016). In fact, they smile almost constantly while singing in contrast to intermittent smiling while talking to infants (see Fig. 3.1). Many mothers also move while they sing—swaying from side to side or bobbing their head—generating multimodal musical performances that can be seen as well as heard. At times, mothers hold or move infants as they sing, adding yet another modality to the mix.

Effects of Maternal Singing

Newborns and older infants are more attentive to singing in the maternal style than to conventional informal singing by the same singer (Masataka, 1999; Trainor, 1996), a finding that parallels the listening preferences of newborns and older infants for infant- over adult-directed speech (Cooper & Aslin, 1990; Fernald, 1985). These listening preferences are generally attributed to the positive vocal tone or happy-sounding quality of infant-directed speech and singing (Corbeil, Trehub, & Peretz, 2013; Singh et al., 2002).

Although infant-directed speech and singing seem to be equally effective for *capturing* infant attention (Corbeil et al., 2013; Costa-Giomi, 2014), they differ in their efficacy for *sustaining* infant attention and regulating emotion. In one study that explored this issue, 7- to 10-month-old infants heard a continuously playing audio recording of a woman singing a children's song or speaking the lyrics in an infant- or adult-directed manner (Corbeil, Trehub, & Peretz, 2016). The question of interest was how long it would take before infants became visibly upset while listening to these materials in a relatively unengaging environment—a dimly lit room with no parent or other person in view. Surprisingly, infants listened to the song more than twice as long as to the speech before showing visible signs of discontent (a cry face) for 4 s (see Fig. 3.2). The presumption is that the regular beat

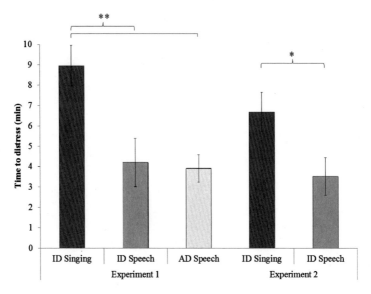

Fig. 3.2 Average time, in minutes, until infants became distressed while listening to speech, infant- or adult-directed, or singing. In Experiment 1, infants listened to a Turkish children's song or the spoken lyrics of that song. In Experiment 2, infants listened to infant-directed singing or speech in their native language (French) (From Corbeil et al. (2016))

of children's songs, which is typically lacking in speech (other than metrical poetry), prolongs infants' attention and relative contentment. If regularity in beat structure is important, then recited nursery rhymes should be more effective than conventional infant-directed speech in delaying infant distress. If the sustained pitches of singing are also relevant, then sung nursery rhymes should be even more effective than rhythmic recitations.

It is important to note that the stimuli in the aforementioned studies featured the voices of unfamiliar speakers and singers, either actors who simulated the maternal or non-maternal style or mothers of other infants who were recorded in previous natural interactions. The impact of such stimuli is likely to be enhanced by familiar voices and also by the opportunity to see as well as hear singers and speakers. Indeed, audiovisual recordings of maternal singing (own mother recorded in previous interactions with infants) are considerably more engaging to 6-month-old infants than comparable recordings of maternal speech (Nakata & Trehub, 2004). Moreover, the intensity of infants' engagement is evident not only from their extended visual fixations on the image of their singing mother but also in infants' physical stillness, another index of attention capture and engagement (Bacher & Robertson, 2001).

Even with unfamiliar singers and speakers, infants exhibit greater attentiveness to audiovisual versions of singing than to audiovisual versions of speech (Costa-Giomi, 2014). The temporal regularity of songs, the steady beat in particular, is likely to be implicated. There is suggestive evidence that infants use the beat of infant-directed singing to listen in a predictive manner, as revealed by systematic eye movements to the singer's eyes in anticipation of the beat (Lense & Jones, 2016).

Audiovisual singing with familiar (maternal) and unfamiliar (maternal style) singers could be compared in future research. One would expect maternal singing to be advantageous because of many familiar elements aside from the mothers' familiar voice and face. As noted, mothers use a relatively small repertoire of songs that they sing repeatedly (Trehub et al., 1997), and they sing songs almost identically on different occasions (Bergeson & Trehub, 2002). Familiarity increases the appeal of music for adults (Szpunar, Schellenberg, & Pliner, 2004), and it is likely to do so for infants as well.

Live maternal singing has the potential for even greater infant engagement because of the possibility of performances attuned to infant feedback (Trehub et al., 2016). In fact, such singing, even in the absence of physical contact, modulates the arousal levels of contented 5- to 7-month-olds, as reflected in their salivary cortisol levels (Shenfield, Trehub, & Nakata, 2003). After maternal singing episodes, the arousal levels of infants converge relative to pretest levels. For example, infants with initially low arousal levels exhibit slight elevations, and those with initially higher levels exhibit slight reductions, reflecting a potential convergence on optimal arousal levels.

The aforementioned affect-regulatory consequences of audio versions of infant-directed singing (Corbeil et al., 2016) and the arousal-modulating effects of live maternal singing (Shenfield et al., 2003) were demonstrated with infants who were calm and contented, at least initially. To investigate the relative efficacy of multimodal maternal speech and singing (vocal, visual, and tactile stimulation) for reversing distress in 10-month-old infants, Ghazban (2013) used a version of the still-face procedure (Mesman, van IJzendoorn, & Bakermans-Kranenburg, 2009) that featured an initial play phase (60 s); a brief stress-induction phase (15 s) in which mothers were silent, immobile, and unresponsive while facing infants; and a final reunion phase (90 s) in which mothers interacted freely with infants except for their vocalizations being restricted to singing on some trials and to speech on others. The stress-induction manipulation was successful in the sense that infants' arousal levels rose substantially (i.e., elevated skin conductance levels), as did their negative facial and vocal expressions. In the reunion phase, maternal singing was considerably more successful than maternal speech in reducing covert (arousal) and overt (facial and vocal) signs of infant distress (see also Trehub, Ghazban, & Corbeil, 2015).

What factors could account for the efficacy of multimodal maternal singing in reversing infant distress? By singing songs that they usually sing at home, probably in a similar manner (Bergeson & Trehub, 2002), mothers provided highly familiar, rhythmically regular melodies and lyrics, supplemented at times with rhythmic movement. Presumably, the predictable style and content of maternal singing would be a source of comfort for infants who were experiencing stress. Although mothers spoke in an infant-directed manner, they did not have the advantage of scripted material, as when singing songs. Multimodal speech and singing both featured the familiar maternal voice, but the singing episodes featured the same songs sung regularly at home, possibly performed in a similar manner (Bergeson & Trehub, 2002). In other words, the singing episodes provided greater overall familiarity than the speaking episodes, reassuring infants who were upset about their previously unresponsive mother. Moreover, the predictable timing of maternal singing (Nakata & Trehub, 2011) would support covert entrainment which, in turn, facilitates positive engagement with a social partner (Lense & Jones, 2016).

In short, the maternal voice, in song as in speech, is a powerful signal that helps forge and maintain emotional ties between mother and infant. As the maternal voice becomes more and more familiar over time, it becomes an increasingly potent source of security, comfort, and guidance for infants. To date, however, discussions of the mother (or primary caregiver) as an attachment figure and secure base for infants (e.g., Bowlby, 1998) have focused largely on maternal sensitivity in general, with little attention to maternal vocal sensitivity. The maternal voice, with or without accompanying facial expressions, touch, and movement (Corbeil et al., 2016; Ghazban, 2013), makes powerful contributions to infant emotional regulation and, ultimately, to emotional, social, and cognitive development. Undoubtedly, maternal singing affects the singer as well as the listener, but the consequences on mothers have not been explored to date. Nevertheless, the historical and cross-cultural record is consistent with the view that singing to infants, to others, and even to oneself has favorable consequences on the singer's well-being (Norton, 2016).

Implications for Prematurely Born Infants

Parenting is challenging at the best of times, but the birth of a premature infant presents a host of unexpected challenges. With high levels of uncertainty about the immediate and more distant future, it is not surprising that mothers of prematurely born infants experience greater levels of depression and anxiety than do mothers of full-term infants (Gray, Edwards, O'Callaghan, Cuskelly, & Gibbons, 2013; Miles, Holditch-Davis, Schwartz, & Scher, 2007). In too many cases, the result is enduring negative effects on mother-infant interaction (Forcada-Guex, Borghini, Pierrehumbert, Ansermet, & Muller-Nix, 2011) and infant emotional development (Voigt et al., 2013).

Maternal speech and singing are no panacea for the challenges of parenting a prematurely born infant, but they may provide a modicum of assistance in the NICU and beyond. If mothers understood that their tiny infant has functional hearing and the capacity to recognize their voice and to become familiar with their songs or recited nursery rhymes (Moon, Chap. 2, this volume), they might be motivated to begin nurturing the dyadic relationship by vocal means. In time, they could complement their vocalizations with other modalities of stimulation (e.g., touch, movement). If they understood that these interactions were likely to reduce the incidence of adverse medical events and promote calm, alert states in their fragile infants (Filippa, Devouche, Arioni, Imberty, & Gratier, 2013), and promote more positive outcomes thereafter, they might be gratified by the opportunity to participate actively in their infant's care. Obviously, any such interventions in the NICU and at home must be tailored not only to the infant's health status and psychological needs but also to maternal psychological needs and patterns of distress (Holditch-Davis et al., 2015).

> **Key Messages**
> - Infants are sensitive to subtle differences in pitch and timing patterns and to the expressive nuances of maternal speech and singing.
> - Mothers smile much more when they sing than when they speak to infants, which enhances the impact of maternal singing.
> - Although infant-directed speech and singing have comparable efficacy in *capturing* infant attention, infant-directed singing is more effective in *sustaining* infant attention, delaying infant distress, and ameliorating infant distress.
> - In view of the demonstrable benefits of maternal vocal behavior, it is important to find productive means of bringing some of those benefits to residents of the NICU.

References

Bacher, L. F., & Robertson, S. S. (2001). Stability of coupled fluctuations in movement and visual attention in infants. *Developmental Psychobiology, 39*, 99–106.

Barker, B. A., & Newman, R. S. (2004). Listen to your mother! The role of talker familiarity in infant streaming. *Cognition, 94*, B45–B53.

Belin, P., Zatorre, R. J., & Ahad, P. (2002). Human temporal-lobe response to vocal sounds. *Cognitive Brain Research, 13*, 17–26.

Bergeson, T. R., & Trehub, S. E. (2002). Absolute pitch and tempo in mothers' songs to infants. *Psychological Science, 13*, 71–74.

Bergeson, T. R., & Trehub, S. E. (2006). Infants' perception of rhythmic patterns. *Music Perception, 23*, 345–360.

Bergeson, T. R., & Trehub, S. E. (2007). Signature tunes in mothers' speech to infants. *Infant Behavior & Development, 30*, 648–654.

Blasi, A., Mercure, E., Lloyd-Fox, S., Thomson, A., Brammer, M., Sauter, D., … Murphy, D. G. M. (2011). Early specialization for voice and emotion processing in the infant brain. *Current Biology, 21*, 1220–1224.

Bowlby, J. (1998). *A secure base: Parent-child attachment and healthy human development.* New York, NY: Basic Books.

Brandt, A., Gebrian, M., & Slevc, L. R. (2012). Music and early language acquisition. *Frontiers in Psychology, 3*, 327.

Carral, V., Huotilainen, M., Ruusuvirta, T., Fellman, V., Näätänen, R., & Escera, C. (2005). A kind of auditory "primitive intelligence" already present at birth. *European Journal of Neuroscience, 21*, 3201–3204.

Chang, H. W., & Trehub, S. E. (1977a). Auditory processing of relational information by young infants. *Journal of Experimental Child Psychology, 24*, 324–331.

Chang, H. W., & Trehub, S. E. (1977b). Infants' perception of temporal grouping in auditory patterns. *Child Development, 48*, 1666–1670.

Chong, S. C. F., Werker, J. F., Russell, J. A., & Carroll, J. M. (2003). Three facial expressions mothers direct to their infants. *Infant and Child Development, 12*, 211–232.

Cirelli, L. K., Einarson, K. M., & Trainor, L. J. (2014). Interpersonal synchrony increases prosocial behavior in infants. *Developmental Science, 17*, 1003–1011.

Cirelli, L. K., Wan, S. J., & Trainor, L. J. (2016). Social effects of movement synchrony: Increased infant helpfulness only transfers to affiliates of synchronously moving partners. *Infancy, 21*, 807–821.

Cooper, R., & Aslin, R. (1990). Preference for infant-directed speech in the first month after birth. *Child Development, 61*, 1584–1595.

Corbeil, M., Trehub, S. E., & Peretz, I. (2013). Speech vs. singing: Infants choose happier sounds. *Frontiers in Psychology, 4*, 372.

Corbeil, M., Trehub, S. E., & Peretz, I. (2016). Singing delays the onset of infant distress. *Infancy, 21*, 373–391.

Costa-Giomi, E. (2014). Mode of singing affects infants' preferential attention to singing and speech. *Music Perception, 32*, 160–169.

DeCasper, A. J., & Fifer, W. P. (1980). Of human bonding: Newborns prefer their mothers' voices. *Science, 208*, 1174–1176.

Esposito, G., Yoshida, S., Ohnishi, R., Tsuneoka, Y., del Carmen Rostagno, M., … Kuroda, K. O. (2013). Infant calming responses during maternal carrying in humans and mice. *Current Biology, 23*, 739–745.

Ferber, S. G., Feldman, R., & Makhoul, I. R. (2008). The development of maternal touch across the first year of life. *Early Human Development, 84*, 363–370.

Fernald, A. (1985). Four-month-old infants prefer to listen to motherese. *Infant Behavior & Development, 8*, 181–195.

Fernald, A. (1989). Intonation and communicative intent in mothers' speech to infants: Is the melody the message? *Child Development, 60*, 1497–1510.

Fernald, A. (1992). Meaningful melodies in mothers' speech to infants. In H. Papoušek & U. Jürgens (Eds.), *Nonverbal vocal communication: Comparative and developmental approaches* (pp. 262–282). New York, NY: Cambridge University Press.

Fernald, A. (1993). Approval and disapproval: Infant responsiveness to vocal affect in familiar and unfamiliar languages. *Child Development, 64*, 657–674.

Fernald, A., Marchman, V. A., & Weisleder, A. (2013). SES differences in language processing skill and vocabulary are evident at 18 months. *Developmental Science, 16*, 234–248.

Fernald, A., & Simon, T. (1984). Expanded intonation contours in mothers' speech to newborns. *Developmental Psychology, 20*, 104–113.

Fernald, A., Taeschner, T., Dunn, J., Papousek, M., de Boysson-Bardies, B., & Fukui, I. (1989). A cross-language study of prosodic modifications in mothers' and fathers' speech to preverbal infants. *Journal of Child Language, 16*, 477–501.

Field, T., Diego, M., & Hernandez-Reif, M. (2006). Prenatal depression effects on the fetus and newborn: A review. *Infant Behavior & Development, 29*, 445–455.

Filippa, M., Devouche, E., Arioni, C., Imberty, M., & Gratier, M. (2013). Live maternal speech and singing have beneficial effects on hospitalized preterm infants. *Acta Paediatrica, 102*, 1017–1020.

Forcada-Guex, M., Borghini, M., Pierrehumbert, B., Ansermet, F., & Muller-Nix, C. (2011). Prematurity, maternal posttraumatic stress and consequences on the mother–infant relationship. *Early Human Development, 87*, 21–26.

Frota, S., Butler, J., & Vigário, M. (2014). Infants' perception of intonation: Is it a statement or a question? *Infancy, 19*, 194–213.

Ghazban, N. (2013). *Emotion regulation in infants using maternal singing and speech* (Unpublished doctoral dissertation). Ryerson University, Toronto, Canada.

Gray, P. H., Edwards, D. M., O'Callaghan, M. J., Cuskelly, M., & Gibbons, K. (2013). Parenting stress in mothers of very preterm infants: Influence of development, temperament and maternal depression. *Early Human Development, 89*, 625–629.

Grossmann, T., Oberecker, R., Koch, S. P., & Friederici, A. D. (2010). The developmental origins of voice processing in the human brain. *Neuron, 65*, 852–858.

Hannon, E. E., & Trehub, S. E. (2005). Metrical categories in infancy and adulthood. *Psychological Science, 16*, 48–55.

Hart, B., & Risley, T. R. (1995). *Meaningful differences in the everyday experience of young American children*. Baltimore, MD: Brookes Publishing Co.

Herrera, E., Reissland, N., & Shepherd, J. (2004). Maternal touch and maternal child-directed speech: Effects of depressed mood in the postnatal period. *Journal of Affective Disorders, 81*, 29–39.

Hoff, E. (2003). The specificity of environmental influence: Socioeconomic status affects early vocabulary development via maternal speech. *Child Development, 74*, 1368–1878.

Holditch-Davis, D., Santos, H., Levy, J., White-Traut, R., O'Shea, T. M., … David, R. (2015). Patterns of psychological distress in mothers of preterm infants. *Infant Behavior & Development, 41*, 154–163.

Hurtado, N., Marchman, V., & Fernald, A. (2007). Spoken word recognition by Latino children learning Spanish as their first language. *Journal of Child Language, 34*, 227–249.

Ilari, B. (2015). Rhythmic engagement with music in early childhood: A replication and extension. *Journal of Research in Music Education, 62*, 332–343.

Jean, A. D. L., Stack, J. M., & Fogel, A. (2009). A longitudinal investigation of maternal touching across the first six months of life: Age and context effects. *Infant Behavior & Development, 32*, 344–349.

Kim, H. I., & Johnson, S. P. (2014). Detecting 'infant-directedness' in face and voice. *Developmental Science, 17*, 621–627.

Kirschner, S., & Tomasello, M. (2009). Joint drumming: Social context facilitates synchronization in preschool children. *Journal of Experimental Child Psychology, 102*, 299–314.

Kirschner, S., & Tomasello, M. (2010). Joint music-making promotes prosocial behavior in 4-year-old children. *Evolution and Human Behavior, 31*, 354–364.

Kitamura, C., & Burnham, D. (1998). The infant's response to maternal vocal affect. In C. Rovee-Collier, L. Lipsitt, & H. Hayne (Eds.), *Advances in infancy research* (vol. 12, pp. 221–236). Stamford, CT: Ablex Publishing Corp.

Kitamura, C., & Burnham, D. (2003). Pitch and communicative intent in mothers' speech: Adjustments for age and sex in the first year. *Infancy, 4*, 85–110.

Kitamura, C., & Lam, C. (2009). Age-specific preferences for infant-directed affective intent. *Infancy, 14*, 77–100.

Kitamura, C., Thanavisuth, C., Luksaneeyanawin, S., & Burnham, D. (2002). Universality and specificity in infant-directed speech: Pitch modifications as a function of infant age and sex in a tonal and non-tonal language. *Infant Behavior & Development, 24*, 372–392.

Kondaurova, M. V., Bergeson-Dana, T., Zu, H., & Kitamura, C. (2015). Affective properties of mothers' speech to infants with hearing impairment and cochlear implants. *Journal of Speech, Language, and Hearing Research, 58*, 590–600.

Leerkes, E. M., Supple, A. J., O'Brien, M., Calkins, S. D., Haltigan, J. D., Wong, M. S., & Fortuna, K. (2015). Antecedents of maternal sensitivity during distressing tasks: Integrating attachment, social information processing, and psychobiological perspectives. *Child Development, 86*, 94–111.

Lense, M., Jones, W. (2016, July). Beat-based entrainment during infant-directed singing supports social engagement. Paper presented at 14th biennial meeting of the International Conference on Music Perception and Cognition, San Francisco, CA.

Mampe, B., Friederici, A. D., Christophe, A., & Wermke, K. (2009). Newborns' cry melody is shaped by their native language. *Current Biology, 19*, 1994–1997.

Masataka, N. (1999). Preference for infant-directed singing in 2-day-old hearing infants of deaf parents. *Developmental Psychology, 35*, 1001–1005.

McAuley, J. D., Jones, M. R., Holub, S., Johnston, H. M., & Miller, N. S. (2006). The time of our lives: Life span development of timing and event tracking. *Journal of Experimental Psychology: General, 135*, 348–367.

Mehr, S. A., Song, L. A., & Spelke, E. S. (2016). For 5-month-old infants, melodies are social. *Psychological Science, 27*, 486–501.

Mesman, J., van IJzendoorn, M. H., & Bakermans-Kranenburg, M. J. (2009). The many faces of the still-face paradigm: A review and metaanalysis. *Developmental Review, 29*, 120–162.

Miles, M. S., Holditch-Davis, D., Schwartz, T. A., & Scher, T. (2007). Depressive symptoms in mothers of prematurely born infants. *Journal of Developmental and Behavioral Pediatrics, 28*, 36–44.

Nakata, T., & Trehub, S. E. (2004). Infants' responsiveness to maternal speech and singing. *Infant Behavior & Development, 27*, 455–464.

Nakata, T., & Trehub, S. E. (2011). Expressive timing and dynamics in infant-directed singing. *Psychomusicology: Music, Mind and Brain, 21*, 45–53.

Narayan, C. R., & McDermott, L. C. (2016). Speech rate and pitch characteristics of infant-directed speech: Longitudinal and cross-linguistic observations. *Journal of the Acoustical Society of America, 139*, 1272–1281.

Norton, K. (2016). *Singing and wellbeing: Ancient wisdom, modern proof*. New York, NY: Routledge.

Nygaard, L. C., Sommers, M. S., & Pisoni, D. B. (1994). Speech perception as a talker-contingent process. *Psychological Science, 5*, 42–46.

Phillips-Silver, J., & Trainor, L. J. (2005). Feeling the beat: Movement influences infant rhythm perception. *Science, 308*, 1430.

Pickens, J., & Bahrick, L. E. (1995). Infants' discrimination of bimodal events on the basis of rhythm and tempo. *British Journal of Developmental Psychology, 13*, 223–236.

Plantinga, J., & Trainor, L. J. (2005). Memory for melody: Infants use a relative pitch code. *Cognition, 98*, 1–11.

Raby, K. L., Roisman, G. I., Fraley, R. C., & Simpson, J. A. (2015). The enduring predictive significance of early maternal sensitivity: Social and academic competence through age 32 years. *Child Development, 86*, 695–708.

Ryalls, B. O., & Pisoni, D. B. (1997). The effect of talker variability on word recognition in preschool children. *Developmental Psychology, 33*, 441–452.

Segal, J., & Newman, R. S. (2015). Infant preferences for structural and prosodic properties of infant-directed speech in the second year of life. *Infancy, 20*, 339–351.

Shenfield, T., Trehub, S. E., & Nakata, T. (2003). Maternal singing modulates infant arousal. *Psychology of Music, 31*, 365–375.

Singh, L., Morgan, J. L., & Best, C. T. (2002). Infants' listening preferences: Baby talk or happy talk? *Infancy, 3*, 365–394.

Soderstrom, M., Ko, E. S., & Nevzorova, U. (2011). It's a question? Infants attend differently to yes/no questions and declaratives. *Infant Behavior & Development, 34*, 107–110.

Soto-Faraco, S., Navarra, J., Weikum, W. M., Vouloumanos, A., Sebastián-Gallés, N., & Werker, J. F. (2007). Discriminating languages by speech-reading. *Perception & Psychophysics, 69*, 218–231.

Stefanics, G., Háden, G. P., Sziller, I., Balázs, L., Beke, A., & Winkler, I. (2009). Newborn infants process pitch intervals. *Clinical Neurophysiology, 120*, 304–308.

Stern, D. N., Spieker, S., Barnett, R. K., & Mackain, K. (1983). The prosody of maternal speech: Infant age and context related changes. *Journal of Child Language, 10*, 1–15.

Szpunar, K. K., Schellenberg, E. G., & Pliner, P. (2004). Liking and memory for musical stimuli as a function of exposure. *Journal of Experimental Psychology: Learning, Memory, and Cognition, 30*, 370–381.

Trainor, L. J. (1996). Infant preferences for infant-directed versus non infant-directed playsongs and lullabies. *Infant Behavior & Development, 19*, 83–92.

Trainor, L. J., Austin, C. M., & Desjardins, R. (2000). Is infant-directed speech prosody a result of the expression of emotion? *Psychological Science, 11*, 188–195.

Trainor, L. J., Clark, E. D., Huntley, A., & Adams, B. A. (1997). The acoustic basis of preferences for infant-directed singing. *Infant Behavior & Development, 20*, 383–396.

Trainor, L. J., & Trehub, S. E. (1992). A comparison of infants' and adults' sensitivity to western musical structure. *Journal of Experimental Psychology: Human Perception and Performance, 18*, 394–402.

Trainor, L. J., & Trehub, S. E. (1993). What mediates infants' and adults' superior processing of the major over the augmented triad? *Music Perception, 11*, 185–196.

Trainor, L. J., Wu, L., & Tsang, C. D. (2004). Long-term memory for music: Infants remember tempo and timbre. *Developmental Science, 7*, 289–296.

Trehub, S. E. (2016). Infant musicality. In S. Hallam, I. Cross, & M. Thaut (Eds.), *The Oxford handbook of music psychology* (2nd ed.pp. 387–397). Oxford, UK: Oxford University Press.

Trehub, S. E., Ghazban, N., & Corbeil, M. (2015). Musical affect regulation in infancy. *Annals of the New York Academy of Sciences, 1337*, 186–192.

Trehub, S. E., & Gudmundsdottir, H. R. (2015). Mothers as singing mentors for infants. In G. F. Welch, J. Nix, & D. Howard (Eds.), *Oxford handbook of singing*. Oxford: Oxford University Press/Advance online publication. doi:10.1093/oxfordhb/9780199660773.013.25

Trehub, S. E., & Hannon, E. E. (2009). Conventional rhythms enhance infants' and adults' perception of musical patterns. *Cortex, 45*, 110–118.

Trehub, S. E., Plantinga, J., Brcic, J., & Nowicki, M. (2013). Cross-modal signatures in maternal speech and singing. *Frontiers in Psychology, 4*, 811.

Trehub, S. E., Plantinga, J., & Russo, F. A. (2016). Maternal vocal interactions with infants: Reciprocal visual influences. *Social Development, 25*, 665–683.

Trehub, S. E., Schellenberg, E. G., & Kamenetsky, S. B. (1999). Infants' and adults' perception of scale structure. *Journal of Experimental Psychology: Human Perception and Performance, 25*, 965–975.

Trehub, S. E., & Thorpe, L. A. (1989). Infants' perception of rhythm: Categorization of auditory sequences by temporal structure. *Canadian Journal of Psychology, 43*, 217–229.

Trehub, S. E., Thorpe, L. A., & Morrongiello, B. A. (1985). Infants' perception of melodies: Changes in a single tone. *Infant Behavior & Development, 8*, 213–223.

Trehub, S. E., Thorpe, L. A., & Morrongiello, B. A. (1987). Organizational processes in infants' perception of auditory patterns. *Child Development, 58*, 741–749.

Trehub, S. E., & Trainor, L. J. (1998). Singing to infants: Lullabies and play songs. *Advances in Infancy Research, 12*, 43–77.

Trehub, S. E., Unyk, A. M., Kamenetsky, S. B., Hill, D. S., Trainor, L. J., Henderson, J. L., & Saraza, M. (1997). Mothers' and fathers' singing to infants. *Developmental Psychology, 33*, 500–507.

Trehub, S. E., Unyk, A. M., & Trainor, L. J. (1993). Maternal singing in cross-cultural perspective. *Infant Behavior & Development, 16*, 285–295.

Voigt, B., Brandl, A., Pietz, J., Pauen, S., Kliegel, M., & Reuner, G. (2013). Negative reactivity in toddlers born prematurely: Indirect and moderated pathways considering self-regulation, neonatal distress and parenting stress. *Infant Behavior & Development, 36*, 124–138.

Volkova, A., Trehub, S. E., & Schellenberg, E. G. (2006). Infants' memory for musical performances. *Developmental Science, 9*, 584–590.

Vongpaisal, T., Trehub, S. E., Schellenberg, E. G., van Lieshout, P., & Papsin, B. C. (2010). Children with cochlear implants recognize their mother's voice. *Ear and Hearing, 31*, 555–566.

Vouloumanos, A., & Curtin, S. (2014). Foundational tuning: How infants' attention to speech predicts language development. *Cognitive Science, 38*, 1675–1686.

Vouloumanos, A., & Werker, J. F. (2007). Listening to language at birth: Evidence for a bias for speech in neonates. *Developmental Science, 10*, 159–164.

Weikum, W. M., Vouloumanos, A., Navarro, J., Soto-Faraco, S., Sebastián-Gallés, N., & Werker, J. F. (2007). Visual language discrimination in infancy. *Science, 316*, 1159.

Weisleder, A., & Fernald, A. (2013). Talking to children matters: Early language experience strengthens processing and builds vocabulary. *Psychological Science, 24*, 2143–2152.

Werker, J. F., & McLeod, P. J. (1989). Infant preference for both male and female infant-directed talk: A developmental study of attentional and affective responsiveness. *Canadian Journal of Psychology, 43*, 230–246.

Winkler, I., Háden, G. P., Ladinig, O., Sziller, I., & Honing, H. (2009). Newborn infants detect the beat in music. *Proceedings of the National Academy of Sciences USA, 106*, 2468–2471.

Wolff, P. H. (1963). Observations on the early development of smiling. In B. Foss (Ed.), *Determinants of infant behaviour, II* (pp. 113–167). London, England: Methuen.

Zatorre, R. J., & Baum, S. R. (2012). Musical melody and speech intonation: Singing a different tune. *PLoS Biology, 10*, e1001372.

Zentner, M., & Eerola, T. (2010). Rhythmic engagement with music in infancy. *Proceedings of the National Academy of Sciences USA, 107*, 5768–5773.

Chapter 4
The Development of Infant Participation in Communication

Maya Gratier and Emmanuel Devouche

Abstract *Introduction*: Full-term infants experience human voices in ecological contexts. Transnatal memory of the mother's voice plays a crucial role in guiding infants' first social encounters. On the basis of the earliest interactions with social partners, involving well-coordinated behavior, infants rapidly develop communicative and socio-cognitive skills.

Main aims of the chapter: In this chapter we describe three major transitions in socio-communicative development in the first year of life leading to foundational acquisitions of the end of the first year, such as joint attention, leading to language skills. We aim to highlight developmental continuity between these known transitions and the extent to which various forms of participation in infants, such as intent listening, less focused overhearing, or active production, underlie the seemingly emergent socio-cognitive skills of the end of the first year.

Conclusions: Based on the major breakthroughs of the last decades that have provided detailed understanding of the development of preverbal communication in infancy, it is worth investigating newborn preterm infants' communicative abilities, even while in the NICU, and the ways in which parents may support the earliest forms of participation in social exchange. In this chapter we describe how small-scale ecological change in the NICU can facilitate participatory exchange between a preterm infant and a mother.

M. Gratier (✉)
Laboratoire Ethologie, Cognition, Développement, Université Paris Nanterre, Nanterre, France
e-mail: gratier@gmail.com

E. Devouche
Laboratoire de Psychopathologie et Processus de Santé (LPPS),
Institut de Psychologie – Université Paris Descartes, Paris, France

© Springer International Publishing AG 2017
M. Filippa et al. (eds.), *Early Vocal Contact and Preterm Infant Brain Development*, DOI 10.1007/978-3-319-65077-7_4

Infants are sensitive to social partners from birth and possess the means to indicate their social motivation to engage with them. This chapter traces the development of infant communicative abilities, from birth to the advent of speech, by reviewing studies of infants' participation in everyday, real-life situations with familiar partners. It also presents evidence from experimental research supporting the conclusions drawn from naturalistic studies of parent-infant social interaction. The main argument of this chapter is that experiences of intimacy and closeness between parents and very young infants, rooted in dynamic processes of multimodal behavioral coordination, form the basis of the first protolinguistic semantic system that is shared only with familiar partners and from which conventional and consensual speech arises. In the final part of the chapter, we suggest that even preterm infants may benefit from multimodal attuned behavior from their parents offering them opportunities to be participants in social life from the very start. We provide an illustration of the kind of parental sensitivity to preterm infant's communicative abilities that may be observed in NICU with minor adjustments of its particular ecology.

Prenatal Preparedness for Communication

Newborns are equipped to perceive the world they are born into. Their sensory systems are active since long before birth. They are also highly motivated to seek out the attention and affective engagement of social partners. We have strong evidence today that newborns already perceive others in a holistic way. Indeed they perceive faces and voices together, body movement and tactile stimuli, smells, and shapes. There is reason to believe that the mother's voice plays a major role in driving the intricate intersensory and intermodal connections that are formed and then retained in memory in the first days after birth. Hearing the mother's voice in utero is a salient, coherent, and highly frequent experience that creates continuity between the periods preceding and following birth, despite the drastic changes involved in leaving the uterine environment.

In a series of elegant studies designed to understand the mechanisms underlying newborns' preference for their mothers' face over that of strangers, Sai (2005) found that a preference for the mother's face is guided by recognition of the mother's voice. Indeed only infants who have experience of their mother's face and voice together in real-life situations show a strong preference for the mother's face when it is presented as a static image in an experimental setting. Other transnatal continuities may contribute to guiding the infant toward an integrated multimodal perception of the world such as body movement, taste, and smell. Indeed, research on newborns' sense perception has shown that they can recognize smells of substances they experienced in utero, including their own amniotic fluid, as well as smells experienced very soon after birth (Marlier, Schaal, & Soussignan, 1998). It is thus very likely that smell is rapidly associated in memory with maternal voice and face. It will be important in the future for researchers to identify more specifically how voice, movement, or taste become patterned signatures so powerfully retained in the earliest formed memories.

We also have evidence today that neonates are capable of engaging in social interaction, especially with their mothers. Dominguez, Devouche, Apter, and Gratier (2016) have recently shown that mothers speak affectionately and responsively to their neonates who in turn respond with subtly timed vocalizations. Furthermore, analysis of the content of mothers' speech reflects an implicit attribution of both a social stance and mental states to their newborn infant, specifically when they are in a quiet alert state and not when they are drowsy or asleep (Dominguez, Gratier, Martel, Apter, & Devouche, submitted). T.B. Brazelton was a pioneer in discovering how efficiently and forcefully newborns engage with social partners, and he and his colleagues have proven, over the years, that they are well equipped to do so.

When interacting with their mothers, newborns experience their faces moving in synchrony with the changing qualities of their voices, and they experience tactile stimulation, warmth, odors, and taste from the milk the mother provides. They also experience their own body moving with the mother's body, and proprioceptive experience is perhaps rooted in the perception of being moved by another, as it is already the case in utero. Neonates in fact show a sense of proprioception guided by vision, suggesting they coordinate sensory-motor feedback from their own body with visual information from the external world (Van der Meer, Van der Weel, & Lee, 1995). All of these experiences, in the real-life settings of the ordinary yet specialized encounters they have with caring adults, may indeed lay the ground for early cross-modal learning and modes of perception that are more and more refined and adapted to their growing needs and developing motives.

The Ecological Niche of the Neonate

Studies of neonatal psychology do not sufficiently take into account the degree to which the social world becomes organized around the infant so that there is an immediate adaptation of the context the child lives within to its own motives and abilities. The newborn does not merely encounter the outside world when it is born; its sights, sounds, and smells are not merely taken up by the active sense perception of the infant. What the newborn encounters is a world closing in on its own specific presence, tuning in to provide not only the material but also the psychological conditions that will enable its development. Around the world, newborns are met by caring adults who carry in their minds theories of what they need and can do and of how they will develop and what they should achieve. Material props, such as cribs, slings, and strollers, have been invented in support of these theories. Protective spaces are created for the infant, and adults filter out from these spaces certain stimuli, such as heat, light, or volatile substances, an excess of which is thought to perturb or harm the newborn. All infants adapt to the variety of ways in which caring adults around the world hold them, talk or sing to them, and rock and manipulate them. Super and Harkness (1986) have described these combined physical, social, and material environmental adaptations as a child's "developmental niche," and this is a most useful concept. However, more and more recent evidence from developmental psychology supports a theory of mutual adaptation between infants and the "natural" contexts that enable their development. The infant's active role, from birth, in shaping the kind of care it receives, most evidently in terms of socio-affective involvement, is today widely accepted. Infants respond to the adapted environment they are born into and by doing so alter the way adults tune in to their specific needs and motives. The mutual relationship between the infant and its social environment has been the subject of some study in the last decades, some of which will be reviewed in the following paragraphs.

The Infant as Participant

Irving Goffman (1981) has described how "participation frameworks" emerge in verbal interactions between adults, providing opportunities for participants to display their relationship and their roles within it. Participants take on alternating roles as speakers and hearers with respect to the unfolding topic of their conversation. A hearer contributes to communication largely through nonverbal behavioral feedback. By extension, when a nonverbal infant attends to a social partner, through gaze, for example, a framework for communication is set up, and the partner is encouraged to uphold it by producing communicative behavior an infant can take in.

Today, evidence is available to support the claim that neonates seek out social partners and attend to them in specific ways. Farroni, Csibra, Simion, and Johnson (2002) have shown that, when presented with pairs of static photographs, newborns look longer and orient more frequently to a face with direct gaze than to a face with averted gaze. Even more interestingly, newborns have been found to associate the experience of being talked to, in infant-directed speech, to that of being looked at (Guellai & Streri, 2011). In this study, neonates were familiarized with videos of unfamiliar talking faces with either direct or averted gaze. When tested with photographs of the previously seen face and a new one, infants looked longer at the face that had previously spoken to them but only when it had been associated with direct gaze.

It has been known for a few decades now that young infants are sensitive to the appropriateness of the communicative behavior of social partners. Using the ingenious double video-replay procedure, Murray and Trevarthen (1985) and later Nadel and Tremblay-Leveau (1999) showed that 2-month-olds rapidly react when their mother's behavior becomes noncontingent in relation to their own behavior. They thus have clear expectations of the *way* speakers should be attending to them but also of the *kinds* of behaviors they should be directing to them. Experiments using the still-face procedure (Cohn & Tronick, 1989) have shown that very young infants make active attempts to reengage inattentive partners, and it appears that even newborns react with decreased eye contact and negative emotion to the sudden interruption of infant-directed communication when an unfamiliar partner adopts a "still face" (Nagy, 2008). It is quite clear from these studies then that not only do very young infants perceive being the object of others' attention (Reddy, 2008) but also that they attend more to people attending to them. This clearly lays the ground for mutually negotiated social interaction. There is still scope for further research on the process of setting up mutual attention, giving rise to the earliest forms of participation frameworks between adults and infants. For example, in verbal conversation, distinctions have been drawn between participants' roles based on their intent and degree of interest. Are infants sensitive to the degree of attention a social partner displays toward them? Is their attention to others always focused or do they also rely on a diffused mode of attention?

Young infants show different reactions to people and to objects (Legerstee, 1991; Rönnqvist & von Hofsten, 1994). They direct communicative attempts to other people (Legerstee, Pomerleau, Malcuit, & Feider, 1987; Reddy, Hay, Murray, & Trevarthen, 1997) and discriminate communicative attempts of people and of animated dolls (Legerstee, 2005). Indeed, by 5 months infants respond to intentional actions performed by a human hand but not by a mechanical claw (Woodward, 1998). Furthermore, infants aged 3–4 months imitate people but not objects (Legerstee, 1991). Imitative behavior in infants from birth has been identified as a strong marker of social initiative and motivation (Kugiumutzakis, 1998, 1999; Meltzoff & Moore, 1977). Imitation of facial expressions, gestures, and vocalizations, both in spontaneous social interaction and in controlled studies where models perform actions affording imitation, shows that infants are well equipped to display their role as active participants in social interchange. Indeed, Nagy and Molnar's (2004) study of neonatal imitation shows that when infants initiate actions they previously imitated, in order to establish a reciprocal gestural turn taking, their heart rate decreases, whereas when they imitate the action of the partner, their heart rate increases. Young infants' participation in being picked up, evidenced by anticipatory body movement that has been measured using pressure captors (Reddy, Markova, & Wallot, 2013), provides further proof of their readiness to be participants in coordinated interpersonal communication.

Careful naturalistic observation of infants with caring adults directing attention to them, through gaze, touch, or bodily handling, has shown that from the earliest moments of life out of the womb, they are active partners, listening intently and expressing interest in others with knit-brow expressions and "pre-speech" mouth movements (Trevarthen, 1977), calling and responding with vocalizations that acquire resonance and well-formed intonation contours (Dominguez et al., 2016; Gratier & Devouche, 2011), and smiling and adjusting their posture in a coordinated process of matching emotion (Markova & Legerstee, 2006). Infants' participation is multimodal, and recent studies are offering exciting insights into the complex organization of sense perception it is rooted in.

Multimodal Experiences

It seems that at birth, infants are already tuned to perceive human expressions of emotion and intention through various modalities. They are known to prefer the more musical sounds of infant-directed speech (IDS) over the faster, more clipped utterances adults direct to each other. Infant-directed speech contains elongated vowels that afford melodic modulation, as well as onomatopoeia that often have an iconic relation to the emotions or concepts being expressed. It is associated with facial expressions that match its intent and intensity: an elongated vowel sound is synchronous with a mouth held open, rounded eyes, and raised eyebrows. There is recent evidence showing that 8-month-olds and even newborns extract prosodic information from voice and from head and face kinematics (Guellaï, Streri, Chopin, Rider, & Kitamura, 2016; Kitamura, Guellaï, & Kim, 2014). Newborn infants look longer at faces of people who have spoken to them than at faces of people who looked at them silently (Guellai & Streri, 2011) suggesting that multimodal experiences are particularly salient for them.

Most social and nonsocial situations infants encounter call upon multiple sensory modalities. How the senses are integrated – or differentiated – in infancy is the subject of much research and debate. Some interesting intermodal perceptual abilities are well established today. At 5 weeks, infants recognize a visual shape that they have experienced through oral sucking, suggesting a connection between visual and tactile perception (Meltzoff & Borton, 1979). Two- to three-month-olds can transfer information from a haptic to a visual experience, but it is not until 5 months of age that vision to touch transfers become possible (Streri, 1987, 1991). Numerous studies have shown that young infants perceive amodal relations between events presented in different modalities (Lewkowicz & Lickliter, 1995). They detect the temporal synchrony in the common rhythm and durations of tones and flashing lights (Lewkowicz, 1986). They also show surprising perception of cross-sensory correspondences, such as associations between auditory pitch and visual height or visual sharpness (Walker et al., 2009). Auditory pitch has been found to be associated with visual brightness, thinness, and size (Asano et al., 2015; Dolscheid, Hunnius, Casasanto, & Majid, 2014).

In everyday contexts, sounds, smells, and shapes blend to provide whole experiences of other people, pleasurable events, and anticipated feelings. Do infants sense the world they live in before they make sense of it? When they hear the musically expressive modulations of affectionate social partners' voices, speaking to them or to others, do they conjure up a host of other feelings that begin to connect them with their past and anticipated future? Could the process of sensing increasingly familiar patterns of intermodal experience, repeated and varied over time, constitute infants' first experience of culture?

Finding a Voice and Picking Up Intentions

By 6–8 weeks after birth, all infants start producing cooing sounds, although some infants are more vocal than others. These sounds are interpreted by adults as intentional and responsive or attention seeking (Bloom, 1988; Gratier, Devouche, Bobin-Bègue, Apter, & Lacheret, 2015). Coos are often coordinated with directed gaze and smiles, and the increased frequency of these behaviors around the second month of life explains why this period is characterized by frequent and prolonged social interaction with various partners, often termed "protoconversation" (Lavelli & Fogel, 2013; Trevarthen, 1977, 1993). Indeed, adults respond more frequently to longer, more melodic, and resonant infant vocalizations, reinforcing the production of vocal sounds that appear to be more similar to human speech (Bloom, Russell, & Wassenberg, 1987). Interactions at these ages are also characterized by a high degree of interpersonal coordination marked by turn taking, particularly in the vocal modality (Gratier Devouche, Guellai, Infanti, Yilmaz, & Parlato-Oliveira 2015).

Social interaction, which involves reciprocity in the form of turn taking and matching expressions or imitation, can be considered an important locus of developmental change. Its earliest forms are perhaps rooted in innate dispositions or rudimentary habits acquired in utero. A few researchers suggest that very young human infants share this turn-taking ability with other species, such as monkeys or songbirds (Masataka, 2003; Takahashi, Narayanan, & Ghazanfar, 2013). In human development, the emergence of crucial socio-cognitive skills such as joint attention and social referencing are dependent on the quality of social interactions. It has been found, for example, that when parents are responsive and emotionally attuned to infants in social interactions, infants have more adaptive relational abilities (secure attachment) (Isabella & Belsky, 1991) and develop more complex forms of babbling before they learn to speak (Goldstein, King, & West, 2003). Even in 3-month-olds, intonational contours of infant vocalizations produced in the context of dyadic face-to-face engagement are scaffolded by maternal vocal imitation (Gratier & Devouche, 2011) suggesting that very young infants acquire new vocal skills in the course of interacting with adult partners. Recent evidence shows that vocal development is also shaped by social interaction in marmoset monkeys (Takahashi et al., 2016) and in zebra finches (Chen, Matheson, & Sakata, 2016).

The initial period of dyadic mutual engagement described as a period of "primary intersubjectivity" (Trevarthen, 1977, 1993) is followed by a phase characterized by increasingly formatted or conventional interactive routines (Bruner, 1985), including culturally transmitted repertoires of songs and games. Infants' motives develop from an interest centered on others, to interest in objects and how others treat them, and to interest in sharing curiosity about objects, events, and practices with others. The sharing of experience directed toward participating in a world of common knowledge, or common sense, is described as "secondary intersubjectivity" (Trevarthen & Hubley, 1978).

Social interaction between preverbal infants and adults can be considered an important precursor to language development in at least three respects. First, it serves to socialize infants to communication formats, such as turn taking, common to preverbal and verbal interaction. Second, it is likely to enable to development of socio-cognitive skills oriented to the perception of intentionality and common reference, known to be inextricable from typical language development (Rochat, Querido, & Striano, 1999). Third, social interaction conveys meaning to infants, which is rooted in multisensory experiences of communicative behavior, well before they can grasp the meaning of words (Gratier, Devouche, Dominguez, & Apter, 2015; Trevarthen, 1989).

There is evidence, mostly from cross-cultural studies of social interaction between adults and infants, that infants behave according to culture-specific communicative conventions already by the third month of life (Gratier, 2003; Keller, Otto, Lamm, Yovsi, & Kärtner, 2008). Parent-infant interactions are organized around different predominant modalities in different cultures. Mutual gaze and vocalization are preferred communicative modalities in the so-called WEIRD (Western, educated, industrialized, rich, and democratic) cultures, whereas in non-WEIRD cultures, interactions are more tactile and kinesthetic (Stork, 1986). Young infants' preference for communicative behavior that is directed to them suggests they can perceive being the object of someone else's attention. Reddy (2008) suggests the experience of being the object of attention, in the first months of life, is foundational for the development of the socio-cognitive skills that guide relationship formation and learning processes from the end of the first year onwards. Indeed, the development of attention deserves greater attention from researchers, especially in the period between the predominantly dyadic mutual attention of adult-infant interaction and the emergence of joint attention, when infants engage in complex patterns of alternating attention to persons, object, or events. The development of attention supports anticipatory processes, which in turn facilitates the perception of intentional or purposeful behavior in others.

By the end of the first year, infants show clear signs of a readiness to use symbolic communication, and indeed some infants already produce their first "words" at this age. Looking back at the history of intense daily social interactions they have experienced with diverse partners in various contexts, and at the particular qualities of these interactions as they develop (polysensory, emotional, regulated, improvised, embodied, etc.), it appears that the so-called readiness for language is synonymous with a rich-acquired expertise in communication rooted in innate and precocious abilities for communication.

From Meaning Making to the Addition of Language

Chomsky insisted on the uniqueness of language, proposing that it's appearance during the second year of life was based on innate knowledge of the potential structures of human languages. Chomsky's error was to neglect the psychological continuity between meaning shared on the basis of coordinated sensorimotor experience and meaning shared on the basis of common symbolic and grammatical systems. Indeed, the idea that language "emerges" in development is not so accurate nor is the idea that language is "acquired." Much research on language development provides evidence that language is in fact *fabricated* by infants involved in cooperative situations with adults and older children. Indeed, infants do not suddenly begin to speak by pronouncing intelligible *first words* that get to be combined with gestures and other sounds to produce rule-governed sentences. First words are part of the mythology of WEIRD families.

Michael Halliday (1975) was probably the first researcher to highlight the existence of protolanguages between infants and their familiar, intimate partners. Protolanguage covers a whole spectrum of meaningful, context-dependent sounds and bodily expressions, ranging from vocalizations that defy transcription to well-formed words. Parents, and older siblings, must learn the child's protolanguage in order to maintain and enrich the quality of communication that characterizes preverbal stages. More recently, using vast amounts of daily video and audio recordings of one child's entry into language, Deb Roy (2009) has shown just how densely intertwined context, shared understanding, and early language production are. It is thus on the basis of established, often idiosyncratic, shared understanding that infants learn to reshape sounds and bodily expression that are already meaningful (to the people most important to them) in order to render them accessible to a wider group of social partners.

Perspectives on Supporting Multimodal Experience in the NICU

Interactions between mothers and premature infants are often less than optimal, involving lower maternal adaptation to infant signals, leading to decreased maternal touch, vocalization, and gaze (Minde, Whitelaw, Brown, & Fitzhardinge, 1995). Mothers of preterm infants have been noted to provide a less responsive and stimulating home environment as compared with mothers of full-term infants (Barrera et al., 1987). Suitable for consistent and reciprocal interaction, skin-to-skin practice is currently the only relational multisensory care method offered to both partners, immediately after birth in a majority of NICUs in the Western world.

Buil et al.'s (2016) work illustrates how a new practice can emerge from the kind of research described in this chapter. In the NICU where she worked with preterm infants, A. Buil was facing numerous mothers' complaints about the difficulty of establishing face-to-face exchanges with their infants. Indeed, kangaroo positioning is usually vertical on the mother's chest, inside her clothes, and does not particularly favor eye-to-eye contact (cf. Fig. 4.1). Therefore, mothers sometimes preferred an arm-holding cuddle. To address this issue of early mother-infant communication, Buil et al. (2016) decided to implement a new positioning and to test the effects of adopting a frontal semi-reclined position for the infant, on the parent's belly and off center on the chest and with a flexed posture around the mother's nipple. This posture was based on a naturally asymmetrical tonic neck posture (ATNP) (Bullinger, 2004; Casaer, 1979) and involves the use of a stretchy baby wrap to maintain the infant's position without compressing its body. This type of positioning is being referred to as "supported diagonal flexion" (SDF) kangaroo positioning. So far, it has been tested on 15 very premature infants (age at birth between 26 and 32 weeks gestation), including ten infants with a need of respiratory support. The skin-to-skin session occurred between 1 and 3 days after birth and with all premature infants in a physiologically stable condition.

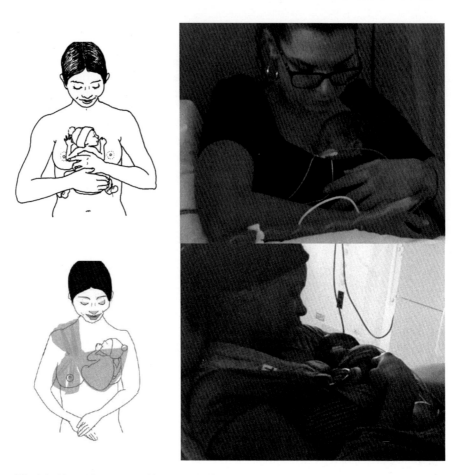

Fig. 4.1 *Above.* Kangaroo position extracted from Kangaroo Mother Care: A Practical Guide (World Health Organization [WHO], 2003) and a picture illustrating the generally recommended vertical kangaroo positioning, which has special focus on the importance to ensure free airways. *Under.* Schema illustrating the kangaroo FDS positioning and a picture illustrating the kangaroo FDS positioning. It is a novel way to apply SSC in order to enhance multimodal communication between mother and infant. However, it needs further careful exploration before it can be recommended for general use since there are obvious concerns regarding the safeguarding of patent airways in the more immature infants or if the mother falls asleep (Reprint with the permission of A. Buil)

Buil et al. (2016) observed that, compared to the usual vertical positioning, the kangaroo SDF positioning technique improves early mother-baby communication and positive emotion of both partners. Indeed, mothers pay more visual attention to the infant's face and tend to vocalize and smile more. Moreover, results show there are less disorganized gestures or negative vocalizations in infants in the SDF positioning and that SDF even fosters better regulatory states by diminishing drowsiness in favor of more deep sleep. SDF positioning also positively impacts the duration of skin-to-skin sessions, and mothers in the kangaroo SDF group appear to feel more comfortable in face-to-face exchanges, the former probably being a consequence of the latter.

More recently, in a submitted paper, Buil et al. (submitted) also revealed that SDF also impacted the spontaneous touch of mothers from the very first skin-to-skin session at 30 weeks GA. The mothers in this study practiced kangaroo care for the first time in the SDF position, yet they immediately manifested more active touch, as well as greater feeling of security. The ecology of the SDF positioning thus offers preterm infants the opportunity to take on a role they seem ready for, the role of participant in a social interaction. The kangaroo SDF positioning technique is a novel way to apply SSC in order to enhance multimodal communication between mother and infant, and although it was found to be physiologically safe in Buil et al. (2016) study, it needs further careful exploration before it can be recommended for general use.

These early results suggest parents are prepared to interact with premies in the NICU. Indeed, recognizing their infant as a participant must be a transformative experience for any expectant parent. These results also support the idea that the ecological niche of the preterm baby living in the NICU can be sensitively, efficiently, and quite simply shaped to resemble more closely the ecological niche of a term neonate.

Conclusion

In this paper we have highlighted research that provides, over the last few decades, an increasingly clearer picture of the roles infants play in setting up the conditions for their own development. The process of mutual adaptation between the infant and its environment, which is largely social, has not been sufficiently studied. Yet detailed insight into this process is likely to help practitioners better identify optimal conditions for infants requiring more controlled and structured intervention from the environment for their survival, such as preterm infants. Full-term infants by nature require intervention from able adults, and in this sense it is not useful to oppose the "natural" lives of term infants with the "unnatural" lives of hospitalized infants. Environments are constructed around infants, but most importantly infants participate from the earliest moments of life in this construction, and they are well equipped to do so. The ways in which they participate develop rapidly over the first year, from strong markers of social interest manifested early on (such as gaze orientation) to expressive language. The roles and status others agree to bestow on them evolve accordingly. This mutual positioning is the condition for the development of a communication that grows creatively and meaningfully between infants and social partners through a historical time into which are woven emotions and stories, shared hope, and past anxieties. We know today that preterm infants respond to their environment. It is more and more urgent that their environments in turn respond to them.

Key Messages
- Infants seek participation in social encounters from the first moments after birth.
- Full-term infants are well equipped to communicate with social partners from birth onwards. They can coordinate facial, vocal, and postural behavior with those of others. Communicative abilities develop with support and affectionate encouragement from attentive adults.
- By the time infants are ready to speak, they already have precise knowledge that is shared with multiple social partners and have acquired expertise in making themselves understood by others.
- It is worth exploring forms of social interaction, including maternal voice, between preterm infants and adults in the NICU, and their potential benefits for cognitive development.

References

Asano, M., Imai, M., Kita, S., Kitajo, K., Okada, H., & Thierry, G. (2015). Sound symbolism scaffolds language development in preverbal infants. *Cortex, 63*, 196–205.

Barrera, M. E., Rosenbaum, P. L., & Cunningham, C. E. (1987). Corrected and uncorrected Bayley scores: Longitudinal developmental patterns in low and high birth weight preterm infants. *Infant Behavior and development, 10*(3), 337–346.

Bloom, K. (1988). Quality of adult vocalizations affects the quality of infant vocalizations. *Journal of Child Language, 15*(03), 469–480.

Bloom, K., Russell, A., & Wassenberg, K. (1987). Turn taking affects the quality of infant vocalizations. *Journal of Child Language, 14*, 211–227.

Bruner, J. (1985). The role of interaction formats in language acquisition. In *Language and social situations* (pp. 31–46). New York, NY: Springer.

Buil, A., Carchon, I., Apter, G., Laborne, F. X., Granier, M., & Devouche, E. (2016). Kangaroo supported diagonal flexion positioning: New insights into skin-to-skin contact for communication between mothers and very preterm infants. *Archives de Pédiatrie, 23*(9), 213–220.

Buil, A., Fillon-Devys, D., Granger, A., Roger, K., Thomas, N., Apter, G., & Devouche, E. (submitted). Impact de l'installation en Flexion Diagonale Soutenue sur le maternage tactile spontané lors de la première séance de peau-à-peau en réanimation néonatale.

Bullinger A. (2004). *Le développement sensori-moteur de l'enfant et ses avatars* (Un parcours de recherche). Toulouse: Erès.

Casaer, P. (1979). Postural behavior in newborn infant. In W. Heinenmann (Ed.), *Clinics in developmental medicine*. London, England: Spastics International Medical Publications, Medical Book.

Chen, Y., Matheson, L. E., & Sakata, J. T. (2016). Mechanisms underlying the social enhancement of vocal learning in songbirds. *Proceedings of the National Academy of Sciences, 113*(24), 6641–6646.

Cohn, J. F., & Tronick, E. (1989). Specificity of infants' response to mothers' affective behavior. *Journal of the American Academy of Child & Adolescent Psychiatry, 28*(2), 242–248.

Dolscheid, S., Hunnius, S., Casasanto, D., & Majid, A. (2014). Prelinguistic infants are sensitive to space-pitch associations found across cultures. *Psychological Science, 25*(6), 1256–1261.

Dominguez, S., Devouche, E., Apter, G., & Gratier, M. (2016). The roots of turn-taking in the neonatal period. *Infant and Child Development, 25*(3), 240–255.

Dominguez, S., Gratier, G., Martel, K., Apter, G., & Devouche, E. (submitted). Aux origines de la personne : Quand la mère parle à son nouveau-né. *Neuropsychatrie de l'enfant et de l'adolescent.*

Farroni, T., Csibra, G., Simion, F., & Johnson, M. H. (2002). Eye contact detection in humans from birth. *Proceedings of the National Academy of Sciences, 99*(14), 9602–9605.

Goffman, E. (1981). *Forms of talk.* Philadelphia, PA: University of Pennsylvania Press.

Goldstein, M. H., King, A. P., & West, M. J. (2003). Social interaction shapes babbling: Testing parallels between birdsong and speech. *Proceedings of the National Academy of Sciences, 100*(13), 8030–8035.

Gratier, M. (2003). Expressive timing and interactional synchrony between mothers and infants: Cultural similarities, cultural differences, and the immigration experience. *Cognitive Development, 18,* 533–554.

Gratier, M., & Devouche, E. (2011). Imitation and repetition of prosodic contour in vocal interaction at 3 months. *Developmental Psychology, 47*(1), 67.

Gratier, M., Devouche, E, Bobin-Bègue, A., Apter, G. & Lacheret, A. (2015). *Judgments of emotion and communicative intent in infant vocalization at 1 and 5 months.* Poster presented at the International Conference on Infant Studies, New Orleans, 25–28 May 2015.

Gratier, M., Devouche, E., Dominguez, S., & Apter, G. (2015). What words can't tell. In U. M. Ludtke (Ed.), *Emotion in language: Theory–research–application.* Amsterdam, The Netherlands/Philadelphia, PA: John Benjamins Press.

Gratier, M., Devouche, E., Guellai, B., Infanti, R., Yilmaz, E., & Parlato-Oliveira, E. (2015). Early development of turn-taking in vocal interaction between mothers and infants. *Frontiers in Psychology, 6*(1167), 10–3389.

Guellai, B., & Streri, A. (2011). Cues for early social skills: Direct gaze modulates newborns' recognition of talking faces. *PLoS One, 6*(4), e18610.

Guellaï, B., Streri, A., Chopin, A., Rider, D., & Kitamura, C. (2016). Newborns' sensitivity to the visual aspects of infant-directed speech: Evidence from point-line displays of talking faces. *Journal of Experimental Psychology: Human Perception and Performance, 42*(9), 1275–1281.

Halliday, M. A. K. (1975). *Learning how to mean. Explorations in the development of language.* London, England: Edward Arnold.

Isabella, R. A., & Belsky, J. (1991). Interactional synchrony and the origins of infant-mother attachment: A replication study. *Child Development, 62*(2), 373–384.

Keller, H., Otto, H., Lamm, B., Yovsi, R. D., & Kärtner, J. (2008). The timing of verbal/vocal communications between mothers and their infants: A longitudinal cross-cultural comparison. *Infant Behavior & Development, 31*(2), 217–226.

Kitamura, C., Guellaï, B., & Kim, J. (2014). Motherese by eye and ear: Infants perceive visual prosody in point-line displays of talking heads. *PLoS One, 9*(10), e111467.

Kugiumutzakis, G. (1998). Neonatal imitation in the intersubjective companion space. In S. Braten (Ed.), *Intersubjective communication and emotion in early ontogeny* (pp. 63–88). Cambridge, UK: Cambridge University Press.

Kugiumutzakis, G. (1999). Genesis and development of early infant mimesis to facial and vocal models. In J. Nadel & G. Butterworth (Eds.), *Imitation in infancy* (pp. 36–59). Cambridge, UK: Cambridge University Press.

Lavelli, M., & Fogel, A. (2013). Inter dyad differences in early mother–infant face-to-face communication: Real-time dynamics and developmental pathways. *Developmental Psychology, 49,* 2257–2271.

Legerstee, M. (1991). The role of person and object in eliciting early imitation. *Journal of Experimental Child Psychology, 51*(3), 423–433.

Legerstee, M. (2005). *Infants' sense of people: Precursors to a theory of mind.* Cambridge, UK/ New York, NY: Cambridge University Press.

Legerstee, M., Pomerleau, A., Malcuit, G., & Feider, H. (1987). The development of infants' responses to people and a doll: Implications for research in communication. *Infant Behavior & Development, 10*(1), 81–95.

Lewkowicz, D. J. (1986). Developmental changes in infants' bisensory response to synchronous durations. *Infant Behavior & Development, 9*(3), 335–353.

Lewkowicz, D. J., & Lickliter, R. (1995). A dynamic systems approach to the development of cognition and action. *Journal of Cognitive Neuroscience, 7*(4), 512–514.

Markova, G., & Legerstee, M. (2006). Contingency, imitation, and affect sharing: Foundations of infants' social awareness. *Developmental Psychology, 42*(1), 132.

Marlier, L., Schaal, B., & Soussignan, R. (1998). Neonatal responsiveness to the odor of amniotic and lacteal fluids: A test of perinatal chemosensory continuity. *Child Development, 69*(3), 611–623.

Masataka, N. (2003). *The onset of language* (Vol. 9). Cambridge, UK: Cambridge University Press.

Meltzoff, A. N., & Borton, R. W. (1979). Intermodal matching by human neonates. *Nature, 28*, 403–404.

Meltzoff, A. N., & Moore, M. K. (1977). Imitation of facial and manual gestures by human neonates. *Science, 198*(4312), 75–78.

Minde, K., Whitelaw, A., Brown, J., & Fitzhardinge, P. (1995). Developmental outcome as a function of the goodness of fit between the infant's cry characteristics and the mother's perception of her infant's cry. *Pediatrics, 95*, 516–521.

Murray, L., & Trevarthen, C. (1985). Emotional regulation of interactions between two-month olds and their mothers. In T. A. Field & N. A. Fox (Eds.), *Social perception in infants* (pp. 177–197). Norwood, NJ: Ablex Publishers.

Nadel, J., & Tremblay-Leveau, H. (1999). Early perception of social contingencies and interpersonal intentionality: Dyadic and triadic paradigms. In P. Rochat (Ed.), *Early social cognition: Understanding others in the first months of life* (pp. 189–212). Mahwah, NJ: Erlbaum.

Nagy, E. (2008). Innate intersubjectivity: Newborns' sensitivity to communication disturbance. *Developmental Psychology, 44*(6), 1779.

Nagy, E., & Molnar, P. (2004). Homo Imitans or homo provocans? Human imprinting model of neonatal imitation. *Infant Behavior & Development, 27*(1), 54–63.

Reddy, V. (2008). *How infants know minds*. Cambridge, MA Harvard University Press.

Reddy, V., Hay, D., Murray, L., & Trevarthen, C. (1997). Communication in infancy: Mutual regulation of affect and attention. In G. J. Bremner, A. Slater, & G. Butterworth (Eds.), *Infant development: Recent advances* (pp. 247–273). Hove, UK: Psychology Press.

Reddy, V., Markova, G., & Wallot, S. (2013). Anticipatory adjustments to being picked up in infancy. *PLoS One, 8*(6), e65289.

Rochat, P., Querido, J. G., & Striano, T. (1999). Emerging sensitivity to the timing and structure of protoconversation in early infancy. *Developmental Psychology, 35*, 950–957.

Rönnqvist, L., & von Hofsten, C. (1994). Neonatal finger and arm movements as determined by a social and an object context. *Early Development and Parenting, 3*(2), 81–94.

Roy, D. (2009). *New horizons in the study of child language acquisition*. Proceedings of Interspeech 2009, Brighton, England.

Sai, F. Z. (2005). The role of the mother's voice in developing mother's face preference: Evidence for intermodal perception at birth. *Infant and Child Development, 14*(1), 29–50.

Stork, H. E. (1986). *Enfances indiennes*. Paris, France: Bayard Éditions-Païdos-Le Centurion.

Streri, A. (1987). Tactile discrimination of shape and intermodal transfer in 2-to 3-month-old infants. *British Journal of Developmental Psychology, 5*(3), 213–220.

Streri, A. (1991). *Voir, atteindre, toucher. Les relations entre la vision et le toucher chez le bébé*. Paris, France: Presses Universitaires de France.

Super, C. M., & Harkness, S. (1986). The developmental niche: A conceptualization at the interface of child and culture. *International Journal of Behavioral Development, 9*(4), 545–569.

Takahashi, D. Y., Narayanan, D. Z., & Ghazanfar, A. A. (2013). Coupled oscillator dynamics of vocal turn-taking in monkeys. *Current Biology, 23*(21), 2162–2168.

Takahashi, D. Y., Fenley, A. R., & Ghazanfar, A. A. (2016). Early development of turn-taking with parents shapes vocal acoustics in infant marmoset monkeys. *Philosophical Transactions of the Royal Society B, 371*(1693), 20150370.

Trevarthen, C. (1977). Descriptive analysis of infant communicative behavior. In H. Schaffer (Ed.), *Studies in mother-infant interaction* (pp. 227–270). New York, NY: Academic.

Trevarthen, C. (1989). Signs before speech. In T. A. Sebeok & J. Umiker-Sebeok (Eds.), *The semiotic web* (pp. 689–755). Berlin, Germany/New York, NY/Amsterdam, The Netherlands: Mouton de Gruyter.

Trevarthen, C. (1993). The self born in intersubjectivity: An infant communicating. In U. Neisser (Ed.), *The perceived self: Ecological and interpersonal sources of self-knowledge* (pp. 121–173). New York, NY: Cambridge University Press.

Trevarthen, C., & Hubley, P. (1978). Secondary intersubjectivity: Confidence, confiding and acts of meaning in the first year. In A. Lock (Ed.), *Action, gesture, and symbol: The emergence of language* (pp. 183–227). New York, NY: Cambridge University Press.

Van der Meer, A. L. H., Van der Weel, F. R., & Lee, D. N. (1995). The functional significance of arm movements in neonates. *Science, 267*(5198), 693.

Walker, P., Bremner, J. G., Mason, U., Spring, J., Mattock, K., Slater, A., & Johnson, S. P. (2009). Preverbal infants' sensitivity to Synaesthetic cross-modality correspondences. *Psychological Science, 21*(1), 21–25.

Woodward, A. L. (1998). Infants selectively encode the goal object of an actor's reach. *Cognition, 69*(1), 1–34.

World Health Organization. (2003). *Kangaroo mother care: A practical guide.* Department of Reproductive Health and Research, Geneva, Switzerland.. ISBN 92 4 1590351.

Chapter 5
Brain Mechanisms in Emotional Voice Production and Perception and Early Life Interactions

Didier Grandjean

Abstract *Introduction.* The understanding of social human interactions through vocalizations, especially at an early stage of development, necessitates characterization of the brain mechanisms that produce the mother's emotional vocalizations and of perception, that is, how the brain is able to perceive emotion in the mother's vocalizations.

Main aims. In this chapter, we review how emotions can impact on voice production during social interactions, as described in peripheral and central neurophysiological studies. We discuss how emotions are characterized by peripheral reactions modulating the vocal tractus, thus influencing the way people vocalize with others. The perception of emotion in the voice has been extensively studied in adult populations, and the neuronal networks involved in the different stages of emotion perception, categorization, and valuation are discussed in this chapter.

Conclusions. On the basis of empirical evidence in adults and infants, as well as in newborns, the mechanisms of emotional perception in the voice and its development are discussed and extended to an early stage of development, including in premature newborns.

How Emotion Affects Vocal Production

The main goal of this chapter is to present an integrated framework from the production of emotion in the voice to its perception, including how emotion can impact on vocalizations; how these vocalizations, emotionally connoted, are processed at the brain level by the auditory system; and how they affect interpersonal communication. Of course, this dynamic view of human interaction through the auditory

D. Grandjean (✉)
Department of Psychology and Educational Sciences and Swiss
Center for Affective Sciences, University of Geneva,
Geneva, Switzerland
e-mail: didier.grandjean@unige.ch

© Springer International Publishing AG 2017   71
M. Filippa et al. (eds.), *Early Vocal Contact and Preterm Infant Brain Development*, DOI 10.1007/978-3-319-65077-7_5

sensory system is not restricted to adults but evolves from the early stages beginning in pregnancy to later stages of development. For example, mothers or fathers talking to their newborns produce what is called infant-directed speech or baby talk, exaggerating the prosodic aspects in order to help segmentation or recruit the attention of the newborn. Like the other interactive sensory systems, such as vision or a sense of touch, that allow humans to develop an ensemble of representations, the auditory domain is crucial for emotional and social development.

Emotions can be defined as massive temporally organized changes (e.g., through synchronization) of the five different organismic components (Grandjean, Sander, & Scherer, 2008; Sander, Grandjean, & Scherer, 2005; Scherer, 1984a, 1984b): (i) the cognitive or appraisal component through modulations in the central nervous system that allow the organism to process information and integrate it in a series of representations or as a unified representation – whether consciously accessible or not (Grandjean et al., 2008); (ii) the autonomic component, which is functionally related to homeostasis; (iii) the expressive component (facial, vocal, gestural, and postural aspects); (iv) the motivational component, especially related to action tendencies and performed actions; and finally (v) the so-called feeling component. The latter component has been conceptualized as an integrated representation or a series of representations that are potentially consciously accessible and can be verbally expressed (Grandjean et al., 2008). Feelings can also be a way to modulate or regulate emotions, for example, by controlling one or several components (e.g., controlling facial expression in a specific social context) or by reevaluating events, that is, what researchers have defined as reappraisal (e.g., reevaluating a specific context). Reappraisal is thought to be characterized as a different way of appraising events, for example, changing the interpretation or the agency of a negative event. If your newborn has a crisis of rage, you can interpret it as "his or her will to manipulate me to obtain something" or "he or she is suffering and needs something"; these different ways of understanding and conceptualizing the same event induce very different emotions (K. R. Scherer, Dan, & Flykt, 2006; Smith & Ellsworth, 1985) and related actions.

When you are exposed to a difficult situation, the way you appraise it affects the different components related to emotions mentioned earlier (van Reekum et al., 2004). The domain of vocalization is directly related to the expressive component. When you express vocalizations, different organismic systems are involved. The respiratory, phonatory, and articulatory systems are the main systems (Fig. 5.1) that can be modulated by emotions in the vocal domain, which in turn modify the vocalizations produced (e.g., P. J. Davis, Zhang, Winkworth, & Bandler, 1996). Typically, the intensity, that is, the loudness, of your vocalization is strongly influenced by the quantity of air that you are able to expel through your vocal tract. The vibration of the vocal chords is directly related to phonation. Finally, all the muscles in the lower part of your face and throat allow you to articulate and then organize the bursts of air that you expel from your body. All of these systems can be affected by emotions, especially through the autonomic system, which can affect, for example, the phonatory system and your ability to control the air that you expel. As an example, in stressful situations, humans have the tendency to breathe superficially and more rapidly compared with how they breathe in a relaxed state (e.g., Boiten, 1998; Butler, Wilhelm, & Gross, 2006).

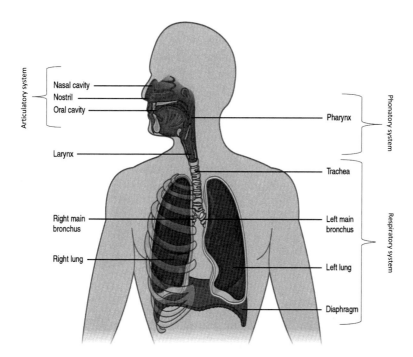

Fig. 5.1 Three main body systems are involved in vocalization: (i) the respiratory system, (ii) the phonatory system, and (iii) the articulatory system

Mechanisms Involved in the Production of Affective Vocalizations

The production of emotional vocalizations is a complex phenomenon involving a series of mechanisms at different levels, including the peripheral and central systems. These components of vocalization production can be described in at least three different interacting peripheral systems: (i) the respiratory system, mainly related to the energy of production through the level of subglottal air pressure; (ii) the phonation system, defined as how and at which frequency the vocal chords vibrate and structure the airflow, mainly related to vocal frequency, type of phonation, and register of the voice; and (iii) the articulatory system, which contributes to the shape and variance of the vocal tract (e.g., length, volume), impacting on voice quality and resonance (e.g., organization of the formants) (Banse & Scherer, 1996); see Fig. 5.1. All of these peripheral systems can be modulated by direct or indirect influences of the sympathetic and parasympathetic systems, which are strongly modulated by emotional processes. More specifically, respiratory characteristics have been shown to be affected by emotion (e.g., Etzel, Johnsen, Dickerson, Tranel, & Adolphs, 2006). The phonatory and articulatory systems can also be modulated by the emotional state of the speaker. In cats, for example, as shown from periaqueductal gray stimulations, every specific call or vocalization induces complex specific muscle patterning, allowing the animal to produce specific prototypical vocalizations (Subramanian, Arun, Silburn, & Holstege, 2016). During an emotional episode, all of these subsystems are influenced by the impact of brain regions known to be crucial in emotion, such as the amygdala and the orbitofrontal regions, which modulate the areas involved in the control or regulation of respiration, phonation, and articulation.

Two main brain motor systems are thought to be crucial for the generation of vocalization; the first system is composed of the mesencephalic periaqueductal gray matter, and the second involves the motor and premotor cortical areas and the subcortical nuclei, especially the basal ganglia (Fruhholz, Klaas, Patel, & Grandjean, 2015; Holstege & Subramanian, 2016); see Fig. 5.2. While the periaqueductal gray

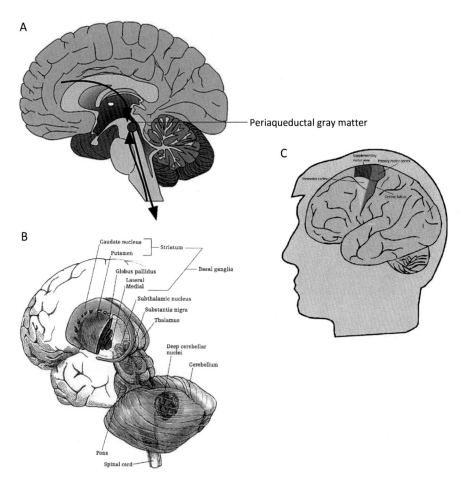

Fig. 5.2 Two main brain systems are involved in vocalization: the periaqueductal gray matter (**a**) and the basal ganglia (**b**), as well as cortical regions, including the primary motor cortex, the supplementary motor area, and the premotor cortex (**c**)

matter is essential for prototypical and automatized vocal production, the cortical areas are more related to planned and controlled motor actions. The periaqueductal gray matter is influenced by limbic and cortical regions such as the amygdala, anterior cingulate cortex, insula, and orbitofrontal cortical areas and constitutes a neuronal network involved in emotional vocalizations. This region impacts strongly on the caudal medullary nucleus retroambiguus. It has direct access to the motor neurons involved in vocalization innervating the upper part of the vocal tract, including the soft palate, pharynx, and larynx, as well as the muscle groups in the lower part of the body, including the diaphragm and the intercostal, abdominal, and pelvic floor muscles. All of these systems determine the muscle configuration related to intra-abdominal, intrathoracic, and subglottic pressure, which is necessary for generating vocalization (Holstege & Subramanian, 2016).

To date, only a few brain imaging studies have investigated the brain regions involved in emotional vocalization production in humans. The first evidence about the role of the different brain regions involved in emotional prosody decoding comes from brain lesion studies. In these studies, the authors have shown that a right hemispheric lesion impacts strongly on the production of emotional prosody, inducing a syndrome called dysprosodic or aprosodic production (Blonder et al., 2005; Cancelliere & Kertesz, 1990; Grela & Gandour, 1998; Guranski & Podemski, 2015; Nakhutina, Borod, & Zgaljardic, 2006; Schirmer, Alter, Kotz, & Friederici, 2001). Other brain lesions can also greatly impact on the production of vocalization and prosody, such as those in the periaqueductal gray matter (P. J. Davis et al., 1996), medial frontal cortex (Frysztak & Neafsey, 1991), and basal ganglia (Blonder, Pickering, Heath, Smith, & Butler, 1995; Cohen, Riccio, & Flannery, 1994). Using functional magnetic resonance imaging, Pichon and Kell (Pichon & Kell, 2013) showed that during the preparation of emotional vocalization, the bilateral ventral striatum is more activated than it is during the preparation of nonemotional vocalization. They also highlighted that these specific basal ganglia ventral regions are functionally connected to the temporal poles and the insular cortices; see Fig. 5.2. In addition, they demonstrated that the dorsal parts of the striatum are more involved in the preparation and production of cognitive and motor components of emotional vocalization production and that these dorsal regions are more connected to the motor network of speech production. These authors also discussed how emotional prosody processing involved the right posterior part of the temporal sulcus and gyrus, proposing that the classic view of right lateralization of emotional prosody production might be related to the ability of these right lateralized neuronal populations to process slow acoustical changes through the ventral cortical pathway. In one study comparing repeated and evoked angry and neutral production (Fruhholz et al., 2015), we revealed that angry voice production, compared to neutral production, induced an increased *bold* signal in the temporal voice-sensitive areas, including the left middle superior temporal gyrus (STG) and posterior STG, right STG, anterior cingulate cortex, bilateral basal ganglia (left putamen and right caudate nucleus), and bilateral inferior frontal gyri (IFG). We also showed a significant increase in amygdala response for the angry-evoked condition compared to angry repetition or neutral productions. In a follow-up study (Klaas, Fruhholz, & Grandjean, 2015)

investigating functional connectivity patterns during emotional vocalization production, we revealed an increase in functional connectivity between the bilateral
auditory cortices during affective vocalizations, which points to a bilateral exchange
of relevant acoustic information of produced vocalizations. We also showed that
bilateral motor cortices involved in the control of vocal motor behavior revealed
functional connectivity to the right IFG and right STG. Moreover, we confirmed
that different parts of the basal ganglia presented both positive and negative modula-
tory connectivity with the anterior cingulate cortex and the IFG, as well as with
different parts of the STG.

The studies investigating the production of affective vocalizations and affective prosody in newborns are scarce even though the ability of newborns to produce affective bursts starts at birth. For example, Stewart and collaborators
(Stewart et al., 2013) have shown significant correlations between autonomic
markers (reductions in heart period and respiratory sinus arrhythmia) and the
acoustical characteristics of affective vocalizations in newborns, highlighting the
possible early coupling between the reactivity of the autonomic system and the
maxima and minima of prosodic cues. These results favor a functional role for the
vocalizations produced by newborns during emotional states (as marked by autonomic reactions) to induce phasic reactions in parental care (attentional focus
toward the baby's state) in order to promote actions to reduce the newborn's negative emotional states (i.e., distress), for example, related to a hungry condition.
These kinds of early distress vocalizations are thought to be mainly associated
with the periaqueductal gray system. An interesting study done by Mampe and
collaborators has revealed that early vocalizations such as cries are influenced by
the surrounding spoken language, probably by passive exposure during the last
3 months of pregnancy (Mampe, Friederici, Christophe, & Wermke, 2009). They
analyzed 60 crying patterns of newborns (2–5 days of life), 30 French and 30
German, revealing that French newborns produced a pattern of rising melodies,
whereas German newborns preferentially produced a falling melodic contour, like
those produced by the respective adults (French versus German) in everyday life
in terms of usual prosodic contours. During development, newborns, and later on
infants, learn progressive modulations of this periaqueductal gray system in order
to increase control of their vocalizations as a result of the complex relationships
between motor cortical areas and the basal ganglia systems promoting, in the
context of vocalization, what scientists call "habits". Two main components have
been proposed as being crucial to the control of vocalization, also called the "principle of efficient modulation". The first is the vertical component described in the
frame/content theory in which MacNeilage and collaborators proposed that the
first training for vocalization control is related to mandibular oscillation (i.e.,
openness/closing mouth movements; B. L. Davis, MacNeilage, & Matyear, 2002;
MacNeilage, 1998a, 1998b), allowing newborns to progressively use a more fine-
tuned way to shape their vocal production. The second component, described as
the horizontal component, has been called "constriction control" in which fine
control of the upper part of the vocal tract allows newborns/infants to shape the
resonances useful for speech production (Boe et al., 2013). Such progressive con-

trol and instrumentalization of vocalizations in newborns is, of course, contingent on early life interactions in the context of child caring by adults.

To summarize, the studies about emotional prosody production have revealed that depth structures, especially the periaqueductal gray matter, are essential in the context of automatic vocalization production, often occurring in the context of emotions. During their development, children progressively take control of their vocalization in more structured communication contexts as a result of different cortical areas, including not only the pre-supplementary motor area, supplementary motor area, and motor cortices but also the ventro-dorsal prefrontal cortex (Aboitiz & Garcia, 2009), the subcortical areas such as the basal ganglia nuclei for habits (Graybiel, 2008; Peron, Fruhholz, Verin, & Grandjean, 2013), and the basic periaqueductal gray system. As mentioned earlier, these systems are also functionally connected to the auditory system (including the primary auditory cortex, STG, and superior temporal sulcus (STS), especially for auditory feedback) and to different structures involved in emotion such as the amygdala, insula, and anterior cingulate cortex, among others. Finally, the role of the inferior frontal areas is also crucial in speech production and emotional categorization in the context of prosodic modulations (Fruhholz et al., 2015; Klaas et al., 2015).

Relationships Between Produced Emotional Vocalizations and Their Perception

The perception of emotional prosody can be described in a systematic fashion, as Brunswik (Brunswik, 1956) has suggested for other mechanisms of human characteristic attribution (e.g., intelligence), by using a dedicated model between the speaker and the listener and taking into consideration different processing steps. In an adapted Brunswik model for the perception of the emotional voice (Grandjean, Banziger, & Scherer, 2006), we have proposed that the perception of emotion in vocalization is related to a kind of schemata recognition based on the probability that specific acoustic features are specifically correlated to specific states, as has been shown by the systematic analysis of acoustical profiles of different emotions (Banse & Scherer, 1996); see Fig. 5.3.

The initial step is about the production and how the vocal message is encoded – unintentionally or intentionally – from the speaker's perspective. This means that in a specific emotional state, the different components of emotion affect the way that the speaker produces a specific vocalization. At the end of the speaker's vocal tract, one can systematically characterize the acoustic features for a specific vocalization. This available information can be used by the listener's cognitive system in order to build up a representation of this vocal percept. As in the other sensory domains, our auditory perceptions do not correspond one on one with how researchers can characterize the produced vocalizations at the physical level (i.e., objective). For example, we are more sensitive to intensity level (i.e., energy) in high frequencies compared with low frequencies, meaning that our sensory and cognitive systems are

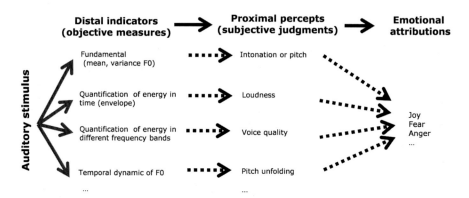

Fig. 5.3 Adapted Brunswik's model for the perception of emotional prosody (Adapted from Grandjean et al. (2006))

not linearly sensitive to intensity and frequency. Physical analysis of the fundamental frequency of a sound (f0) does not correspond perfectly to the perceived f0, called pitch. This perception step has been conceptualized in a Brunswikian approach as the first stage of decoding from the listener's perspective. Of course, the environment in which a specific vocalization is produced can also have a large impact on perception, for example, in the context of a noisy situation such as that experienced by premature babies in neonatology environments. This first stage of perception is thought to be followed by a process of percept integration in order to build up a dynamic integrated percept, such as that categorized as a human voice, or corresponding to the sound produced by a specific object, such as a glass breaking on the floor. The so-called perceived auditory object is also the subject of a third processing step that we can describe as the processing of categorization. In emotion recognition, it is related to a series of processes, based on a probabilistic approach, to characterize the percept as a sign of joy or irritation, for example. It is also related to the ability of the cognitive system to extract the invariants between sensory information and inferences based on past experiences; these inferences are also used by humans and other animals such as apes to attribute emotional mental states of others (Gruber & Grandjean, 2017).

A large corpus of literature has been developed to systematically study how the human brain is able to extract emotional information from voice signals. Our auditory peripheral system is characterized by a series of mechanisms, from air pressure to the vibration of the tympanic membrane to a mechanical structure comprising three ossicles (malleus, incus, and stapes). The last part of this mechanical system is able to modulate the vibration of the little oval membrane in our inner ear, which in turn produces movement of the liquid contained in the cochlear system. The waves of this liquid induce movement of the specific appendages of nerve cells, the so-called hair cells. A metabolic cascade, the so-called transduction phenomenon (not described here in detail) produces the first neural signal in our nervous system. The firing of these neurons entrains a series of brain processes along what is called the ascending auditory pathway. This neural pathway is organized into several cerebral structures, starting from the ventral and dorsal cochlear nuclei located in the brain stem and projecting to the superior olivary complex and the inferior colliculus, respectively. The latter projects to the medial geniculate nuclei of the thalamus, which then projects to the primary auditory cortical regions. Brain imaging studies that investigated the perception of emotional prosody have revealed a complex neuronal network. This network is composed of different parts of temporal areas, including the STG and the STS. These voice-sensitive areas, described primarily by Belin and collaborators (Belin, Zatorre, Lafaille, Ahad, & Pike, 2000), are modulated by emotional prosody (Ceravolo, Fruhholz, & Grandjean, 2016a, 2016b; Ethofer et al., 2006, 2012; Ethofer, De Ville, Scherer, & Vuilleumier, 2009; Fruhholz, Ceravolo, & Grandjean, 2012; Fruhholz & Grandjean, 2013a; Fruhholz et al., 2016; Grandjean et al., 2005; Sander et al., 2005; Wiethoff et al., 2008; Wildgruber et al., 2005) even in the context of unvoiced emotional prosody, that is, whispered voicing (Fruhholz, Trost, & Grandjean, 2016), which is often used in the context of intimate communication. These temporal regions are thought to be crucial in building up complex auditory objects and are significant in the context of emotional communication. The amygdala complex is also thought to be essential in emotional prosody decoding, especially for rapid reaction to such emotional signals and for organization of the emotional response to such relevant positive or negative auditory stimuli, as evidenced by brain imaging (Bach et al., 2008; Fruhholz et al., 2012; Fruhholz & Grandjean, 2012a; Johnstone, van Reekum, Oakes, & Davidson, 2006; Sander et al., 2005; Schirmer et al., 2008; Wiethoff, Wildgruber, Grodd, & Ethofer, 2009; Wildgruber, Ackermann, Kreifelts, & Ethofer, 2006) and amygdala lesion studies (Dellacherie, Hasboun, Baulac, Belin, & Samson, 2011; Fruhholz et al., 2015; Scott et al., 1997). These temporal and subcortical regions are parts of a distributed neural network also involving the frontal regions, especially the inferior frontal regions (IFG) and the orbitofrontal regions (OFC). Although the right IFG is thought to be especially important for discrimination and categorization of emotional prosody that is based on dynamic acoustic invariants (Beaucousin et al., 2007; Buchanan et al., 2000; Ethofer et al., 2006, 2012; Eviatar & Just, 2006; Fruhholz et al., 2012; Fruhholz & Grandjean, 2012b, 2013b; Fruhholz, Gschwind, & Grandjean, 2015; Johnstone et al., 2006; Leitman et al., 2010; Mizuno & Sugishita, 2007; Tzourio-Mazoyer et al., 2007; Wildgruber et al., 2004; 2006), the OFC is especially important for contextual valuation of emotional auditory stimuli such as in the case of sarcasm (Paulmann, Seifert, & Kotz, 2010; Sander et al., 2005; Schirmer & Kotz, 2006; Schirmer et al., 2008; Wildgruber et al., 2006); see Fig. 5.4.

Empirical evidence for auditory emotional perception at an early stage of life is scarce. It has been demonstrated, using behavioral measures, that newborns have a preference for the human voice compared to nonvocal auditory stimuli (EcklundFlores & Turkewitz, 1996; Hutt, Vonbernu, Lenard, Hutt, & Prechtl, 1968). Using electro-encephalography and mismatch negativity, an event-related component elicited in the context of specific rule violations, Cheng and collaborators showed in 1- to 5-day-old newborns that, compared to neutral or to matched control stimuli, happy, angry, and fearful intonations (using the word "dada") elicited a significant stronger

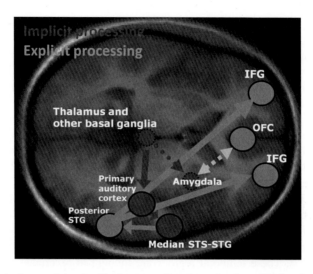

Fig. 5.4 Cerebral network involved in the processing of emotional vocalization: implicit processing (*red*), including the thalamus and other basal ganglia (e.g., subthalamic nucleus, striatum),
primary auditory cortex, median superior temporal sulcus (*STS*) and superior temporal gyrus
(*STG*), and amygdala complex, and explicit processing (*green*), including mainly the posterior
STG, inferior frontal gyri (*IFG*), and orbitofrontal cortex (*OFC*). The median STS and STG are
parts of the sensitive voice regions described by Belin et al. in 2000 (Belin et al., 2000) (Adapted
from Wildgruber, Ethofer, Grandjean, and Kreiflets, 2009)

mismatch response in the right hemisphere (Cheng, Lee, Chen, Wang, & Decety,
2012). Furthermore, Mastropieri and Turkewitz showed that happy intonations more
often elicited open-eye behaviors when newborns were exposed to a typical mother
speech pattern, which was not the case for a foreign language (Mastropieri &
Turkewitz, 1999). This observation is compatible with the concept of sensitivity of
language context during pregnancy (see also Chap. 2 by Moon). The early ability to
react to the mother's voice has also been documented in premature newborns. Filippa
and collaborators (Filippa, Devouche, Arioni, Imberty, & Gratier, 2013) showed that
the physiological state of a premature newborn is significantly modulated during
exposure to the mother's live voice compared to situations without such exposure.
Furthermore, they showed that exposure to the mother's voice significantly decreases
the number of critical events during this challenging period of development. Using
functional magnetic resonance imaging, Abrams and colleagues (Abrams et al.,
2016) showed that at a later stage of development, exposure of infants to the biological mother's voice (around 10 years), compared to other unknown mothers' voices,
induced an increase in activity (*bold* signal) in a large neuronal network, including
the primary auditory network in the midbrain and cortical regions, the voice-sensitive temporal areas (STG/STS), and a series of regions known for their implications
in emotional processes, including the amygdala, nucleus accumbens (in the ventral
part of the striatum), OFC, and anterior insula and cingulate. They also demonstrated the implications of the fusiform gyrus, especially the part known to be modulated by face perception; the authors interpreted this finding in the context of facial

mental imagery related to the perception of infants to their own mother's voice. The brain connectivity patterns have also revealed significant correlations between the infant's social communication skills and the strength of brain connectivity between the voice-sensitive areas (especially the STS) and the amygdala, nucleus accumbens, OFC, dorsal part of the cingulate, and anterior insula.

The Concept of Scheme of Production and Perception in the Context of Social Communication

One important issue in the developmental perspective is how the cognitive system and, by extension, the brain mechanisms are able to evolve in ontogenetic time to at least be a representative part of reality and then render the organism able to interact with his/her complex environment, not only at the physical level but also at the social and emotional levels. Based on genetic and early epigenetic influences and related phylogenetic determinants, the brain and other body systems (e.g., muscular, skeletal, sensory systems) have to be able to learn how to guide behavior in order to achieve numerous different goals, the first being to survive. In order to stabilize the relationships between environmental features, interoceptive and proprioceptive states, and the interactions with motor actions and related explicit or implicit goals, the system has to be able to extract the invariants at different levels. Several researchers have proposed that a Bayesian approach might be a way to explain this ability of biological systems to build up stable coupling between internal states, representations, and actions. One brain system seems to be an excellent candidate to achieve this: the complex system formed by the dynamic interactions between the basal ganglia, other subcortical structures (such as hippocampal formation), and cortical territories. The basal ganglia are a complex system that include the brain origins of the dopaminergic system through the ventral tegmental area and the substantia nigra. These regions are characterized by a huge number of dopaminergic neurons that impact on the rest of the brain. Different nuclei comprise the basal ganglia system: the subthalamic nucleus, globus pallidus, striatum composed of the nucleus accumbens and the caudate nucleus, and thalamus. These nuclei have numerous connections with other subcortical structures such as the amygdala, hippocampal formation, claustrum, and colliculus, among others. Graybiel (2008) has proposed that this system is crucial to build up what she called a chunking process. This concept, chunking, from our point of view, seems crucial to explain how, starting from a hyperconnected and relatively unstructured system, which is the state of the early brain-body system in newborns, the system is able to extract invariants between the sensory and motor systems and environmental elements. Chunking is defined as a series of simple steps, with processing action becoming a kind of integrated series of evaluation-representation-actions able to achieve a specific function, for example, grasping an object. In this case, the coupling of sensory/representation/action is simple, but the concept has been extended to more complex behavior such as that involved in complex learning, for example, being able to drive a car automatically (i.e., after learning to drive, it is no longer necessary to think effortfully about each action for driving). Graybiel has proposed the concept of habits, which is opposed to what researchers have defined as goal-oriented actions. We think that the early ability to perceive the world is not very different in terms of the mechanisms involved to what we described for learning to drive. This means that the system has to learn and then extract the invariants between sensory information and representation/action related to them. From such a perspective, the ability of the newborn to learn about this environment and how to interact with it necessitates automatization of some procedures involving specific brain region interactions and then the progressive shaping of the neuronal system through the synaptic weights, which is a kind of crystallization of neuronal networks to achieve specific functions. The learning of social communication, especially through the vocal system, can be understood in this context of learning habits, both at the production and the perception levels. The central nervous system of the newborn is then able to learn progressively, by systematic invariant extraction in the context of action/perception, how to produce specific vocalizations and adapt them to the interpersonal context. With the systematic repetition or special relevance of some situations, the neural connectivity pattern, thanks to the basal ganglia system and its interaction with cortical areas, is progressively shaped to respond to specific functions, for example, social functions, both at the production and the perception levels.

In light of the studies performed in adults and newborns in the vocal domain, we can reasonably predict that during early parental emotional vocal interactions, similar brain regions are involved in both newborns and adults. Of course, the ability of newborns to extract invariants for both production and perception levels is progressively shaped by their experience. Early life interactions are crucial to promote the best functioning of the newborn and to shape the complex brain-body systems for the best adaptation of the physical environment but also, and perhaps even more crucially, for the social context.

The investigation of the brain mechanisms involved in the production and perception of emotional voice processing at an early stage of development, including in premature populations, should be extended and developed further. Such studies may better characterize how and when future interventions, such as exposure to the mother's live voice, have the best impact on promoting the development of the social brain during this crucial period, which is strongly characterized by brain maturation processes, and on long-term effects on the development of social skills.

Key Messages

• The production of reflex-like vocalizations at an early stage of development is mainly related to the periaqueductal gray matter. Progressively, newborns learn to control the production of emotional vocalization through interactions between this brain region as well as the subcortical nuclei, especially the basal ganglia, and motor cortical areas. This progressive control is essential in the social life of newborns and later on during childhood.

- The perception of emotion in the voice involves a series of specific brain mechanisms, mainly including the voice-sensitive areas (superior temporal regions), basal ganglia, amygdala, orbitofrontal regions, and inferior frontal regions.
- The development of habits for emotional voice processing involves complex functional neuronal loops between the basal ganglia and other subcortical and cortical areas, both at the production and the perception level, and is crucial for social communication skills.

References

Aboitiz, F., & Garcia, R. (2009). Merging of phonological and gestural circuits in early language evolution. *Reviews in the Neurosciences, 20*(1), 71–84.

Abrams, D. A., Chen, T. W., Odriozola, P., Cheng, K. M., Baker, A. E., Padmanabhan, A., … Menon, V. (2016). Neural circuits underlying mother's voice perception predict social communication abilities in children. *Proceedings of the National Academy of Sciences of the United States of America, 113*(22), 6295–6300.

Bach, D. R., Grandjean, D., Sander, D., Herdener, M., Strik, W. K., & Seifritz, E. (2008). The effect of appraisal level on processing of emotional prosody in meaningless speech. *NeuroImage, 42*(2), 919–927.

Banse, R., & Scherer, K. R. (1996). Acoustic profiles in vocal emotion expression. *Journal of Personality and Social Psychology, 70*(3), 614–636.

Beaucousin, V., Lacheret, A., Turbelin, M. R., Morel, M., Mazoyer, B., & Tzourio-Mazoyer, N. (2007). FMRI study of emotional speech comprehension. *Cerebral Cortex, 17*(2), 339–352.

Belin, P., Zatorre, R. J., Lafaille, P., Ahad, P., & Pike, B. (2000). Voice-selective areas in human auditory cortex. *Nature, 403*(6767), 309–312.

Blonder, L. X., Heilman, K. M., Ketterson, T., Rosenbek, J., Raymer, A., Crosson, B., … Roth, L. G. (2005). Affective facial and lexical expression in aprosodic versus aphasic stroke patients. *Journal of the International Neuropsychological Society, 11*(6), 677–685.

Blonder, L. X., Pickering, J. E., Heath, R. L., Smith, C. D., & Butler, S. M. (1995). Prosodic characteristics of speech pre- and post-right hemisphere stroke. *Brain and Language, 51*(2), 318–335.

Boe, L. J., Badin, P., Menard, L., Captier, G., Davis, B., MacNeilage, P., … Schwartz, J. L. (2013). Anatomy and control of the developing human vocal tract: A response to Lieberman. *Journal of Phonetics, 41*(5), 379–392.

Boiten, F. A. (1998). The effects of emotional behaviour on components of the respiratory cycle. *Biological Psychology, 49*(1–2), 29–51.

Brunswik, E. (1956). *Perception and the representative design of psychological experiments* (2nd ed.). Berkeley, CA: University of California Press.

Buchanan, T. W., Lutz, K., Mirzazade, S., Specht, K., Shah, N. J., Zilles, K., & Jancke, L. (2000). Recognition of emotional prosody and verbal components of spoken language: An fMRI study. *Brain Research. Cognitive Brain Research, 9*(3), 227–238.

Butler, E. A., Wilhelm, F. H., & Gross, J. J. (2006). Respiratory sinus arrhythmia, emotion, and emotion regulation during social interaction. *Psychophysiology, 43*(6), 612–622.

Cancelliere, A. E., & Kertesz, A. (1990). Lesion localization in acquired deficits of emotional expression and comprehension. *Brain and Cognition, 13*(2), 133–147.

Ceravolo, L., Fruhholz, S., & Grandjean, D. (2016a). Modulation of auditory spatial attention by angry prosody: An fMRI auditory dot-probe study. *Frontiers in Neuroscience, 10*, 216.

Ceravolo, L., Fruhholz, S., & Grandjean, D. (2016b). Proximal vocal threat recruits the right voice-sensitive auditory cortex. *Social Cognitive and Affective Neuroscience, 11*(5), 793–802.

Cheng, Y. W., Lee, S. Y., Chen, H. Y., Wang, P. Y., & Decety, J. (2012). Voice and emotion processing in the human neonatal brain. *Journal of Cognitive Neuroscience, 24*(6), 1411–1419.

Cohen, M. J., Riccio, C. A., & Flannery, A. M. (1994). Expressive aprosodia following stroke to the right basal ganglia: A case report. *Neuropsychology, 8*(2), 242–245.

Davis, B. L., MacNeilage, P. F., & Matyear, C. L. (2002). Acquisition of serial complexity in speech production: A comparison of phonetic and phonological approaches to first word production. *Phonetica, 59*(2–3), 75–107.

Davis, P. J., Zhang, S. P., Winkworth, A., & Bandler, R. (1996). Neural control of vocalization: Respiratory and emotional influences. *Journal of Voice, 10*(1), 23–38.

Dellacherie, D., Hasboun, D., Baulac, M., Belin, P., & Samson, S. (2011). Impaired recognition of fear in voices and reduced anxiety after unilateral temporal lobe resection. *Neuropsychologia, 49*(4), 618–629.

EcklundFlores, L., & Turkewitz, G. (1996). Asymmetric headturning to speech and nonspeech in human newborns. *Developmental Psychobiology, 29*(3), 205–217.

Ethofer, T., Anders, S., Erb, M., Herbert, C., Wiethoff, S., Kissler, J., ... Wildgruber, D. (2006). Cerebral pathways in processing of affective prosody: A dynamic causal modeling study. *NeuroImage, 30*(2), 580–587.

Ethofer, T., Anders, S., Wiethoff, S., Erb, M., Herbert, C., Saur, R., ... Wildgruber, D. (2006). Effects of prosodic emotional intensity on activation of associative auditory cortex. *Neuroreport, 17*(3), 249–253.

Ethofer, T., Bretscher, J., Gschwind, M., Kreifelts, B., Wildgruber, D., & Vuilleumier, P. (2012). Emotional voice areas: Anatomic location, functional properties, and structural connections revealed by combined fMRI/DTI. *Cerebral Cortex, 22*(1), 191–200.

Ethofer, T., De Ville, D. V., Scherer, K., & Vuilleumier, P. (2009). Decoding of emotional information in voice-sensitive cortices. *Current Biology, 19*(12), 1028–1033.

Etzel, J. A., Johnsen, E. L., Dickerson, J., Tranel, D., & Adolphs, R. (2006). Cardiovascular and respiratory responses during musical mood induction. *International Journal of Psychophysiology, 61*(1), 57–69.

Eviatar, Z., & Just, M. A. (2006). Brain correlates of discourse processing: An fMRI investigation of irony and conventional metaphor comprehension. *Neuropsychologia, 44*(12), 2348–2359.

Filippa, M., Devouche, E., Arioni, C., Imberty, M., & Gratier, M. (2013). Live maternal speech and singing have beneficial effects on hospitalized preterm infants. *Acta Paediatrica, 102*(10), 1017–1020.

Fruhholz, S., Ceravolo, L., & Grandjean, D. (2012). Specific brain networks during explicit and implicit decoding of emotional prosody. *Cerebral Cortex, 22*(5), 1107–1117.

Fruhholz, S., & Grandjean, D. (2012a). Amygdala subregions differentially respond and rapidly adapt to threatening voices. *Cortex, 49*, 1394–1403.

Fruhholz, S., & Grandjean, D. (2012b). Towards a fronto-temporal neural network for the decoding of angry vocal expressions. *NeuroImage, 62*(3), 1658–1666.

Fruhholz, S., & Grandjean, D. (2013a). Multiple subregions in superior temporal cortex are differentially sensitive to vocal expressions: A quantitative meta-analysis. *Neuroscience and Biobehavioral Reviews, 37*(1), 24–35.

Fruhholz, S., & Grandjean, D. (2013b). Processing of emotional vocalizations in bilateral inferior frontal cortex. *Neuroscience and Biobehavioral Reviews, 37*(10 Pt 2), 2847–2855.

Fruhholz, S., Gschwind, M., & Grandjean, D. (2015). Bilateral dorsal and ventral fiber pathways for the processing of affective prosody identified by probabilistic fiber tracking. *NeuroImage, 109*, 27–34.

Fruhholz, S., Hofstetter, C., Cristinzio, C., Saj, A., Seeck, M., Vuilleumier, P., & Grandjean, D. (2015). Asymmetrical effects of unilateral right or left amygdala damage on auditory cortical processing of vocal emotions. *Proceedings of the National Academy of Sciences of the United States of America, 112*(5), 1583–1588.

Fruhholz, S., Klaas, H. S., Patel, S., & Grandjean, D. (2015). Talking in fury: The cortico-subcortical network underlying angry vocalizations. *Cerebral Cortex, 25*(9), 2752–2762.

Fruhholz, S., Trost, W., & Grandjean, D. (2016). Whispering – The hidden side of auditory communication. *NeuroImage, 142*, 602–612.

Fruhholz, S., van der Zwaag, W., Saenz, M., Belin, P., Schobert, A. K., Vuilleumier, P., & Grandjean, D. (2016). Neural decoding of discriminative auditory object features depends on their socio-affective valence. *Social Cognitive and Affective Neuroscience, 11*(10), 1638–1649.

Frysztak, R. J., & Neafsey, E. J. (1991). The effect of medial frontal cortex lesions on respiration, "freezing," and ultrasonic vocalizations during conditioned emotional responses in rats. *Cerebral Cortex, 1*(5), 418–425.

Grandjean, D., Banziger, T., & Scherer, K. R. (2006). Intonation as an interface between language and affect. *Progress in Brain Research, 156*, 235–247.

Grandjean, D., Sander, D., Pourtois, G., Schwartz, S., Seghier, M. L., Scherer, K. R., & Vuilleumier, P. (2005). The voices of wrath: Brain responses to angry prosody in meaningless speech. *Nature Neuroscience, 8*(2), 145–146.

Grandjean, D., Sander, D., & Scherer, K. R. (2008). Conscious emotional experience emerges as a function of multilevel, appraisal–driven response synchronization. *Conscioussness and Cognition, 17*(2), 484–495.

Graybiel, A. M. (2008). Habits, rituals, and the evaluative brain. *Annual Review of Neuroscience, 31*, 359–387.

Grela, B., & Gandour, J. (1998). Locus of functional impairment in the production of speech rhythm after brain damage: A preliminary study. *Brain and Language, 64*(3), 361–376.

Gruber, T., & Grandjean, D. (2017). A comparative neurological approach to emotional expressions in primate vocalizations. *Neuroscience and Biobehavioral Reviews, 73*, 182–190.

Guranski, K., & Podemski, R. (2015). Emotional prosody expression in acoustic analysis in patients with right hemisphere ischemic stroke. *Neurologia i Neurochirurgia Polska, 49*(2), 113–120.

Holstege, G., & Subramanian, H. H. (2016). Two different motor systems are needed to generate human speech. *The Journal of Comparative Neurology, 524*(8), 1558–1577.

Hutt, C., Vonbernu, H., Lenard, H. G., Hutt, S. J., & Prechtl, H. F. R. (1968). Habituation in relation to state in human neonate. *Nature, 220*(5167), 618–620.

Johnstone, T., van Reekum, C. M., Oakes, T. R., & Davidson, R. J. (2006). The voice of emotion: An FMRI study of neural responses to angry and happy vocal expressions. *Social Cognitive and Affective Neuroscience, 1*(3), 242–249.

Klaas, H. S., Fruhholz, S., & Grandjean, D. (2015). Aggressive vocal expressions-an investigation of their underlying neural network. *Frontiers in Behavioral Neuroscience, 9*, 121.

Leitman, D. I., Wolf, D. H., Ragland, J. D., Laukka, P., Loughead, J., Valdez, J. N., ... Gur, R. C. (2010). "It's not what you say, but how you say it": A reciprocal temporo-frontal network for affective prosody. *Frontiers in Human Neuroscience, 4*, 19.

MacNeilage, P. F. (1998a). The frame/content theory of evolution of speech production. *Behavioral and Brain Sciences, 21*(4), 499–511.

MacNeilage, P. F. (1998b). The frame/content view of speech: What survives, what emerges. *Behavioral and Brain Sciences, 21*(4), 532–546.

Mampe, B., Friederici, A. D., Christophe, A., & Wermke, K. (2009). Newborns' cry melody is shaped by their native language. *Current Biology, 19*(23), 1994–1997.

Mastropieri, D., & Turkewitz, G. (1999). Prenatal experience and neonatal responsiveness to vocal expressions of emotion. *Developmental Psychobiology, 35*(3), 204–214.

Mizuno, T., & Sugishita, M. (2007). Neural correlates underlying perception of tonality-related emotional contents. *Neuroreport, 18*(16), 1651–1655.

Nakhutina, L., Borod, J. C., & Zgaljardic, D. J. (2006). Posed prosodic emotional expression in unilateral stroke patients: Recovery, lesion location, and emotional perception. *Archives of Clinical Neuropsychology, 21*(1), 1–13.

Paulmann, S., Seifert, S., & Kotz, S. A. (2010). Orbito-frontal lesions cause impairment during late but not early emotional prosodic processing. *Social Neuroscience, 5*(1), 59–75.

Peron, J., Fruhholz, S., Verin, M., & Grandjean, D. (2013). Subthalamic nucleus: A key structure for emotional component synchronization in humans. *Neuroscience and Biobehavioral Reviews, 37*(3), 358–373.

Pichon, S., & Kell, C. A. (2013). Affective and sensorimotor components of emotional prosody generation. *Journal of Neuroscience, 33*(4), 1640–1650.

Sander, D., Grandjean, D., Pourtois, G., Schwartz, S., Seghier, M. L., Scherer, K. R., & Vuilleumier, P. (2005). Emotion and attention interactions in social cognition: Brain regions involved in processing anger prosody. *NeuroImage, 28*(4), 848–858.

Sander, D., Grandjean, D., & Scherer, K. R. (2005). A systems approach to appraisal mechanisms in emotion. *Neural Networks, 18*(4), 317–352.

Scherer, K. R. (1984a). Emotions – Functions and components. *Cahiers De Psychologie Cognitive-Current Psychology of Cognition, 4*(1), 9–39.

Scherer, K. R. (1984b). On the nature and function of emotion. A component process approach. In K. R. Scherer & P. Ekman (Eds.), *Approaches to emotion* (pp. 293–317). Hillsdale, MI: Erlbaum.

Scherer, K. R., Dan, E. S., & Flykt, A. (2006). What determines a feeling's position in affective space? A case for appraisal. *Cognition & Emotion, 20*(1), 92–113.

Schirmer, A., Alter, K., Kotz, S. A., & Friederici, A. D. (2001). Lateralization of prosody during language production: A lesion study. *Brain and Language, 76*(1), 1–17.

Schirmer, A., Escoffier, N., Zysset, S., Koester, D., Striano, T., & Friederici, A. D. (2008). When vocal processing gets emotional: On the role of social orientation in relevance detection by the human amygdala. *NeuroImage, 40*(3), 1402–1410.

Schirmer, A., & Kotz, S. A. (2006). Beyond the right hemisphere: Brain mechanisms mediating vocal emotional processing. *Trends in Cognitive Sciences, 10*(1), 24–30.

Scott, S. K., Young, A. W., Calder, A. J., Hellawell, D. J., Aggleton, J. P., & Johnson, M. (1997). Impaired auditory recognition of fear and anger following bilateral amygdala lesions. *Nature, 385*(6613), 254–257.

Smith, C. A., & Ellsworth, P. C. (1985). Patterns of cognitive appraisal in emotion. *Journal of Personality and Social Psychology, 48*(4), 813–838.

Stewart, A. M., Lewis, G. F., Heilman, K. J., Davila, M. I., Coleman, D. D., Aylward, S. A., & Porges, S. W. (2013). The covariation of acoustic features of infant cries and autonomic state. *Physiology & Behavior, 120*, 203–210.

Subramanian, H. H., Arun, M., Silburn, P. A., & Holstege, G. (2016). Motor organization of positive and negative emotional vocalization in the cat midbrain periaqueductal gray. *The Journal of Comparative Neurology, 524*(8), 1540–1557.

Tzourio-Mazoyer, N., Beaucousin, V., Lacheret, A., Turbelin, M. R., More, M., & Mazoyer, B. (2007). FMRI study of emotional speech comprehension. *Cerebral Cortex, 17*(2), 339–352.

van Reekum, C. M., Johnstone, T., Banse, R., Etter, A., Wehrle, T., & Scherer, K. R. (2004). Psychophysiological responses to appraisal dimensions in a computer game. *Cognition & Emotion, 18*(5), 663–688.

Wiethoff, S., Wildgruber, D., Grodd, W., & Ethofer, T. (2009). Response and habituation of the amygdala during processing of emotional prosody. *Neuroreport, 20*(15), 1356–1360.

Wiethoff, S., Wildgruber, D., Kreifelts, B., Becker, H., Herbert, C., Grodd, W., & Ethofer, T. (2008). Cerebral processing of emotional prosody – Influence of acoustic parameters and arousal. *NeuroImage, 39*(2), 885–893.

Wildgruber, D., Ackermann, H., Kreifelts, B., & Ethofer, T. (2006). Cerebral processing of linguistic and emotional prosody: fMRI studies. *Progress in Brain Research, 156*, 249–268.

Wildgruber, D., Ethofer, T., Grandjean, D., & Kreiflets, B. (2009). A cerebral network model of speech prosody comprehension. *International Journal of Speech-Language Pathology, 11*(4), 277–281.

Wildgruber, D., Hertrich, I., Riecker, A., Erb, M., Anders, S., Grodd, W., & Ackermann, H. (2004). Distinct frontal regions subserve evaluation of linguistic and emotional aspects of speech intonation. *Cerebral Cortex, 14*(12), 1384–1389.

Wildgruber, D., Riecker, A., Hertrich, I., Erb, M., Grodd, W., Ethofer, T., & Ackermann, H. (2005). Identification of emotional intonation evaluated by fMRI. *NeuroImage, 24*(4), 1233–1241.

Part II
The NICU Acoustic Environment and the Preterm Infant's Auditory System Development

Chapter 6
The Sound Environments and Auditory Perceptions of the Fetus and Preterm Newborn

M. Kathleen Philbin

Abstract This critical review of the literature of the sound environment and auditory perception of the fetus and preterm newborn considers classic and contemporary studies.

This chapter aims to examine animal studies as a starting point and stimulus for knowledge of fetal and preterm infant auditory perception and behavior development. It also appraises listening conditions in a newborn intensive care unit (NICU) as these affect perception of the mother's voice. Practices intended to augment fetal and preterm listening environments are considered. An understanding of sound measurement is intended to improve the validity of research and effectiveness of clinical practices regarding exposure to mother's voice.

The chapter concludes that the fetus perceives its environment as quiet but complex and that the mother's voice is a prominent signal but heartbeat sounds are not. Strong vibroacoustic stimulation of no benefit and possible harm includes some workplaces and sports, transport vehicles, and speakers attached to the belly or inserted in the vagina.

Although ambient sound equivalent levels may be low and hard, reverberant surfaces in old and new NICUs produce startling, distracting, and disturbing individual sounds for infants and adults. The amount of auditory experience "good enough" for perception and language development is unknown. Perception of frequency alone is a minor component of language competence. A holistic view of the infant suggests that "sound deprivation" may be a misnomer if some live speech and singing are available. Skin-to-skin holding with speech provides an effective basis for language development in the NICU environment.

M.K. Philbin, RN, PhD (✉)
Independent Researcher, Moorestown, NJ, USA
e-mail: kathleenphilbin@comcast.net

© Springer International Publishing AG 2017
M. Filippa et al. (eds.), *Early Vocal Contact and Preterm Infant Brain Development*, DOI 10.1007/978-3-319-65077-7_6

Animal and Human Models of Fetal Hearing

Science teaches skepticism in applying the results of animal studies to humans. However, some questions about humans cannot be answered directly by humans. They can, however, be approached in carefully designed and conducted animal studies. Conversely animal studies can suggest avenues of understanding that can only be pursued with humans.

Philbin, Lickliter, and Graven (2000) and Lickliter and Bahrick (2000) make the case for pursuing human and animal studies citing well-tested parallels of human fetal hearing and behavioral responsiveness to sound shown in several animal models. However, some recent literature has dismissed the relevance of one of the most studied models of the fetal sound environment, the pregnant ewe (e.g., Lahav, 2015). The purpose of this section, therefore, is to give a few brief examples of established concordance and to outline the back and forth between questions and answers that make animal studies invaluable for advancing knowledge about both humans and animals.

Sheep Model of Fetal Development Ewe and human have a similar size fetus and pregnant uterus. There are also "similarities in the physics of transmission and early development of inner ear function prenatally" (Abrams & Gerhardt, 2000). Older but still valid studies using this model (e.g., Gerhardt & Abrams, 2000; Abrams & Gerhardt, 2000; Armitage, Baldwin, & Vince, 1980) show, for example, that sounds available to the head of a fetal sheep are similar to those recorded by hydrophone near the neck of a human fetus at term (Richards, Frentzen, Gerhardt, McCann, & Abrams, 1992). Using a hydrophone (designed for use in fluid) shows both a slight but significant reduction in intrauterine sound levels (perceived as loudness/quietness and measured as decibels (dB) of airborne, external sounds) and a slight but significant amplification of internal sounds, particularly the maternal voice. Both show a varied intrauterine sound environment of internal and external sounds, including voices surrounding the mother.

Avian Models The science of hearing *development* has been furthered in major respects with the use of avian models. Mammals are closely related to humans but not with respect to developmental psychoacoustics. However, avian hearing development is like human in that it is precocial, developing in many ways in a fluid environment before hatching or birth. Most mammals, by contrast, are born with relatively undeveloped hearing that subsequently matures in air. Additional advantages are that avians develop quickly, are readily available, and are easily manipulated in the shell. Many studies of the bobwhite quail and ducks show discrimination of and approach behavior toward the calls of the chick's specific mother hen compared with other hens as well as the disruption of psychoacoustic development by other sensory stimuli (e.g., Harshaw & Lickliter, 2011). Rubel et al. (1984) developed an avian model of the physical development of the cochlea and hair cells and their related brain structures. Following on these findings Philbin, et al. used the native (untrained) peeping of the domestic chick to describe the development of many psychoacoustic abilities found in the human neonate including disruption of habituation (Philbin, Ballweg, & Gray, 1994).

Research in habituation illustrates the ability of an animal model to answer questions suggested by human studies and, in turn, to provide a platform for furthering human research. Habituation is important because it enables an organism to discriminate the novel from the typical, thus improving safety, the location of food, and other complex learning. The ability to habituate or decrease responding to repeated sounds is used as a marker of neurobehavioral development in the widely accepted newborn and preterm human infant neurobehavioral development assessments designed by Brazelton, et al. (1987), Als et al. (2005), and Lester et al. (2004). However, while most healthy term newborns habituate to repeated sounds and other stimuli, most preterm newborns do not. The scientific question is whether the newborn intensive care unit (NICU) environment might have an influence on preterm infants' development of habituation.

Hatchlings of the domestic chicken show a very sturdy ability to habituate. Many studies make use of this ability to document attention to novel events in the acoustic environment. To answer the question of habituation abilities suggested by the human developmental assessments, Philbin et al. (1994) exposed chick embryos to tape recordings of NICU sound while keeping all other sensory experience the same as that of a control group. Unexpectedly, the experimental group of hatchlings, unlike the controls, did not habituate reliably to repeated bursts of white noise. A more recent animal study using brain mapping via functional magnetic resonance imaging (fMRI) shows that environmental noise, such as might make up a NICU sound environment, retards auditory cortical development (e.g., Chang & Merzenich, 2003).

Findings such as these lead back to the question about preterm humans and their environments. Is there a difference in habituation to sound between preterm infants cared for in a noisy NICU and those in a quiet one? Stated another way, is the unreliable habituation found in preterm humans a product of nature or nurture? With the advent of very quiet, single-patient rooms and the continued use of crowded, noisy ones, this question could now be asked and perhaps answered with human infants. An answer in the positive would then suggest a line of research regarding the effect of newborn intensive care on preterm infants responses to the other stimuli well described in neurobehavioral testing.

The Development of Sound Perception: Developmental Psychoacoustics

Hearing is developing actively by the 20th week of gestation, and the fetus is shown to respond to sound by 24th week (*National Institute of Occupational Health and Safety* – NIOSH). The development of species-typical perception is complex. It occurs in conjunction with the particularly specialized acoustic environment of the uterus. In the inner ear, physical vibrations are translated to nerve conduction by the hair cells of the cochlea and from there to the auditory centers of the brain.

The Development of the Perception of Frequency: Tonotopic Organization Sound frequencies are initially registered as different but without an ordered pattern, distinct but disorganized. With maturation and experience, as each hair cell in the cochlea becomes associated with a specific counterpart in the auditory brain centers, the individual frequencies are organized precisely in both inner ear and brain, just as the keys on a piano (Gray, 1991; Appler & Goodrich, 2011). Similar organization occurs with the physical registration and central nervous system organization of level, rhythm, duration, and other attributes of sound perception.

The phenomenon of hair cell maturation, the *place principle*, was first described by Rubel et al. (1984). Low-frequency sounds are the earliest to register at the large end of the basilar membrane near the oval window that connects the middle and inner ears (Querleu, Verspy, & Vervoort, 1988; review Gerhardt & Abrams, 2000). Sound and vibration from both the external and internal maternal environments have been recorded in the pregnant ewe near term from 60 Hz (i.e., very low) to 8000 Hz, the high end of the frequencies of speech. As its complex structures develop, the basilar membrane becomes increasingly flexible and capable of moving the emerging hair cells further toward the apex. The registration of lower frequencies moves along simultaneously, leaving the large end to register ever-higher frequencies (Rubel et al., 1984). Stated another way, the hair cells that once registered lower-frequency sounds eventually register higher-frequency sounds until, at some point in early infancy, the entire membrane and all hair cells and their related central functions are developed. While the exact timing of this progression is known in avian, ewe, and other models, it is not well known in humans.

This development of lower frequencies first is advantageous for fetal hearing development as the sounds most available in the uterine environment are also in the lower frequencies due to the loss of energy of higher frequencies in the transition through the maternal tissue and amniotic fluid barrier. However, high-energy (i.e., high decibel; loud) sounds of all frequencies transit into and through the uterus with less loss of energy and affect the fetus at all frequencies it is capable of perceiving.

Perception of Sound Level: The Development of Hearing Acuity During fetal life the ossicles (three small bones) of the middle ear cannot perform their amplifying, translational functions because outer, middle, and inner ear are all fluid filled. At this time the hair cells of the inner ear are stimulated directly by vibrations of the fetal skull. Bone-conducted stimulation of the cochlear hair cells produces actual hearing and is not a "separate sense" as stated in some contemporary publications. The consequence of transmission of sound waves in this manner is similar to an adult hearing loss of about 40 dBA. (Note: dBA refers to a particular, nonlinear decibel conversion – the A scale – that represents sound levels as they are perceived by humans. The dBC scale does not make a conversion and is seldom used in reports relative to human hearing. dB usually refers to dBA if the topic relates to humans.) The relatively quiet world of the uterus is biologically compatible with the development of fetal ear and auditory centers during maturation. The ability to perceive sound level develops over time in utero and after full-term birth (Rabinowitz, Willmore, Schnupp, & King, 2011). Considering this, one must use caution in deciding what constitutes auditory deprivation for a preterm infant as the same levels of 40 dBA to 60 dBA are common in new, not crowded, or single-room NICUs.

Perception of a Signal in Noise A signal can be any distinct stimulus. In the case of hearing, it is usually a sound with characteristics that set its intelligibility apart from the rest of the ambient environment. While most aspects of hearing mature at a rapid pace during the first and second years of life, the perception of a signal in noise is not adult-like until late childhood or early adolescence, depending on the test used. The lateness of this ability has broad implications for all children's environments including child care centers and schools.

The immature auditory system (end organ and brain) is best able to detect a sound signal if parts of it are at a higher frequency (perceived as pitch) and level (perceived as loud/quiet) and more varied frequency pattern, or if it has different tonal qualities than other sounds. A high signal-to-noise ratio occurs in utero fairly often with respect to the maternal voice because it is different in these aspects from other sounds.

The Effect of the Predictability of the Sound Environment on Attention and Distraction Attention to a sound signal varies with the predictability or orderliness of the background. Infants and children require a more orderly ambient sound environment than adults in order to maintain attention (Gray & Philbin, 2004). This is to say, prior to adulthood distractibility increases and, therefore, attention decreases as predictability of the acoustic environment and age decrease. An environment perceived as predicable (and, therefore, not distracting) by an adult may be unpredictable and distracting for children and even more so for an infant. These differences between infant and adult perception make adults' poor judgment of sound signals intelligible to preterm infants. This is important in considering the required orderliness of the sound environment enabling a preterm infant to discriminate the mother's voice, music, or other environmental sounds.

The Acoustic Environment and Auditory Perception of the Fetus

The acoustic environment of the fetus consists of a closed chamber filled with a fetal body and fluid more dense than ocean water. The chamber wall provides a solid but flexible boundary with the approximate density of muscle that changes in shape, thickness, and tautness with fetal movement and growth in body size. Prior to the engagement in the pelvis, the head can be in any location (review: Abrams & Gerhardt, 2000). These multiple changes result in variable deflective and absorptive acoustic properties and a variable acoustic environment for the fetus.

Intrauterine sounds originate in three sources. *Internally generated sounds* originate in the maternal organs, voice, and movement. They are conducted via tissue and bone through the body, cross the uterine wall, and travel through intrauterine fluid directly stimulating the hair cells of the cochlea via vibratory compression of the fetal head. They lose little energy in the process of transmission through the body and uterus and can even amplify (Richards et al., 1992). *Externally generated sounds* are conducted via air and must cross the maternal-uterine tissue barrier, losing considerable energy in the process if levels are only moderately loud. Sounds in the uterus are usually of low frequency, but sounds of any frequency can pass through if the level is high enough. However, these high frequencies may not be perceived by the fetus because of the gradual development of perception of frequencies described above. (The same restrictions on perception are the case for young preterm infants; high frequencies in the NICU may not be perceived.) The third sound source is *external vibroacoustic stimulation* (VAS) by mechanical objects making physical contact with the maternal body.

Maternal Heartbeat Sounds and the Maternal Voice Some researchers, clinicians, and laymen believe that heartbeat sounds dominate the uterine sound environment (Panagiotidis & Lahav, 2010; Salk, 1960, 1962). The purpose of this section is to examine the science supporting the belief.

The theory of prominent intrauterine heartbeat sounds originated in 1960 with Lee Salk, a psychiatrist in Queens, New York (Salk, 1960, 1962). Although it seems quaint now, this nearly 70-year-old theory of imprinting was persuasive and consistent with science at the time (e.g., Hess, 1959; Moltz, 1960). The idea came to him during a visit to the Central Park Zoo in Manhattan, an old-style zoo of mostly isolated animals in small cages. He does not cite methods of primate behavior research but simply asserts that in 40 out of 42 of his own observations, a single rhesus monkey carried her infant against her left side ("closest to her heart"). The entire theory of heartbeat sounds was based on the way in which mother monkeys and newly delivered women held their infants.

Salk's idea caught on and is so emotionally attractive that it perhaps will require a type of scientific revolution – a fundamental shift in thinking – to see past the data that don't support it and thus dislodge it from popular and scientific culture (Kuhn, 2012). There have been few studies based on the singular experience of imprinting to heartbeat sounds although DeCasper and Singafoos (1983) present a literature review of work emphasizing a broader picture of imprinting and the effects of fetal auditory experience.

Overreaching his data, Salk asserted that imprinting by intrauterine heartbeat sounds was "the basis of all later learning" (Salk, 1962, p. 762) and persisted into adulthood. The rhythms of music and dance are given as examples of the "universal" and "biological tendency [of man]" to seek proximity to a heartbeat sound because it "has survival value … [and] involves mutual satisfaction" (p. 762). He proposed that a monkey or human mother holds her infant so that she can hear *her own* heart because she then had "the sensation of her own heartbeat reflected back" (p. 762). In other words, her own imprinting to heartbeat sounds leads her to hold the next-generation infant in such a way that it too will imprint to heartbeat sounds.

Salk tested his imprinting theory by comparing group (whole room) responses of healthy toddlers in cribs in a hospital for orphans. Individual infants were not tested, and groups did not serve as their own controls. In his several studies, each of the two groups received only the experimental (heartbeat) or a very different control stimulus (e.g., unspecified lullaby or room sounds, including sounds made by other infants/toddlers).

A methodological error in these studies, as well as in some contemporary studies (e.g., Panagiotidis & Lahav, 2010; Ullal-Gupta, Van den Bosch der Nederlanden, Tichko, Lahav, & Hannon, 2013) is that the experimental and control stimuli are *too* different from one another; there were too many variables to isolate the discrimination of heartbeats specifically. For example, one variable, e.g., the voice, may be of a significantly higher frequency or level than heartbeat (e.g., Panagnostakis & Lahav, 2010). In other studies, the more simple heartbeat sound could attract the infant's attention simply because it has fewer tone changes and is more rhythmic than, say, the "no control" of random room sounds (e.g., Doheny, Hurwitz, Insoft, Ringer, & Lahav, 2012; Rand & Lahav, 2014).

It is possible that any two sounds with features similar to heartbeat could elicit attention or orientation equally. For example, a rhythmic waltz beat (lub dub-dub, lub dub-dub) as well as the quarter time beat of the heart itself (lub dub pause pause, lub dub pause pause) could both be attracting stimuli. If, for example, *both* heartbeat-like conditions showed clinically significant, lower heart rates than no stimulus – all in a very quiet acoustic chamber – the infant listener would be responding to the rhythmic nature or some other feature of the signals rather than to heartbeat *per say*.

It is reasonable to assume that preterm and term infants could make fine discriminations between heartbeat-like sounds. Shahidullah and Hepper (1994) showed that fetuses at 27–35 weeks gestational ages could discriminate between "baba" and "bibi." Moon et al. (2013) showed that newly born infants could discriminate subtle differences in sounds of the same vowel in two languages. DeCasper and Fifer (1980) showed that newborns could discriminate between their mother's voice and the voice of other women. DeCasper and Prescott (1984) showed that they can discriminate between female and male voices, and Spence and deCasper (1987) showed discrimination between different frequencies of the same words. If preterm and term infants can make these fine discriminations, surely they could discriminate between "lub dub-dub, lub dub-dub" and "lub dub pause pause, lub dub pause pause."

Following from the work of Salk, Bench (1968) measured heartbeat sounds from pregnant women prior to the onset of labor. The state of consciousness of the women is not given, and there is no information about the presence of the maternal voice. These studies are now recognized as invalid because a microphone (not hydrophone – designed to function in fluid) was covered with a rubber sleeve, thereby made inaccurate. It was passed through the cervix and moved around the inside of the uterus before and after rupturing membranes. The researchers particularly tried for placement over the ear of the unborn infant whose head was engaged in the pelvis.

Probably because of placement of the microphone, only heartbeat and other cardio-vascular sounds could be identified and were reported to be loud. Bench concluded, and the scientific and lay communities accepted, that these measurements represented acoustic conditions throughout fetal life.

Grimwade et al. (1970) also attempted to measure intrauterine sounds. It is important to understand this and the Bench studies because the findings are at times the rationale for the levels and frequencies produced by speakers attached to the belly and inserted in the vagina. Their study included 16 pregnant women, at term but not in active labor, before and after rupture of the membranes. Again, the microphone was positioned near the fetal head engaged in the pelvis. It also included seven nonpregnant women undergoing uterine curettage. For both groups of subjects, the covered microphone was passed through the cervix, and the vagina was packed with gauze for the purpose of excluding extrauterine room sounds. However, it is uncertain from the report whether this packing was effective. The state of consciousness of the women is not given, and the emphasis is on measuring noise and using other studies to interpret it as primarily the sounds of pulse.

The microphone was calibrated to 55 dB and above and between 100 and 1000 Hz, the mid-dB range of comfortable sound levels, and very low to low, mid-frequency range of sounds perceptible by humans. The authors assumed that this calibration guaranteed accuracy at other levels and frequencies. The capabilities of the microphone and its calibration appear to guarantee exclusion of more quiet and high-frequency sounds. Using complex calculations based on the actual measurements, the authors conclude that sound levels in the pregnant uterus have an arithmetic mean of 95 dB – very loud – for sounds assumed to be the maternal pulse. (See Section 6.6 for the inaccuracy involved in calculating an arithmetic mean for decibels.) The authors speculated that these sounds were important for sensory development.

In 1980, Armitage et al. (1980) specifically addressed the Bench studies using a hydrophone (designed for measurement in fluid) inside the amniotic sac of pregnant ewes and a tested methodology. Their methodology and equipment were well established. They report:

> ...we have found that the sounds of the mother's eating, drinking, rumination, breathing, and muscular movements were discernable, as also were sounds from outside the mother; external sounds were attenuated by 30 dB on average. Sounds from the cardiovascular system were not perceptible, however. (p. 1173)

All sounds between 100 and 1000 Hz were recorded at 40 dB or less, many within the likely acuity level of fetal hearing.

In 1992, Richards et al. (1992) studied intrauterine sounds of conscious women with a spinal block in early stage labor. They used a hydrophone passed through the cervix and had very different findings than Bench's and Walker, Grimwade, and Woods' high sound level intrauterine environments (Richards et al., 1992). Their results were as follows:

> Low-frequency sounds (0.125 kHz) generated outside the mother were reduced by an average of 3.7 dB. There was a gradual increase in attenuation for increasing frequencies, with

a maximum attenuation of 10 dB at 4 kHz, [within the range of human speech].... Intrauterine sound levels of the mother's voice were enhanced by an average of 5.2 dB whereas external male and female voices were attenuated by 2.1 and 3.2 dB, respectively. ....[All] were statistically significant. (p186)

Abrams and Gerhardt (2000), using their well-developed ewe model, also found no evidence of heartbeat sounds but did document a prominent maternal voice. They write,

mother's voice... [is] the most significant and common mode of potential auditory stimulation [by]... non-air-induced acoustic stimulation in the uterus.

Vibroacoustic Stimulation (VAS) VAS may originate in air with enough energy to cross the air-tissue barrier into the uterus or be conducted to the fetal head (and, thereby cochlea) through coupling of the sound source with the woman's body.

Unintentional VAS: Work and Recreation VAS in work and recreation can originate in air and simultaneously through direct coupling of the woman's body via stadium floor and seats, farm vehicle frame and seats, and riflery, leaning against machinery or an instrument (e.g., belly against the piano keyboard, shoulder against the bridge of the double bass), and riding in closed cars with a boom box radio. The National Institute for Occupational Health and Safety (NIOSH, 2016b) advises women to "avoid noise you can feel as a rumble, ... noisy jobs: machines, guns, loud music, crowds of people, sirens, trucks, airplanes." However, professionals are advised to exercise caution in recommending changes in work conditions as this may cause the loss of family income.

For preterm infants in transport vehicles such as helicopters or ambulances (less so in fixed-wing aircraft), directly coupled VAS is delivered via the vehicle body and the attached incubator and ventilator and then to the infant itself, with the head being exposed to the potential for intraventricular hemorrhage. Homemade anti-vibration pads and gel-positioning devises are ill advised as the material can amplify as well as dampen vibration. Accelerometer studies and specifically matched anti-acceleration pads can be made in collaboration with qualified engineers.

Intentional VAS: Commercial and Parental Sources A particular word of caution is offered concerning the practice of attaching audio headphones to the belly of a pregnant woman (Abrams & Gerhardt, 2000; Abrams, Hutchinson, Gerhardt, Evans, & Pendergast, 1987) or, by reasonable extension, of inserting a sound (vibration) source into the vagina (www.Babypod.net/en/babypod). The level at the fetal ear is impossible to control because of acoustic dynamics in the uterine space. Further, objects placed in the vagina have potential for trauma to the urethra and cervix and expose bladder, vagina, and cervix to infection from a foreign body. The purpose is typically teaching or instilling a preference for music or the acquisition of a nonnative language assumed to be advantageous for the child. The practice is promoted for commercial gain and loosely based on the invalid research of Bench and Walker, Grimwade, and Wood reviewed above.

Intentional VAS: Diagnostic Purposes Obstetric clinicians may use VAS from an adapted artificial larynx. The purpose is to assess the well-being of the fetus by stimulating heart rate, gross motor movement, and facial reflexes. Abrams, Gerhardt, Peters, and their associates (e.g., Abrams & Gerhardt, 2000) conducted extensive and still valid studies of VAS by the artificial larynx. They showed that the highest-energy VAS stimuli are in the low-frequency ranges, the frequencies first actively transmitting signal in the developing auditory system. Gagnon found that fetuses between 33 and 40 weeks gestation had an increase in gross movements beginning 10 min after stimulation by an artificial larynx and lasting up to an hour (Gagnon, 1989). Philbin et al. (1996) show heart rate changes including bradycardia and tachycardia in term infants in response to the sounds and low-frequency vibrations of an MRI machine.

See Table 6.1, for a summary of the information in this section.

The Sound Environment, Listening Conditions, and Sound Measurements in Newborn Intensive Care

Frequencies Available in the Acoustic Environment: Questionable Effects on Hearing, Language Development, and Music Perception Frequencies in the environment of the preterm infant are relevant only to their perception; higher frequencies *available in the environment* may be only partially perceived because of the gradual development of the basilar membrane (and, therefore frequency registration) with postmenstrual age. This information is relevant to a current controversy about the nonspecific effects on hearing and language development of the newborn intensive care unit (NICU) frequencies above 500 dB termed "high" (e.g., Lahav, 2015; Lahav & Skoe, 2014). As it happens, there is no authority that defines low, mid, upper mid, and high frequencies. The automotive industry, the National Aeronautics and Space Administration, the audio equipment industry, and the American National Standards Institute (ANSI), all have different definitions (e.g., Smith, 2013). The frequencies of speech are in a range including and well above 500 Hz and are not considered high in most definitions.

See Table 6.2.

Language development and musical abilities are far more complex than frequency perception. They are dependent on the infant's and child's innate capabilities and, equally important, on environmental influences such as the language and music available in the environment and, particularly, on involving interaction. Infant- and child-directed speech is termed *motherese* by some researchers and clinicians. Socialization with children and early childhood education also influence language, social development, and musical ability. Such development occurs over many years in many settings.

Sound Levels Within the Infant Incubator and Mother's Voice The range of sound levels in the *acoustically sealed, empty* infant compartment of a newer-designed

Table 6.1 Effects of the intrauterine environment on the fetus

Intrauterine sound environment	Effects
Biologically expected, natural, not augmented	Necessary, continuous, beneficial
Naturally occurring heartbeat and cardiovascular sounds	Neutral effects, rarely discriminated
Naturally occurring maternal speech	Necessary to development, beneficial, frequent, prominent
Diagnostic vibroacoustic stimulation	Clinically useful but disorganizing for the fetus
High-level, low-frequency work and recreation vibrations in air or coupled to the woman's body	Disorganizing, possibly harmful to fetal hearing
Recorded sound sources attached to belly or vagina	Not beneficial, disorganizing, potential sources of trauma and infection

Table 6.2 Definitions of low to high frequencies used by the automotive industry, the National Aeronautics and Space Administration (NASA), the audio equipment industry, and the American National Standards Institute (ANSI)

Range name	Low end	High end
Low frequencies	250–300 Hz	500 Hz
Mid frequencies (includes voice)	300–400 Hz	2000–3400 Hz
Upper mid frequencies (includes voice) (this category is not in all definitions)	1000–4000 Hz	5000–6000 Hz
High frequencies (the low end of these frequencies is within the range of voice)	1300–4000 Hz	10,000– 20,000 Hz

Note that 500 Hz is not the cut-off point between low and high frequencies

incubator tends to be narrow. Motor noise in such an incubator is an essentially constant broad band of low frequencies of relatively low SPL (about 50 dBA), well tolerated by most preterm infants. However, due to its cubic shape, static size, and stiff shell, the same incubator is a reverberant chamber and effective amplifier of additional low, middle-range, and high-frequency sounds and vibrations. Additionally, sounds of the NICU environment entering through portholes opened many times each day; respiratory equipment inside the shell, and, particularly, the infant's own cry can make the chamber a remarkably high SPL environment with short duration but often occurring levels above 100 dB as measured by this author. The infant is also removed from the incubator many times each day, for example, for feeding, skin care, and procedures. In sum, the infant is living in a very quiet environment only part of the time.

While the mother's voice cannot penetrate a closed incubator with tight seals, she can be heard if her head is close to an open door of an incubator porthole. It is obviously also heard when the mother speaks near the infant's head on an open warmer and when the infant is held. The natural, automatic adjustment of any speaker's vocal effort is based on distance from the listener, background sound levels, speech privacy intentions, and the listener's behavior. This adjustment will likely make a mother's voice level high enough above background to be heard but low enough to be comfortable for the infant. The tonal quality and prosody of the voice will also aid in distinguishing it from other sounds in the environment.

Startling Short-Duration Sound in Old-Style and Newly Designed NICUs High-level, short-duration, unexpected sounds are perceived as sudden and distinct from the background. They are distracting and unpleasant for both adults and infants. At times they evoke a startle response and vital sign changes in both infants and adults (e.g., Philbin et al., 1994). Such sounds can occur in old-design, crowded NICUs, and also in newer designed NICUs with ample space for each bed, including single rooms. These newer yet acoustically unaccommodating NICU rooms typically do not have sound absorptive surfaces on walls and ceiling and impact strike preventive materials for flooring. Such brief sounds are lost in room sound equivalent measurements (L_{eq}), a measure of central tendency, but can be captured by the human ear and verified in measurements of L_{10}, the level exceeded 10% of the time, and L_{max}, the level lasting 1/20 of a second.

Lack of Auditory Deprivation in the NICU All things considered, a very quiet NICU room or incubator may as likely be an advantage as a disadvantage for hospitalized preterm and term infants. In addition to sounds, they are exposed to pain and massive stimulation of other sensory systems (i.e., touch, kinesthetic, vestibular, olfactory, gustatory, and visual) multiple times each day. Looking at the infant holistically, low sound levels may be a respite allowing sleep and recovery from other stimuli.

Regardless of these facts, some investigators and clinicians (e.g., Rand & Lahav, 2014; McMahon, Wintermark, & Lahav, 2012) suggest that a NICU incubator or new NICU single room may be *too quiet* or have *too few* auditory stimuli and constitute conditions of auditory and language deprivation. However, new NICU single-bed rooms with ample sound-absorbing surface materials typically meet the Recommended Standards for Newborn ICU Design, described below. These and other authors propose benefits of adding recorded sound to the acoustic environment. However, studies and standard assessments of the fetus and preterm newborn, such as the NIDCAP, NNNS, and APIB, generally indicate that any purposefully added stimulation must be carefully considered and administered. Additionally, the long- and short-term negative effects of hospital stimuli on infants and parents are unknown; the amount and type of auditory stimulation "good enough" for language and social development are also unknown. The history of the neonatology is rife with examples of attempting to solve a problem without fully understanding it or the proposed solutions.

Mother's Voice and Music: Live Versus Recorded Although the upper frequencies are largely lost in utero, the maternal voice, like external live voices, carries a tonal quality and prosody unlike other sounds, as described above. The same phrase or word is rarely produced in the same way twice but is constantly novel and attracting to attention within the constraints of a single exemplar, the mother. This is the biologically expected manner of exposure, sustained attention, and increasing recognition of the maternal voice and the language and social competence it carries. These stimuli are quite different from recorded sounds.

Repetitious sounds elicit less attention over time if levels are in the low-moderate range. All animals, from the neurologically most simple to the more complex (e.g., newly hatched chicks in Philbin et al., 1994), to the most complex (humans), habituate to repeated, moderately strong stimuli. One might ask whether habituation is the desired effect of exposure to mother's voice and music.

If a tape-recorded voice and music are *not* habituated, one might ask whether the recorded sound is played at high levels, variations in frequency, and tempo to sustain attention long after the infant's response would otherwise be fatigued. One would hope that a live speaker, vocalist, or instrumentalist or person responsible for monitoring recorded sounds would be attentive to the infant and make the necessary adjustments, including stopping, to facilitate behavioral organization and state stability.

NICU Conditions of Auditory Masking and Distraction: Perceptibility of Mother's Voice and Skin-to-Skin Holding The preterm infant's limited ability to discriminate signal from noise means that sounds at significantly high levels in the near environment (e.g., old-style, crowded, reverberant NICU rooms) can mask the mother's voice and cause distraction (Gray & Philbin, 2004). In a crowded, noisy NICU, the voice signal level can be raised by decreasing distance and air transmission time (i.e., bringing mother and baby closer together) and, most effectively, by direct, soft tissue transmission through the mother's body to the infant's body and cochlea with skin-to-skin holding. Staff speaking with the mother during this care are best advised to speak quietly to avoid interrupting the infant's discrimination of the mother's similar voice signal. During skin-to-skin holding, the mother may sleep, rest, or otherwise not talk for periods of time. Many people read in a monotonous tone with less emphasis and rhythm than their speech. However, speech behaviors natural to the mother are the infant's basis for future language acquisition. Clinicians are cautioned to avoid interfering with them.

See Table 6.3, for a summary of the information in this section.

Sound Measurement of Voice and Music: Research and Clinical Interventions

Researchers and clinicians rely on accuracy in the literature and aspire to valid studies and clinical interventions. However, many studies report inaccurate and misleading measurements of sound thereby adding confusion to the literature, failed studies, and ineffective or detrimental clinical interventions. Gray (2000) and Gray and Philbin (2000) provide complete descriptions of the properties of sound and sound measurement in the NICU. A summary of information particular to voice and music is provided here.

Table 6.3 Effects of the intensive care unit sound environment on preterm infants

Intensive care sound environment	Effects
High or low ambient sound equivalent levels (L_{eq}) with high-level sound events. Reverberant surface materials: dry wall, plaster, thin vinyl flooring	Infants: behavior state disruption Infants and adults: physiologic changes, startle, distraction; not beneficial
Recorded sounds (heartbeat, voice, music) not adaptive to changing behaviors and vital signs of the infant	Potential for state/behavior disruption or habituation, questionably beneficial
Periods of quiet in an incubator or NICU room with sound absorptive surfaces accompanied by exposure to speech with caregiving and skin-to-skin care	Possibly a respite from behavior state disruption and multiple strong stimuli of other sensory systems with caregiving
Live, adaptive, sensitive maternal, family, and caregiver voices at moderate sound levels	Potentially beneficial in any behavioral state
Skin-to-skin holding with moderate-level voice sounds – mother and family	Potentially beneficial in any behavioral state

Accuracy of the Equipment Some studies are flawed by the use of inexpensive sound level meters (SLMs) with microphones that collect only a narrow range of frequencies leaving much of the sound unmeasured. One might say that if an intervention or study is worth doing, it is worth having the equipment necessary to do it right. Type II is a designation for a very accurate microphone. Such a microphone is necessary for a valid study or clinical intervention. Type I is a designation for a microphone of extremely fine accuracy of the type needed for measuring the acoustic environments of some scientific equipment. These microphones are unnecessarily sensitive, and expensive, for the more gross measurement of room acoustics. Methods sections of studies and clinical manuals should specify the type of microphone used to ensure that a quality Type II (or Type I) microphone and not an inaccurate toy-type or subprofessional microphone is being used.

Sound Level Measurements The Recommended Standards for Newborn ICU Design *are not intended* to apply to all conditions but only to the design of NICUs (White, Smith, & Shepley, 2013). They are based on studies of the wake-up thresholds of multiple *term* infants (Philbin, Robertson, & Hall, 1999) not to perceptions of individual preterm infants that are best determined by the infant's behavior.

The sound equivalent level (L_{eq}) is a measure of central tendency. It gives a general picture of the sound levels (perceived as loudness or quietness) in a room over a given period of time. The standards (White et al., 2013) define an appropriate L_{eq} for the design of a NICU infant room as 45 dBA *over 1 h*. The Recommended Standards are not particularly useful in evaluating specific sound levels as they affect a specific listener, adult, or infant, at a specific time because they are intended for evaluating general room conditions occurring over an entire given period. For example, an hour is too long to be relevant to conditions during live interventions and some clinical studies.

The level exceeded 10% of the time (L_{10}) indicates the irregular, individual levels higher than 90% of other levels over a given period of time. It is an indicator of the general range of relatively loud sounds. An L_{10} almost never occurs over a sustained length of time in a NICU and is 50 dBA over an hour in the Recommended Standards. These sounds would affect individuals; their sources are worth identifying and eliminating or reducing if the goal is to decrease the L_{eq} and other levels.

Unlike the other two amalgamated levels, L_{max} describes the one highest *individual* sound occurring in a given period of time and lasting 1/20th of a second, a time period easily perceived by humans. There are usually a number of levels close to this one indicator as readily seen on the graphs of time periods of, for example, 1 min, produced by professional grade, Type II dosimeter SLMs. L_{max} is absorbed in L_{eq}, making L_{eq} an inappropriate measurement of individual, annoying, and distracting sounds. If the environment is perceived as noisy despite the L_{eq} and L_{10} being within limits, the sources of L_{max}, individual, sounds are worth locating and eliminating. Human is generally a good detector of these sound sources.

Other Sound Levels of Interest: L_{90} and L_{pk}   The standards are focused on designing against high sound levels. However, the level of quiet is another measure important to research and clinical intervention (Philbin & Gray, 2001). This can be measured as L_{90}, the level exceeded 90% of the time. Old crowded NICUs often have a small difference between the noise floor (e.g., L_{90}) and the L_{eq}; there may never be moments of quiet. Alternatively, a more quiet NICU room could have only a somewhat lower L_{eq} but a much lower L_{90}. In other words, the spread between loud and quiet could be wider, but that reality is hidden in the L_{eq}. A lower L_{90} would indicate a lower noise floor and many episodes of relative quiet. Interesting quality improvement projects can be devised to lower the L_{90}.

Some studies report the *peak level* (L_{pk}), a technical term for the highest individual sound level during a specific period of time. Graphs produced by dosimeter SLMs can include L_{pk}s, and their high levels look dramatic. However, these are instantaneous measurements and may not last long enough to be perceptible. They are not appropriate to descriptions of sound level in a NICU room or available to a particular listener. L_{pk} is available on a SLM for the purpose of protecting delicate instruments sensitive to high-level sounds such as would affect an electron microscope. They are also useful in heavy industry where many brief and high-level sounds could affect hearing acuity (National Institute of Occupational Safety and Health – NIOSH, 2016a, 2016b). No known NICU can produce sounds that reduce hearing acuity, and reporting them in studies of the NICU environment misrepresents the conditions in the room.

The Error of Averaging Sound Level Measurements   A common error in the literature and in practice is to interpret a series of sound level measurements as a mathematical average. However, sound levels are logarithmic measurements; the numbers are multiples of each other. For example, 60 dBA is perceived as twice as loud as 53 or 50 dbA. Mathematical averages of several L_{eq} measurements will always underestimate actual conditions (i.e., indicate the space to be more quiet than it actually is). To arrive at the L_{eq}, a SLM performs complex calculations to equally distribute the energy reflected in the measurements over the specified time period. Therefore, to avoid confusion and misrepresentation of conditions, the L_{eq} should not be thought of, referred to, or summarized as an average. The *range* of L_{eq} measurements taken at the times of interest can serve as a correct representation of the central tendency of room conditions.

Determining Sound Levels for Live and Recorded Speech and Music In order to avoid masking recorded and live music, it must be played at a level perceptible to the infant. Keeping the signal below or at the L_{eq} or L_{10} limits in the standards may make it unintelligible to an infant and conceal positive findings, as may have happened in the study by Dearn and Shoemark (2014). The most appropriate limits for added stimuli should be based on an accurate, sensitive observation of the infant's behavior. This might be done using behavioral observations such as those in the Newborn Individualized Developmental Care and Assessment Program (NIDCAP) (Als & McAnulty, 2014). If one is determined to use the standards for research and clinical purposes, levels of a song or mother's speech might be above L_{10}, (50 dBA in the Recommended Standards), but not above L_{max} (65 dBA in the Recommended Standards).

Location of the Microphone: Sound Levels and Distance Between the SLM Microphone and Listener Some measurements in published studies place the microphone in the center of the room or at an unspecified distance from the infant listener and proceed as if these are the levels at the infant's ear (e.g., Lahav, 2015). However, sound levels increase or decrease over distance, and the change is not linear but geometric. In an open field, sound is reduced by ~6 dB with every doubling of distance from the microphone (e.g., 1 m, 2 m, 4 m, 8 m, etc.) and, conversely, increases ~6 dB every halving of distance (e.g., 64 m, 32 m, 16 m, 8 m, etc.) as it is brought closer to the sound source. The increased decrement in an old-style, crowded NICU with hard, reverberant surfaces varies from this relationship because sound is produced in many places and the room is reverberant; it is not a single sound source in an open field. In such an environment, sound levels and frequencies are best measured close to the infant but not so close as to bump the microphone with normal care activities. In sum, if levels are not measured at a specific distance from the infant, in a room of specific reverberation qualities, the measurements will be uninterpretable.

For example, consider a new NICU with widely spaced beds or single rooms and ample sound absorbent surface materials (i.e., without significant reflections; close to free field conditions). If a L_{eq} of 70 dBA is measured 16 m from a specific infant (e.g., in the center of the room), the level would be about 64 dBA at 8 m (less than L_{max} in the standards), 58 dBA at 4 m, 52 dBA at 2 m, 46 dB at 1 m (less than L_{10} in the Standards), 40 dB at 0.5 m (L_{eq} in the Standards), and 34 dBA at 0.25 m; below most background sounds of the heating, ventilation, and air conditioning (HVAC) system; and probably not perceptible to many preterm infants, depending on the characteristics of the sound. In other words, the center-room level of 70 dB is 34 dBA or less near the infant, depending on how close to the ear the microphone is placed.

SLM instruction manuals can be misleading for NICU room measurements because they are typically written for industry conditions. In industry, measurements are often taken in the center of the room because the point is to safeguard hearing from damage by high, sustained sound levels. Sound conditions at the sound sources may overrepresent the sounds at the workers' ears. Surfaces tend to be hard and reverberant in these conditions and approximately the same throughout the space. These spaces are not relevant to any known NICU or to home conditions.

Placement of the SLM Microphone Many studies and clinical interventions are flawed by placement of the microphone on padding laid atop the infant's bed mattress. A Type I or Type II microphone is designed to collect sound waves from all directions. In a room it should be dangled at least 3 feet from a large reflective surface such as a wall or tall cabinet to avoid including reflections. It should not be suspended beneath an air-handling register to avoid overrepresenting HVAC noise. In an incubator the cable can be taped to the center of the inside top of the shell. Because of the small size of the infant compartment and its reverberant character, sound levels are virtually the same everywhere in an incubator, and there is no need to place the microphone near the infant's head or to use two speakers for delivering sound. In any case the features of stereophonic sound are lost in the reverberant incubator shell.

While the microphone cannot be washed, the high-grade stainless steel of the exterior can be wiped clean with a near-dry alcohol pad. The soft microphone cover is not needed in these conditions if the operators are careful to not bump it and cannot be cleaned effectively for infection control purposes. The operating instructions of the equipment usually specify methods of cleaning.

Summary and Conclusions

Animal models of the development of fetal and newborn sound perception and behavioral responses provide useful information impossible to obtain through direct study of the human. Such studies add knowledge regarding the perceptions of level, frequency, and other characteristics of sound that develop gradually during gestation and infancy. However, the perception of signal in noise is not completely developed until late childhood or early adolescence.

Sounds in the pregnant uterus are of low frequency and low level but nonetheless varied and detectable by the fetus. Sounds received at the fetal cochlea are lower than in the uterus itself. Intrauterine sounds form a mixed ambient background of eating, gastrointestinal activity, breathing, and moderately loud external sounds, including voices. Heartbeat sounds are detected occasionally but are no more distinct than other internal sounds. In some studies they are not detected at all by sensitive intrauterine hydrophones. However, the mother's voice is easily detected by the infant due to its consistent prosody and the relative loudness of the higher frequencies.

It is important to protect fetal hearing by avoiding high-level vibroacoustic stimulation in the workplace, entertainment, and sport and by coupling recorded sounds to the mother's body via speakers attached to the belly or inserted in the vagina. Current, incomplete knowledge suggests caution regarding frequent exposure of the fetus to assessment techniques such as vibroacoustic stimulation.

The ambient sound levels of older-design, highly reverberant NICUs are overstimulating for the preterm infant and interfere with detecting the maternal voice. New-design NICUs, including single-room units, may produce annoying, distracting, and overstimulating brief sounds if the surfaces are hard and reflective even though the ambient sound level (L_{eq}) may be within the limits of the Recommended Standards for Newborn ICU Design. Given the myriad, strong stimuli of all sensory systems experienced by the preterm infant, "sound deprivation" in a new or single-room NICU may be a misnomer. The amount of sound necessary for the development of hearing, other sensory systems, language, and organized neurobehavioral responsiveness is not known. The most likely sound experiences eliciting attention and recognition are those of the mother and family members during skin-to-skin holding. As described in classic and contemporary research, native (not managed) sounds specific to the family are the scaffold upon which future language and social competence build.

Acknowledgements The author thanks Jack B. Evans, P. E., for guidance regarding the acoustic environment and sound level measurement.

Key Messages

- The fetus typically lives in a low sound level (perceived as quiet) environment in which mother's voice is a prominent signal but heartbeat sounds are not.
- Although the ambient sound equivalent level (L_{eq}) of a NICU room may be low and hard, reverberant room surfaces can produce startling, distracting, and annoying individual sounds. These are best measured over brief time periods such as L_{max}.
- Given the numerous strong and disorganizing multisensory experiences of intensive care, "sound deprivation" may be a misnomer if some responsive, live speech and singing are available, particularly, during skin-to-skin holding.
- Natural conversation and singing by family members expose infants to the scaffold on which language acquisition is built.

References

Abrams, R. M., & Gerhardt, K. J. (2000). The acoustic environment and physiological responses of the fetus. *Journal of Perinatology, 20*(8 part 2), S31–S36. doi:10.1038/sp.jp.7200445

Abrams, R. M., Hutchinson, A. A., Gerhardt, K. J., Evans, S. L., & Pendergast, J. (1987). Local cerebral glucost utilization in fetal sheep exposed to noise. *American Journal of Obstetrics and Gynecology, 157*(2), 456–460.

Als, H., Butler, S., & McAnulty, G. (2005). Assessment of preterm infants' behavior (APIB): Furthering the understanding and measurement of neurodevelopmental competence in preterm and full-term infants. *Mental Retardation and Developmental Disabilities Research Reviews, 11*, 94–102.

Als, H., & McAnulty, G. B. (2014). Newborn individualized developmental care and assessment program with Kangaroo Mother Care (KMC): Comprehensive care for preterm infants. *Current Womans Health Review, 7*(3), 288–301. doi:10.2174/157340411796355216

Appler, J. M., & Goodrich, L. V. (2011). Connecting the ear to the brain: Molecular mechanisms and the auditory circuit assembly. *Progress in Neurobiology, 93*, 488–508. doi:10.1016/j-pneurobio.2011.01.004

Armitage, S. E., Baldwin, B. A., & Vince, M. A. (1980). The fetal sound environment of sheep. *Science, 208*(4448), 1173–1174. www.ncbi.nim.nih.gov/pubmed/7375927

Babypod. www.Babypod.net/en/babypod/. Accessed October 21, 2016.

Bench, J. R. (1968). Sound transmission to the human foetus through the maternal abdominal wall. *Journal of Genetic Psychology, 113*, 85–87.

Brazelton, T.B., Nugent J.K., Lester B.M., Osofsky, J.D. (Ed). (1987). Neonatal behavioral assessment scale. Handbook of infant development, 2nd ed., (pp. 780–817). Oxford, England: Wiley., xix, 1391 pp.

Chang, E. F., & Merzenich, M. M. (2003). Environmental noise retards auditory cortical development. *Science, 300*(5618), 498–502.

Dearn, T., & Shoemark, H. (2014). The effect of maternal presence on premature infant response to recorded music. *Journal of Obstetric, Gynecologic, and Neonatal Nursing, 43*, 341–350. doi:10.1111/1552-6909.12303

DeCasper, A. J., Fifer, W. P. 1980 Of human bonding: Newborns prefer their mothers' voices. *Science.* 208(4448). 1174–1176. New Series.

DeCasper, A. J., & Prescott, P. (1984). Lateralized processes constrain auditory reinforcement in human newborns. *Hearing Research, 255*, 135–141.

DeCasper, A. J., & Singafoos, A. D. (1983). Intrauterine heartbeat: A potent reinforcer for newborns. *Infant Behavior & Development, 6*, 19–25.

Doheny, L., Hurwitz, S., Insoft, R., Ringer, S., & Lahav, A. (2012). Exposure to biological maternal sounds improves cardiorespiratory regulation in extremely premature infants. *The Journal of Fetal and Neonatal Medicine, 25*(9), 1591–1594. doi:10.3109/14767058.2011.648237

Gagnon, R. (1989). Stimulation of human fetuses with sound and vibration. *Seminars in Perinatology, 13*, 393–402.

Gerhardt, K. J., & Abrams, R. M. (2000). Fetal exposures to sound and vibroacoustic stimulation. *Journal of Perinatology, 20*(8 Pt 2), S21–S30. www.ncbi.nlm.nih.gov/.../11190697

Gerhardt, K. J., Otto, R., Abrams, R. M., Colle, J. J., Burchfield, D. J., & Peters, A. J. M. (1992). Cochlear microphonics recorded from fetal and newborn sheep. *American Journal of Otolaryngology, 13*(4), 226–233.

Gray, L. (1991). Development of a frequency dimension in chickens (Gallus gallus). *Journal of Comparative Psychology, 105*(1), 85–88.

Gray, L. C. (2000). Properties of sound. *Journal of Perinatology, 20*(8 part 2), S6–S11.

Gray, L. C., & Philbin, M. K. (2000). Measuring sound in hospital nurseries. *Journal of Perinatology, 20*(8 part 2), 100–104.

Gray, L. C., & Philbin, M. K. (2004). Effects of the neonatal intensive care unit on auditory attention and distraction. *Clinics in Perinatology, 31*, 243–260. doi:10.1016/j.clp.2004.04.013

Griffiths, S. K., Brown, W. S., Gerhardt, K. J., Abrams, R. M., & Morris, J. R. (1994). The perception of speech sounds recorded within the uterus of a pregnant sheep. *The Journal of the Acoustical Society of America, 96*, 2055–2063.

Grimwade, J. C., Walker, D. W., & Wood, C. (1970). Sensory stimulation of the human fetus. *Australian Journal of Mental Retardation, 2*, 63–64.

Harshaw, C., & Lickliter, R. (2011). Biased embryos: Prenatal experience and the malleability of species-typical auditory preferences. *Developmental Psychobiology, 53*, 291–302.

Hess, E. H. (1959). Imprinting. *Science, 130*, 133–141.

Kuhn, T. S. (2012) The structure of scientific revolutions: 50th anniversary edition. 4th ed. Chicago, IL: University of Chicago Press. 264. ISBN – 13 978-0226458083.

Lahav, A. (2015). Questionable sound exposure outside the womb: Frequency analysis of environmental noise in the intensive care unit. *Acta Pædiatrica, 104*(1), e14–e19. doi:10.1111/apa 12816 Epub 2014 Oct 27

Lahav, A., & Skoe, E. (2014). An acoustic gap between the NICU and womb: A potential risk for compromised neuroplasticity of the auditory system in preterm infants. *Frontiers in Neuroscience, 8*(381), 1–7. doi:10.3389/fnins.2014.00381

Lester, B.M., Tronick, E.Z., Brazelton, T.B. (2004) The neonatal intensive care unit network neurobehavioral scale procedures. Pediatrics. 113(3 Pt. 2), 641-667. PMID: 14993524.

Lickliter, R., & Bahrick, L. E. (2000). The development of intersensory perception: Advantages of a comparative, convergent operations approach. *Psychology Bulletin, 126*, 260–280.

McMahon, E., Wintermark, P., & Lahav, A. (2012). Auditory brain development in premature infants: The importance of early experience. *Annals of the New York Academy of Sciences, 1252*, 17–24. doi:10.1111/j.1749-6632.2012.0645.X

Moltz, H. (1960). Imprinting: Empirical basis and theoretical significance. *Psychological Bulletin, 57*, 291–314.

Moon, C., Lagercrantz, H., & Kuhl, P. K. (2013). Language experienced *in utero* affects vowel perception after birth: A two-country study. *Acta Pediatrica, 102*, 156–160.

National Institute for Occupational Safety and Health. Reproductive health and the workplace. www.cdc.gov/niosh/docs/99-104/pdfs/99-104.pdf. Accessed October 10, 2016a.

National Institute for Occupational Safety and Health. Workplace safety and health topics > Noise and hearing loss prevention > Publications and tools > Sound meter. URL: www.cdc.gov/niosh /.../noisemeter. Accessed October 10, 2016b.

Panagiotidis, J., & Lahav, A. (2010). Simulation of prenatal maternal sounds in NICU incubators: A pilot safety and feasibility study. *The Journal of Maternal-Fetal and Neonatal Medicine, 23*(S3), 106–109. doi:10.3109/14767058 2010. 512185

Philbin, M. K., Ballweg, D. D., & Gray, L. (1994). The effect of an intensive care unit sound environment on the development of habituation in healthy avian neonates. *Developmental Psychobiology, 27*, 11–21.

Philbin, M. K., & Gray, L. (2001). Changing levels of quiet in an intensive care nursery. *Journal of Perinatology, 22*, 455–460.

Philbin, M. K., Lickliter, R., & Graven, S. N. (2000). Sensory experience and the developing organism: A history of ideas and view to the future. *Journal of Perinatology, 20*, S2–S5.

Philbin, M. K., Robertson, A. F., & Hall, J. W., III. (1999). Recommended permissible noise criteria for occupied, newly constructed or renovated hospital nurseries. *Journal of Perinatology, 19*, 559–563.

Philbin, M. K., Taber, K. H., & Hayman, L. A. (1996). Preliminary report: Changes in vital signs of term newborns during magnetic resonance imaging. *American Journal of Neuroradiology, 17*, 1033–1036.

Querleu, D., Verspy, X. R., & Vervoort, P. (1988). La transmission intra-amniotique des voix humaines. Review. *Francais Gynécologie and Obstétrics, 83*(1), 43–50.

Rabinowitz, N. C., Willmore, B. D., Schnupp, J. W., & King, A. J. (2011). Contrast gain in auditory cortex. *Neuron, 70*, 1178–1191. doi:10.1016/j. Neuron 2011.04.030

Rand, K., Lahav, A. (2014) Impact of the NICU environment on language deprivation in preterm infants. Acta Pædiatrica. 10(3):243–248. doi 10.1111/apa-12481 Epub 2013 Nov 23 PMID 24164604

Richards, D. S., Frentzen, B., Gerhardt, K. J., McCann, M. E., & Abrams, R. A. (1992). Sound levels in the human uterus. *Obstetrics and Gynecology, 89*(2), 186–190.

Rubel, E. W., Lippe, W. R., & Ryals, B. M. (1984). Development of the place principle. *The Annals of Otology, Rhinology, and Laryngology, 93*(6), 609–615.

Salk, L. (1960). The effects of the normal heartbeat sound on the behavior of the newborn infant; implications for mental health. *World Mental Health, 12*, 168–175.

Salk, L. (1962, April) Mother's heartbeat as an imprinting stimulus. *Transactions of the New York Academy of Sciences, 10*, 753–763. PMID: 13991116.

Shahidullah, S., & Hepper, P. G. (1994). Frequency discrimination by the fetus. *Early Human Development, 36,* 13–26.

Smith, S. W. (2013). Scientist and Engineer's guide to digital signal processing (p. 640). New York:Springer. ISBN-13:978-0966017632. ISBN-10:09660117633.

Spence, M., & DeCasper, A. (1987). Prenatal experience with low-frequency maternal-voice sounds influence perception of maternal voice samples. *Infant Behavior & Development, 16,* 133–142.

Ullal-Gupta, S., Van den Bosch der Nederlanden, C. M., Tichko, P., Lahav, A., & Hannon, E. E. (2013). Linking prenatal experience to the emerging musical mind. *Frontiers in Systems Neuroscience, 7,* 48. doi:10.3389/fnsys.2013.00048

White, J. D., Smith, J. A., & Shepley, M. M. (2013). Recommended standards for newborn ICU design. *Journal of Perinatology, 33,* S2–16. doi:10.1038/jp.2013.10

Chapter 7
The Auditory Sensitivity of Preterm Infants Toward Their Atypical Auditory Environment in the NICU and Their Attraction to Human Voices

Pierre Kuhn, André Dufour, and Claire Zores

Abstract *Introduction*: Vulnerable preterm infants (PIs) hospitalized in neonatal intensive care units (NICUs) are exposed to environmental stimuli that differ from the stimuli fetuses encounter in utero. Their auditory environment, in particular, is atypical. This new sensory "milieu" may interfere with their neurodevelopment. *Aims*: This review briefly summarizes the anatomical and functional development of the auditory system. We describe the abilities of preterm infants to perceive sounds emerging from background noise, based on studies appropriately designed to assess their auditory sensitivity to the NICU sound environment. *Conclusions*: Neurophysiological and neuroimaging studies, as well as specific auditory tests, demonstrated the anatomical and functional development of the auditory system of PIs. These infants showed fine auditory capabilities before term-equivalent age. PIs in the NICU react physiologically and behaviorally to sounds exceeding 70 dBA and are able to detect and discriminate among sounds emerging from background noise at a minimum signal-to-noise ratio of 5–10 dBA. PI responses to sound depend on sound source and frequency, as well as on sound pressure levels. Loud, high-frequency, and artificial NICU sounds may alter their well-being and disrupt their sleep. Vocal sounds seem to elicit a different pattern of responses. PIs seem particularly sensitive to the biologically meaningful and attractive sounds of their mothers' voices.

P. Kuhn (✉) • C. Zores
Médecine et Réanimation du Nouveau-né Hôpital de Hautepierre, CHU,
Strasbourg, France

Laboratoire de Neurosciences Cognitives et Adaptatives,
CNRS-Université de Strasbourg, Strasbourg, France
e-mail: pierre.kuhn@chru-strasbourg.fr

A. Dufour
Laboratoire de Neurosciences Cognitives et Adaptatives,
CNRS-Université de Strasbourg, Strasbourg, France

© Springer International Publishing AG 2017
M. Filippa et al. (eds.), *Early Vocal Contact and Preterm Infant Brain Development*, DOI 10.1007/978-3-319-65077-7_7

The ability of PIs' perceptual experience of NICU sound ecology to shape their long-term neurodevelopment has not yet been determined, although associations between their early auditory experience and later ability to communicate have been observed.

Introduction

Despite medical advances, preterm infants (PIs), especially very and extremely PIs, hospitalized in neonatal intensive care units (NICUs) remain at risk of neurodevelopmental impairment. In addition to being at risk for cognitive disorders (Larroque et al., 2008; Marlow, Wolke, Bracewell, Samara, & Group, 2005; Moore et al., 2012), they are at risk for delays in language development (van Noort-van der Spek, Franken, & Weisglas-Kuperus, 2012) and for psychiatric disorders. Although many medical factors account for this higher risk of neurodevelopmental sequelae, environmental factors during critical periods of brain development are also involved (Lagercrantz, 2010). Epigenetic factors are apparently involved in this "environmental shaping of the developing brain" during sensitive periods (see Chap. 16 by Montirosso et al.), as are synaptogenesis and selective elimination of synapses during early stages of brain development (Knudsen, 2004). The postnatal environment of PIs in the NICU differs markedly, in different modalities (Carbajal et al., 2008; Kuhn, Astruc, Messer, & Marlier, 2011), from the environment they should have continued to encounter in utero. This new "naturalistic milieu" exposes PIs to excessive sensory stimulation as well as to sensory deprivation that can alter their well-being and may interfere with their neurodevelopment and growth (Anand & Scalzo, 2000; Philbin, Lickliter, & Graven, 2000). As described in Chap. 6, the acoustic environment in the NICU appears particularly deleterious, with high sound pressure levels and high-pitched sounds occurring frequently. This loud, unorganized, and unpredictable noise can contribute to the neurocognitive burden of preterm birth and may lead to attention deficit disorders (Gray & Philbin, 2004) and/or alterations in early communicative skills (see Chap. 10 by Filippa and Kuhn).

These findings have led to the design of developmental care strategies aimed at adapting the sensory experiences of PIs in the NICU to their sensory expectations and capabilities (Als et al., 2004). Guidelines for permissible noise levels in the NICU have been established to improve the acoustic environment of PIs. These recommendations were designed primarily to reduce the exposure of PIs to noise, thereby reducing the deleterious effects of noise on their developing auditory systems and well-being (Philbin, Robertson, & Hall, 2008; White, Smith, Shepley, & Committee to Establish Recommended Standards for Newborn, 2013). Moreover, these guidelines are important in enhancing the access of PIs to the voices of their own mothers, a stimulus found to be biologically meaningful. To date, however, few studies have evaluated the auditory sensitivity of PIs to the auditory environment of their NICUs.

In analyzing the impact of early auditory contact of PIs with their own mothers' voices, it is crucial to determine the abilities of PIs to perceive the acoustic environment of their NICUs and to analyze the main determinants of PI perception of sounds. To provide further insight into the results of studies evaluating the responses of PIs to their auditory milieu, it is important to first summarize the main stages of the anatomical and functional development of the auditory system in the context of preterm birth. Indeed, the effects of noise on the auditory system and hearing function of neonates depend on maturational factors. Finally, knowledge about the sensitivity of PIs to their auditory hospital environment is essential to guide the implementation of evidence-based strategies/interventions for auditory nurturance in the NICU. It is a prerequisite to better adapt the acoustic environment of PIs to their sensory abilities and preferences.

Auditory Development in Preterm Infants

Although the peripheral and central auditory systems develop concomitantly, it is important to describe each separately.

Development of the Outer, Middle, and Inner Ear

The anatomical structures of the outer and middle ears can first be identified during weeks 5–6 of gestation. The initial development of the external auditory system results in many acoustic consequences:

– Increased conductance of high-pitched sounds, which reach the middle ear at higher amplitudes in newborns than in adults
– Attenuation of the sound propagation during the first days of life, caused by the obstruction of the external auditory meatus in preterm and full-term newborns
– Reduced transmission of sounds at all frequencies, especially low frequencies, due to the immaturity of the middle ear ossicles and the musculo-ligamentary system, altering the acoustic properties of the middle ear

Moreover, the anatomical development of the outer and middle ear is associated with an amplification of high-frequency sounds and an attenuation of low-frequency sounds transmitted by air when compared with similar sounds in adults.

In the inner ear, the structure of the cochlea is mature enough to enable it to start functioning as early as 20 weeks of gestation (Pujol, Blatrix, Le Merre, Pujol, & Chaix, 2009; Werner, 2004). Maturation of both the inner and outer hair cells of the cochlea, however, is not complete until week 22 of gestation, when synapses are established with the auditory nerve. The end of cochlear development, occurring during weeks 30–35 of gestation, is essential for normal auditory sensitivity and good pitch perception and frequency resolution (Hall, 2000). The hair cells are organized tonotopically. There seems to be a conflict between the anatomical maturation of the cochlea, which occurs from the base (mainly sensitive to high-frequency sounds) to the apex (mainly sensitive to low-frequency sounds), and its observed functional maturation. In fetuses, which are protected from exposure to high-frequency sounds by the uterine and abdominal walls, the initial responses are limited to low–middle-frequency sounds, with the frequencies that trigger responses expanding gradually over time (Hall, 2000; Hepper & Shahidullah, 1994; Werner, 2004). However, earlier exposure of very PIs to high-frequency sounds in the NICU may disrupt the normal tonotopic tuning of hair cells and alter the later development of the auditory system (Lahav, 2015).

Ontogeny of the Central Auditory Circuits

The development of the central auditory pathways follows the general development of the brain. At the time of onset of cochlear responses to sounds, responses can be recorded until the primary auditory cortex (Rotteveel, Colon, Stegeman, & Visco, 1987a, 1987b; Rotteveel, de Graaf, Colon, Stegeman, & Visco, 1987; Rotteveel, de Graaf, Stegeman, Colon, & Visco, 1987; Rotteveel, Stegeman, de Graaf, Colon, & Visco, 1987). Neuronal migration begins in the brain stem at the end of the second month of gestation and continues in the cerebral cortex after birth. Synaptogenesis and the elaboration of pre- and postsynaptic circuits in the primary auditory cortex are intense as early as week 28 of gestation and continue during the first years of life. Myelination proceeds from the periphery to the center, with the roots of the auditory nerve being completely myelinated at 24–26 weeks of gestation and the entire auditory pathway being completely myelinated at age of 2 years.

Evaluation of the anatomical maturation of the central circuits relies mainly on functional assays using various neurophysiological approaches. For example, perceptual thresholds at the level of the brain stem can be assessed by measuring auditory brain stem responses (ABRs). Although ABR thresholds at frequencies around 500 Hz are similar in full-term newborns and adults, ABR thresholds at frequencies higher than 4000 Hz are 20–25 dB higher in infants than in adults (Sininger, Abdala, & Cone-Wesson, 1997). The cortical event-related potentials evaluating the responses to middle and long latencies indicate that the maturation of the central auditory pathways starts from the thalamus.

Development of Auditory Function

Studies using otoacoustic emission and ABR techniques to evaluate the anatomical and functional development of the auditory system in PIs have shown that the auditory system is functionally mature at post-menstrual ages (PMAs) of 28–30 weeks (Lary, Briassoulis, de Vries, Dubowitz, & Dubowitz, 1985; Ponton, Moore, &

Eggermont, 1996). Otoacoustic emission, a measure of cochlear function, has been observed as early as PMA 30 weeks and in all newborns at PMA 33 weeks (Morlet et al., 1995). At this age, the thresholds are 10–15 decibels slow response A (dBA) higher than in adults, with amplitudes increasing from 30 to 40 weeks of gestational age (GA). These thresholds for middle frequencies appear at around GA 28 weeks and expand to low (<1000 Hz) and high (up to 6000 Hz) frequencies in full-term newborns (Chabert et al., 2006).

Auditory event-related potentials (AERP) evaluate the global functioning of the auditory pathway, as well as the function from each effector until the cortex. Early AERPs have been recorded in PIs regularly, beginning at GA 28 weeks (Rotteveel et al., 1987b), with thresholds decrease as age increases (Lary et al., 1985).

Taken together, these findings indicate that the auditory system in PIs develops anatomically and functionally long before term-equivalent age enabling PIs to perceive their near auditory environment, and it is the case for other components of their sensory environment (Kuhn, Zores, Astruc, Dufour, & Casper, 2011).

Assessing Responses of Preterm Infants to Auditory Stimuli

The challenges associated with evaluating the perceptual auditory abilities of non-verbal individuals, including PIs, are similar to those associated with determining pain perception and nociception (Slater, Fitzgerald, & Meek, 2007). The ability to perceive a stimulus can be determined by assessing physiologic autonomic responses originating in the brain stem and behavioral responses, including complex mixtures of brain integration and motor responses or changes in arousal/sleep state. Highly integrated perception indicates cortical integration of a stimulus in areas of the brain involved in sensory processing. These responses can be evaluated by measuring electrical brain activity (neurophysiological recordings) and/or hemodynamic responses, using modalities such as functional magnetic resonance imaging (fMRI) and functional near-infrared spectroscopy (fNIRS). These tools differ in invasiveness and practicability but are complementary in providing a broad view of auditory sensitivity. The auditory perceptual competences of PIs can be assessed by determining their ability to detect changes in sound pressure levels, to discriminate human speech sounds from artificial (i.e., non-biological) environmental noise, and to perceive their mothers' voices.

Auditory Sensitivity to Changes in Sound Pressure Levels

Since the first demonstration that noise affects the health of hospitalized PIs (Long, Lucey, & Philip, 1980), many studies have assessed the effects of noise on these infants. Unfortunately, most of these studies used experimental designs rather than evaluating the effects of noise in the NICU. In several of these studies, preterm newborns were exposed to 5 s of high-intensity artificial sound (Field, Dempsey, Hatch, Ting, & Clifton, 1979; Vranekovic, Hock, Isaac, & Cordero, 1974; Wharrad & Davis, 1997), including sound pressure levels (SPL) of 90 dB (Field et al., 1979) and 80–100 dB (Wharrad & Davis, 1997) and to warbling tones of 100 dB (Vranekovic et al., 1974). The most frequent responses included an increase in heart rate (HR) proportional to the SPL of the stimulus (Field et al., 1979; Vranekovic et al., 1974; Wharrad & Davis, 1997) and a tendency toward a decrease in respiratory rate (RR) (Vranekovic et al., 1974). Although a few studies have evaluated the impact of NICU noise on newborns' behavioral and/or physiological stability, some of these assessed acoustic environments different from those in contemporary NICUs (Long et al., 1980) or did not include PIs (Trapanotto et al., 2004) or very PIs (Long et al., 1980). Together, these studies showed that environmental noise >70 dBA Leq could result in behavioral changes and disrupt physiological stability. However, the methodology of these studies partially limited the interpretation of their results. For example, they did not measure background noise levels and/or included a wide range of GAs, resulting in the absence of well-defined study populations (Philbin & Klaas, 2000a; Wachman & Lahav, 2011). Better designed studies performed during the last decade have explored the effect of NICU noise on PIs. For example, a study of eight extremely low birth weight infants found no correlation between moderate NICU noise levels (50–60 dBA) and arterial blood pressure, although HR changes started 25–45 s after noise peaks (Williams, Sanderson, Lai, Selwyn, & Lasky, 2009). Another study found that 11 very PIs exhibited sympathetic arousal, as measured by skin conductance, in response to natural sound >65 dBA and with background noise <55 dBA (Salavitabar et al., 2010). A detailed review of all these studies (Wachman & Lahav, 2011) concluded that loud transient noise has negative short-term effects on the cardiovascular and respiratory systems of PIs. These studies, however, did not fully determine the differential auditory SPL sensitivity (signal-to-noise ratio, SNR) or did not evaluate the precise effects of acoustic changes <70 dBA Leq of SPL on the well-being of very PIs.

In a prospective observational study, we systematically evaluated the physiologic responses (HR, RR, SaO_2, and changes in regional cerebral oxygenation, as assessed by near-infrared spectroscopy [NIRS]) and behavioral responses of 26 very PIs to sound peaks (SPs) emerging from background noise (Kuhn et al., 2012, 2013). Each infant was recorded for 10 h, during which a total of 598 isolated sound peaks occurred when the 26 PIs were in quiet and active sleep states (Prechtl, 1974). Of these sound peaks, 410, 137, and 51 were 5–10, 10–15, and >15 dBA, respectively, above the ambient noise. The median baseline SPLs before sound peaks for newborns breathing room air on nasal continuous airway pressure and on mechanical ventilation were 50.1 (range, 48.8–54.1), 59.3 (range, 54.1–61.3), and 50.4 (range, 48.4–53.7) dBA Leq, respectively. The artificial sound peaks had fundamental frequencies (F_0) ranging from 50 to 2730 Hz. Spectral analysis of some complex noises indicated that the frequencies of the first (F_1) and second (F_2) harmonics were of greater amplitude (see Table 7.1). These results were in accordance with other studies showing that PIs are exposed to a toxic sound environment with high-frequency

Table 7.1 Spectral analysis of main frequencies (F_0, F_1, F_2) of high amplitudes emitted by identified sound sources

Sound sources	First predominating amplitude (Hz)	Second predominating amplitude (Hz)
Motor incubator	100	50
Syringe pump alarm 1	456	1092
Syringe pump alarm 2	2270	4540
Syringe pump alarm 3	2730	5460
Humidifier alarm	4336	6504
Tc pCO$_2$ monitor alarm	2700	–
Monitor alarm	490	980
Ventilator alarm	2400	–
Incubator 1 alarm	420	1700
Incubator 2 alarm	2680	5350

Table 7.2 Mean maximum changes from baseline in physiological and cerebral parameters during the 40 s following sound peaks occurring during quiet and active sleep states according to SNR ranges

	Quiet sleep SNR: 5–10 dBA	Quiet sleep SNR: 10–15 dBA	Active sleep SNR: 5–10 dBA	Active sleep SNR: 10–15 dBA
HR (beats/min)	+4.6 (± 1.2)	−3.1 (± 0.8)	+3.1 (± 0.8)	+4.3 (± 1.6)
RR (cycles/min)	−8.8 (± 1.4)	−12.6 (± 3.2)	−4.6 (± 1)	−7.9 (± 1.9)
SaO$_2$ (%)	+0.8 (± 0.4)	−1.0 (± 0.4)	+0.6 (± 0.2)	−2.7 (± 0.7)
rSO$_2$ (%)	+0.9 (± 0.2)	+1.6 (± 0.5)	+0.6 (± 0.2)	−1.7 (± 0.4)

Results are expressed as mean ± standard error of the mean
Abbreviations: *HR* heart rate, *RR* respiratory rate, *SaO$_2$* blood oxygen saturation, *rSO$_2$* regional cerebral oxygen saturation, *SNR* signal-to-noise ratio

noises (Lahav & Skoe, 2014; Marik, Fuller, Levitov, & Moll, 2012), a finding also discussed in Chap. 6.

Significant physiological changes occurred following these sound peaks (Kuhn et al., 2012), indicating that very PIs can detect small changes in their acoustic environments, with a minimal SNR of 5–10 dBA. Exposure to 10–15 dBA sound peaks during active sleep significantly increased mean HR and decreased mean RR and mean systemic and regional cerebral oxygen saturation relative to baseline. The mean changes in physiological and cerebral oxygenation following sound peaks of 5–10 and 10–15 dBA are summarized in Table 7.2.

These moderate acoustic changes were also able to disrupt the sleep of PIs (Kuhn et al., 2013). The rate of awakenings following the sound peaks was significantly higher than the rate of spontaneous arousals during control periods without sound peaks. Awakenings from an active sleep state were observed following more than one third of exposures to sound peaks of SNR 5–10 dBA and around half of exposures to sound peaks of SNR 10–15 dBA.

The nature of these physiologic responses and their rapid onset indicate a reflexive reaction, mediated by the brain stem (Joseph, 2000) and a stress-mediated defensive response known for higher SPL stimuli (Lagercrantz, Edwards, Henderson-Smart, Hertzberg, & Jeffery, 1990; Salavitabar et al., 2010). The decreases in rSO_2 observed for the highest SPLs during active sleep may also be related to alterations in cerebral blood flow autoregulation. This stress reaction exceeding homeostatic regulatory mechanisms has not been observed for sound peaks of 5 dBA above ambient noise, especially when the infants were in the right lateral position, with a head elevation of 15° (Elser, Holditch-Davis, Levy, & Brandon, 2012). Noise-related awakenings are consistent with sleep disruptions related to hospital noises documented in adults, children, term newborns (Gadeke, Doring, Keller, & Vogel, 1969), and PIs (Zahr & Balian, 1995; Zahr & de Traversay, 1995). The association between sleep disruptions and SPL increments and the concomitant physiologic responses of very PIs to noises emphasizes the auditory sensitivity of these PIs to moderate acoustic changes occurring naturally in their new "ecological niche" in the NICU, in addition to showing that PIs are highly sensitive to environmental disturbances during active sleep.

Taken together, the abovementioned studies indicate that very PIs, from at least 28 weeks PMA, are able to detect increases in sound pressure levels in their nearby environment, with a minimal SNR threshold. NIRS showed cortical activation of a frontotemporal neural pathway in response to sound stimuli in preterm and term infants, of GA 28–41 weeks, indicating that PIs have the ability to integrate changes in sound pressure levels into their auditory brains (Zaramella et al., 2001). These findings indicate that PIs are at least minimally conscious of their environment (Lagercrantz & Changeux, 2009) and that these PIs may have the perceptual ability to extract auditory signals from background noise. Another study, which assessed more complex auditory tasks, evaluated developmental changes in masked thresholds in children, with the youngest being 6 months old, and showed that thresholds declined greatly with age (Schneider, Trehub, Morrongiello, & Thorpe, 1989). More comprehensive studies are required to better understand the ontogeny of this perceptual auditory capability of PIs in the NICU.

Responses According to Sound Sources: Human Voices Versus Artificial Noise

One question of particular interest is whether PIs can perceive human voices (HVs) in an environment of background noise. Sound stimuli in the NICU can arise from several sources, including:

- Artificial environmental noise (AEN), produced mainly by respiratory support equipment, monitoring devices, incubators, running water, and opening of sterile bags
- HVs, including vocal sounds made by medical and/or nursing staff, parents, and other visitors

Studies on noise exposure in the NICU have mainly focused on its loudness, measured on a logarithmic scale and expressed as SPL, or its frequency. Although some of these studies have fully described the nature of the sound sources (mainly noise produced by electrical devices, alarms, respiratory support device, and incubators), they have not examined the specific impact of each type of sound source on the responsiveness of PIs. One study, which evaluated PI responses to natural sound >65 dBA and with background noise <55 dBA in the NICU, described the source of each sound (voice or laughter vs alarm events) and the number of each type of event (Salavitabar et al., 2010). However, that study did not examine the specific reactions of PIs to these sounds. To fill this gap, we further analyzed our data (Kuhn et al., 2012, 2013). Concomitant recordings of the SPL and of the sounds through a microphone on the same time scale enabled further analysis of how the nature of each stimulus influenced the responses of newborns. Of the 430 sound peaks in the 5–10 SNR range occurring when the infants were asleep, 322 (74.9%) originated from AENs and 88 (20.5%) from HVs.

We systematically examined the differential responsiveness of very PIs to these two sources of sound peaks emerging from background noise. The physiological changes experienced by these PIs differed markedly depending on the sound sources, indicating different patterns of response (Fig. 7.1).

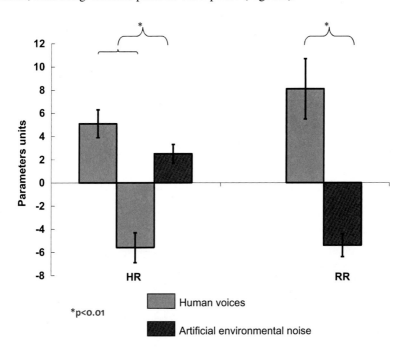

Fig. 7.1 Effects of sound sources on mean maximum variations in heart rate (HR) and respiratory rate (RR) from baseline during the 40 s following exposure to sound peaks 5–10 dBA above background noise, occurring in active sleep state.
HV human voice, *AEN* artificial environmental noise. Bars indicate standard errors, and HR is reported as beats/min and RR as breaths/min. *p value <0.001 between HV and AN sound peaks (Student's t-tests)

Very PIs differed in their physiologic responses to human speech and non-biological NICU sounds. In particular, HVs triggered a significant decrease in HR and a significant increase in RR, whereas AENs triggered a significant increase in HR and a decrease in RR. These opposite cardiorespiratory responses suggest that PIs can discriminate between these two sound sources.

Moreover, HVs had a less detrimental effect on sleep than AENs in the same SNR ranges. Changes in sleep/arousal states were analyzed using previously described methods (Kuhn et al., 2013). Evaluation of rates of sleep disruption during the 40 s following sound peaks showed that these rates differed depending on the sound source. An analysis of all sound peaks from all SNRs (5–10 and 10–15 dBA) occurring during active and quiet sleep states showed that the rate of awakening was significantly higher after sound peaks arising from AENs (36.6%; 95% confidence interval [CI], 28.3%–45.0%) than those arising from HVs (22.8%; 95% CI, 8.3%–37.3%) (Wilcoxon test, $Z_{[13]} = 1.99$, $p = 0.046$).

In summary, the physiologic and behavioral responses of PIs indicate that their well-being is altered mostly by non-biological environmental noise, which could also impede access to HVs. Besides this defensive reaction to AENs, we observed positive responses to HVs. According to the synactive theory of development of the NIDCAP program (Als, 1982), positive responses to HVs can be considered signs of approach. They have already been shown to be possibly triggered by vocal sounds (Philbin & Klaas, 2000b). The responses of PIs to HVs, including increases in RR and decreases in HR without any drop in cerebral oxygenation, suggest that PIs are attracted to these stimuli. The stimulating effects of hedonically positive stimuli on the respiration of PIs have been observed in tactile (Kattwinkel, Nearman, Fanaroff, Katona, & Klaus, 1975), auditory (Fifer & Moon, 1994), and olfactory (Marlier, Schaal, Gaugler, & Messer, 2001) sensory modalities. The reductions in HR are similar to the responses of the orienting cardiac reflex to novel stimuli and stimuli of particular interest (Sokolov, 1963, 1990; Vila et al., 2007) and observed in near-term fetuses exposed to vocal stimuli (Lecanuet, Granier-Deferre, Jacquet, & Busnel, 1992; Lecanuet, Graniere-Deferre, Jacquet, & DeCasper, 2000).

Human speech sounds are unique signals that are essential for the subsequent language development of newborns, especially those born preterm (Caskey, Stephens, Tucker, & Vohr, 2011, 2014). This very well-designed observational study demonstrated that greater exposure to human voices and adult words is correlated with early vocalizations of PIs at 32 and 36 weeks PMA, suggesting that these PIs are able to perceive these stimuli. Indeed, PIs appear able to integrate fine language differences at a cortical level. A functional optical imaging study showed that PIs could distinguish between two syllables ("ba" and "ga") and between two human voices (male and female), beginning at 29 weeks PMA (Mahmoudzadeh et al., 2013), indicating that their cortical circuits could process speech even at an immature stage with incomplete layers of cortical organization. This early ability to activate brain regions involved in linguistic processing can fully explain the different physiologic and behavioral responses PIs display to vocal and nonvocal sounds in the NICU.

Mother's Voice Perception by Preterm Infants

Among human voices, the maternal voice is the most prominent vocal stimulus accessed by full-term newborns. However, the degree of exposure of PIs to their own mothers' voices is highly dependent on implementation of family-centered and developmentally supportive care strategies. The specific preference of a term newborn for its own mother's voice has been well documented (DeCasper & Fifer, 1980). Shortly after birth, a term newborn can distinguish the familiar voice of its mother from that of a stranger (Beauchemin et al., 2011). That electrophysiological study also showed that this auditory processing takes place at both the preattentional and cortical levels.

Many studies have evaluated the benefit of the mother's voice for the well-being of a PI (recently reviewed in Filippa et al., 2017, *Acta Paediatrica*, in press). Most of these studies indicate that a PI can perceive his or her own mother's voice, speaking the mother's native language and using motherese speech, before term-corrected age. Most studies used recorded maternal voices as stimuli, with only a few evaluating the responses of PIs to direct talking or singing (see Chap. 10). As these studies are described elsewhere in this book, we will not further discuss them here. However, the physiologic and behavioral responses to both recorded and live voices indicate that PIs preferentially perceive their own mothers' voices. Despite the differences in recognition capabilities between very PIs and full-term newborns (Therien, Worwa, Mattia, & deRegnier, 2004), the ability to perceive his or her own mother's voice is evidenced in PIs at around 34 weeks of corrected age, based on studies using the mother's voice or sounds as an early intervention (Doheny, Hurwitz, Insoft, Ringer, & Lahav, 2012; Filippa, Devouche, Arioni, Imberty, & Gratier, 2013; Rand & Lahav, 2014). During their first week of life, PIs of PMA 30 ± 2.5 weeks have a lower HR after exposure to maternal sounds than after no exposure (Rand & Lahav, 2014), in agreement with the reduction in HR of fetuses of GA 32–37 weeks in response to the mother's voice (Kisilevsky & Hains, 2011). The specific auditory activation measured with fMRI in fetuses of GA 33 weeks following mother's voice exposure (Jardri et al., 2012) indicated a possible neural basis for this response. Differences in cortical activation were observed in the left and right frontal areas following exposure of PIs of mean GA 30.4 weeks (range, 24.5–35.6 weeks) and mean post-conceptional age of 35–38 weeks to the voices of their mothers and female nurses, suggesting that PIs of this age can discriminate their mothers' voices from the voices of other women (Saito, Fukuhara, Aoyama, & Toshima, 2009). All of these studies indicate that PIs can specifically perceive their mothers' voices prior to their term-corrected age. These PIs are also able to physiologically respond to their mothers' voices at 30 PMA weeks and to integrate these voices at a cortical level from 32 to 34 weeks PMA. Finally, repeated exposure to maternal sounds of PIs of mean GA 30 weeks (range, 25–32 weeks) during the first month of life may enhance the anatomical development of their primary auditory cortex, suggesting an adaptive and experience-dependent brain plasticity specific to maternal sounds (Webb, Heller, Benson, & Lahav, 2015).

Practical Implications

The implementation of efficient sound abatement measures is required to reduce sound pressure levels and to attenuate their variations near PIs in neonatal units. However, this noise-controlled environment should also provide and support continuous access of PIs to human voices, especially to familiar voices like those of their mothers. Eliminating iatrogenic environmental hazards in the NICU appears crucial to promoting positive health outcomes for PIs (Lai & Bearer, 2008). The differential auditory sensitivity of PIs to SPL increments provides evidence for the reinforcement of permissible noise criteria in the NICU and suggests that these recommendations should not only be expressed in terms of hourly Leq or Lmax. Recommendations are important but difficult to implement. Hence, most of the studies evaluating acoustic environments have shown that the recommended targeted SPLs are rarely met.

Various global approaches are available to support a nurturing auditory environment for PIs. These approaches rely first on a systematic evaluation of the acoustic environment and its main determinants in each NICU. Second, the architectural design of each NICU should favor the proximity of infant/parent dyads in the quieter environment of a single family room, as these rooms have been shown to provide long-term benefits to PIs (Lester et al., 2016). Third, the technical equipment in the NICU should be adjusted to the sensory abilities and expectancies of PIs (e.g., reduced sound pressure levels of alarms and limited high-frequency sounds). Fourth, adequate care is required to reduce iatrogenic noise hazards that interfere with sleep. These can include the implementation of a quiet hour (Slevin, Farrington, Duffy, Daly, & Murphy, 2000). The use of a noise sensor light alarm is efficient to sensitize medical and nursing teams and to reduce noise in the NICU (Chang, Pan, Lin, Chang, & Lin, 2006), but the effects of these alarms are transient without repeated and continuous educational programs (Degorre et al., 2017). The use of earplugs on PIs has been shown to reduce their level of exposure to sound pressure (Abou Turk, Williams, & Lasky, 2009). However, further evaluation is required, as earplugs can result in sensory deprivation. Noise protection is required during specific situations with a high risk of noise exposure (e.g., neonatal transport, MRI). Finally, skin-to-skin contact between the child and its mother/father can also enable vocal exposure of the PI and vocal interactions between the mother/father and infant. It should be promoted as it is the best strategy to limit the sensory discontinuity due to preterm birth. The primary recommendation measures are summarized in Fig. 7.2.

Conclusion

Very PIs are sensitive to their auditory environment. They have the capacity to perceive and respond to most of the auditory stimuli present in the NICU. Knowledge about these capabilities of hospitalized newborns should be used to provide them with adequate auditory environments. Future research is required to explore unresolved issues associated with the responses of premature newborns to the sound

Recommended Acoustic Environment

↓ Exposure to deleterous stimulations	↑ Exposure to the maternal/human voices
• Perform a NICU acoustic assessment to follow noise recommendations	• Provide Skin-to-Skin contact in a quiet environment
• Architecture (single family room)	• Parents as primary caregivers encouraged to talk to their infants
• Noise criteria for NICU material/device	
• Change team behaviors	• Direct talking and motherese language
• Auditory protection in special circumstances	

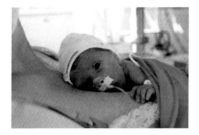

Fig. 7.2 Recommended strategies to provide a nurturing auditory environment for preterm infants

environment of the NICU. Studies in this field are difficult to perform, due to practical limitations and technical and methodological challenges. Studies are needed to evaluate the development of cortical integration of auditory stimuli (especially of familiar voices), to explore the emotional valence that PIs attribute to auditory stimuli and to determine the specific impact of high-frequency noise on the well-being of PIs. As early auditory experience can shape the development of auditory perception, the long-term consequences of auditory experience in early life should be determined further, as it is fundamental to providing more efficient and humane neonatal care.

Key Messages
- Preterm infants detect and discriminate sounds emerging from the background noise in the NICU environment at a minimal signal-to-noise ratio.
- Non-biological environmental NICU sounds can alter the physiological well-being and brain oxygenation of preterm infants and disrupt their sleep.
- Preterm infants display specific patterns of responses and attraction to human voices, especially their own mothers' voices.
- Gaps in knowledge provide opportunities for future research to better understand the development by preterm infants of their abilities to perceive their mothers' voices.

References

Abou Turk, C., Williams, A. L., & Lasky, R. E. (2009). A randomized clinical trial evaluating silicone earplugs for very low birth weight newborns in intensive care. *Journal of Perinatology, 29*(5), 358–363. doi:10.1038/jp.2008.236

Als, H. (1982). Toward a synactive theory of development: promise for the assessment and support of infant individuality. *Infant Mental Health Journal, 3*(4), 229–243.

Als, H., Duffy, F. H., McAnulty, G. B., Rivkin, M. J., Vajapeyam, S., Mulkern, R. V., ... Eichenwald, E. C. (2004). Early experience alters brain function and structure. *Pediatrics, 113*(4), 846–857.

Anand, K. J., & Scalzo, F. M. (2000). Can adverse neonatal experiences alter brain development and subsequent behavior? *Biology of the Neonate, 77*(2), 69–82.

Beauchemin, M., Gonzalez-Frankenberger, B., Tremblay, J., Vannasing, P., Martinez-Montes, E., Belin, P., ... Lassonde, M. (2011). Mother and stranger: An electrophysiological study of voice processing in newborns. *Cerebral Cortex, 21*(8), 1705–1711. doi:10.1093/cercor/bhq242

Carbajal, R., Rousset, A., Danan, C., Coquery, S., Nolent, P., Ducrocq, S., ... Breart, G. (2008). Epidemiology and treatment of painful procedures in neonates in intensive care units. *JAMA, 300*(1), 60–70.

Caskey, M., Stephens, B., Tucker, R., & Vohr, B. (2011). Importance of parent talk on the development of preterm infant vocalizations. *Pediatrics, 128*(5), 910–916. doi:10.1542/peds.2011-0609

Caskey, M., Stephens, B., Tucker, R., & Vohr, B. (2014). Adult talk in the NICU with preterm infants and developmental outcomes. *Pediatrics, 133*(3), e578–e584. doi:10.1542/peds.2013-0104

Chabert, R., Guitton, M. J., Amram, D., Uziel, A., Pujol, R., Lallemant, J. G., & Puel, J. L. (2006). Early maturation of evoked otoacoustic emissions and medial olivocochlear reflex in preterm neonates. *Pediatric Research, 59*(2), 305–308.

Chang, Y. J., Pan, Y. J., Lin, Y. J., Chang, Y. Z., & Lin, C. H. (2006). A noise-sensor light alarm reduces noise in the newborn intensive care unit. *American Journal of Perinatology, 23*(5), 265–271. doi:10.1055/s-2006-941455

DeCasper, A. J., & Fifer, W. P. (1980). Of human bonding: Newborns prefer their mothers' voices. *Science, 208*(4448), 1174–1176.

Degorre, C., Ghyselen, L., Barcat, L., Degrugilliers, L., Kongolo, G., Leke, A., & Tourneux, P. (2017). Noise level in the NICU: Impact of monitoring equipment. *Archives de Pédiatrie, 24*(2), 100–106. doi:10.1016/j.arcped.2016.10.023

Doheny, L., Hurwitz, S., Insoft, R., Ringer, S., & Lahav, A. (2012). Exposure to biological maternal sounds improves cardiorespiratory regulation in extremely preterm infants. *The Journal of Maternal-Fetal & Neonatal Medicine, 25*(9), 1591–1594. doi:10.3109/147670 58.2011.648237

Elser, H. E., Holditch-Davis, D., Levy, J., & Brandon, D. H. (2012). The effects of environmental noise and infant position on cerebral oxygenation. *Advances in Neonatal Care, 12*(Suppl 5), S18–S27. doi:10.1097/ANC.0b013e31826853fe

Field, T. M., Dempsey, J., Hatch, J., Ting, G., & Clifton, R. (1979). Cardiac and behavioral responses to repeated tactile and auditory stimulation by preterm and term neonates. *Developmental Psychology, 15*, 406–416.

Fifer, W. P., & Moon, C. M. (1994). The role of mother's voice in the organization of brain function in the newborn. *Acta Paediatrica. Supplement, 397*, 86–93.

Filippa, M., Devouche, E., Arioni, C., Imberty, M., & Gratier, M. (2013). Live maternal speech and singing have beneficial effects on hospitalized preterm infants. *Acta Paediatrica, 102*(10), 1017–1020. doi:10.1111/apa.12356

Gadeke, R., Doring, B., Keller, F., & Vogel, A. (1969). The noise level in a children's hospital and the wake-up threshold in infants. *Acta Paediatrica Scandinavica, 58*(2), 164–170.

Gray, L., & Philbin, M. K. (2004). Effects of the neonatal intensive care unit on auditory attention and distraction. *Clinics in Perinatology, 31*(2), 243–260. vi. doi:10.1016/j.clp.2004.04.013

Hall, J. W., 3rd. (2000). Development of the ear and hearing. *Journal of Perinatology, 20*(8 Pt 2), S12–S20.

Hepper, P. G., & Shahidullah, B. S. (1994). Development of fetal hearing. *Archives of Disease in Childhood, 71*(2), F81–F87.

Jardri, R., Houfflin-Debarge, V., Delion, P., Pruvo, J. P., Thomas, P., & Pins, D. (2012). Assessing fetal response to maternal speech using a noninvasive functional brain imaging technique. *International Journal of Developmental Neuroscience, 30*(2), 159–161.   ·

Joseph, R. (2000). Fetal brain behavior and cognitive development. *Developmental Review, 20*, 81–98.

Kattwinkel, J., Nearman, H. S., Fanaroff, A. A., Katona, P. G., & Klaus, M. H. (1975). Apnea of prematurity. Comparative therapeutic effects of cutaneous stimulation and nasal continuous positive airway pressure. *The Journal of Pediatrics, 86*(4), 588–592.

Kisilevsky, B. S., & Hains, S. M. (2011). Onset and maturation of fetal heart rate response to the mother's voice over late gestation. *Developmental Science, 14*(2), 214–223.

Knudsen, E. I. (2004). Sensitive periods in the development of the brain and behavior. *Journal of Cognitive Neuroscience, 16*(8), 1412–1425. doi:10.1162/0898929042304796

Kuhn, P., Astruc, D., Messer, J., & Marlier, L. (2011). Exploring the olfactory environment of premature newborns: A French survey of health care and cleaning products used in neonatal units. *Acta Paediatrica, 100*(3), 334–339.

Kuhn, P., Zores, C., Astruc, D., Dufour, A., & Casper, C. (2011). Sensory system development and the physical environment of infants born very preterm. *Archives de Pédiatrie, 18 Suppl 2*, S92–102.

Kuhn, P., Zores, C., Langlet, C., Escande, B., Astruc, D., & Dufour, A. (2013). Moderate acoustic changes can disrupt the sleep of very preterm infants in their incubators. *Acta Paediatrica, 102*(10), 949–954. doi:10.1111/apa.12330

Kuhn, P., Zores, C., Pebayle, T., Hoeft, A., Langlet, C., Escande, B., ... Dufour, A. (2012). Infants born very preterm react to variations of the acoustic environment in their incubator from a minimum signal-to-noise ratio threshold of 5 to 10 dBA. *Pediatric Research, 71*(4 Pt 1), 386–392. doi:10.1038/pr.2011.76

Lagercrantz, H. (2010). *The newborn brain: Neuroscience and clinical applications.* New York, NY: Cambridge University Press.

Lagercrantz, H., & Changeux, J. P. (2009). The emergence of human consciousness: From fetal to neonatal life. *Pediatric Research, 65*(3), 255–260.

Lagercrantz, H., Edwards, D., Henderson-Smart, D., Hertzberg, T., & Jeffery, H. (1990). Autonomic reflexes in preterm infants. *Acta Paediatrica Scandinavica, 79*(8–9), 721–728.

Lahav, A. (2015). Questionable sound exposure outside of the womb: Frequency analysis of environmental noise in the neonatal intensive care unit. *Acta Paediatrica, 104*(1), e14–e19. doi:10.1111/apa.12816

Lahav, A., & Skoe, E. (2014). An acoustic gap between the NICU and womb: A potential risk for compromised neuroplasticity of the auditory system in preterm infants. *Frontiers in Neuroscience, 8*, 381. doi:10.3389/fnins.2014.00381

Lai, T. T., & Bearer, C. F. (2008). Iatrogenic environmental hazards in the neonatal intensive care unit. Clinics in Perinatology, 35(1), 163–181., ix.

Larroque, B., Ancel, P. Y., Marret, S., Marchand, L., Andre, M., Arnaud, C., ... EPIPAGE Study group, EPIPAGE Study group. (2008). Neurodevelopmental disabilities and special care of 5-year-old children born before 33 weeks of gestation (the EPIPAGE study): A longitudinal cohort study. *Lancet, 371*(9615), 813–820. doi:10.1016/S0140-6736(08)60380-3

Lary, S., Briassoulis, G., de Vries, L., Dubowitz, L. M., & Dubowitz, V. (1985). Hearing threshold in preterm and term infants by auditory brainstem response. *The Journal of Pediatrics, 107*(4), 593–599.

Lecanuet, J. P., Granier-Deferre, C., Jacquet, A. Y., & Busnel, M. C. (1992). Decelerative cardiac responsiveness to acoustical stimulation in the near term fetus. *The Quarterly Journal of Experimental Psychology. B, 44*(3–4), 279–303.

Lecanuet, J. P., Graniere-Deferre, C., Jacquet, A. Y., & DeCasper, A. J. (2000). Fetal discrimination of low-pitched musical notes. *Developmental Psychobiology*, *36*(1), 29–39.

Lester, B. M., Salisbury, A. L., Hawes, K., Dansereau, L. M., Bigsby, R., Laptook, A., ... Padbury, J. F. (2016). 18-month follow-up of infants cared for in a single-family room neonatal intensive care unit. *The Journal of Pediatrics*, *177*, 84–89. doi:10.1016/j.jpeds.2016.06.069

Long, J. G., Lucey, J. F., & Philip, A. G. (1980). Noise and hypoxemia in the intensive care nursery. *Pediatrics*, *65*(1), 143–145.

Mahmoudzadeh, M., Dehaene-Lambertz, G., Fournier, M., Kongolo, G., Goudjil, S., Dubois, J., ... Wallois, F. (2013). Syllabic discrimination in premature human infants prior to complete formation of cortical layers. *Proceedings of the National Academy of Sciences of the United States of America*, *110*(12), 4846–4851. doi:10.1073/pnas.1212220110

Marik, P. E., Fuller, C., Levitov, A., & Moll, E. (2012). Neonatal incubators: A toxic sound environment for the preterm infant? *Pediatric Critical Care Medicine*, *13*(6), 685–689. doi:10.1097/PCC.0b013e31824ea2b7

Marlier, L., Schaal, B., Gaugler, C., & Messer, J. (2001). Olfaction in premature human newborns: Detection and discrimination abilities two months before gestational term. In A. Marchlewska-Koj, J. Lepri, & D. Müller-Schwarze (Eds.), *Chemical signals in vertebrates* (vol. Vol. 9, pp. 205–209). New York, NY: Kluwer Academic/Plenum Publisher.

Marlow, N., Wolke, D., Bracewell, M. A., Samara, M., & Group, E. P. S. (2005). Neurologic and developmental disability at six years of age after extremely preterm birth. *The New England Journal of Medicine*, *352*(1), 9–19. doi:10.1056/NEJMoa041367

Moore, T., Hennessy, E. M., Myles, J., Johnson, S. J., Draper, E. S., Costeloe, K. L., & Marlow, N. (2012). Neurological and developmental outcome in extremely preterm children born in England in 1995 and 2006: The EPICure studies. *BMJ*, *345*, e7961. doi:10.1136/bmj.e7961

Morlet, T., Collet, L., Duclaux, R., Lapillonne, A., Salle, B., Putet, G., & Morgon, A. (1995). Spontaneous and evoked otoacoustic emissions in pre-term and full-term neonates: Is there a clinical application? *International Journal of Pediatric Otorhinolaryngology*, *33*(3), 207–211.

Philbin, M. K., & Klaas, P. (2000a). Evaluating studies of the behavioral effects of sound on newborns. *Journal of Perinatology*, *20*(8 Pt 2), S61–S67.

Philbin, M. K., & Klaas, P. (2000b). Hearing and behavioral responses to sound in full-term newborns. *Journal of Perinatology*, *20*(8 Pt 2), S68–S76.

Philbin, M. K., Lickliter, R., & Graven, S. N. (2000). Sensory experience and the developing organism: A history of ideas and view to the future. *Journal of Perinatology*, *20*(8 Pt 2), S2–S5.

Philbin, M. K., Robertson, A., & Hall, J. W., 3rd. (2008). Recommended permissible noise criteria for occupied, newly constructed or renovated hospital nurseries. *Advances in Neonatal Care*, *8*(5 Suppl), S11–S15.

Ponton, C. W., Moore, J. K., & Eggermont, J. J. (1996). Auditory brain stem response generation by parallel pathways: Differential maturation of axonal conduction time and synaptic transmission. *Ear and Hearing*, *17*(5), 402–410.

Prechtl, H. F. (1974). The behavioural states of the newborn infant (a review). *Brain Research*, *76*(2), 185–212.

Pujol, R., Blatrix, S., Le Merre, S., Pujol, T., & Chaix, B. (2009). *Voyage au centre de l'Audition*. Retrieved from http://www.cochlea.org/

Rand, K., & Lahav, A. (2014). Maternal sounds elicit lower heart rate in preterm newborns in the first month of life. *Early Human Development*, *90*(10), 679–683. doi:10.1016/j.earlhumdev.2014.07.016

Rotteveel, J. J., Colon, E. J., Stegeman, D. F., & Visco, Y. M. (1987a). The maturation of the central auditory conduction in preterm infants until three months post term. I. Composite group averages of brainstem (ABR) and middle latency (MLR) auditory evoked responses. *Hearing Research*, *26*(1), 11–20.

Rotteveel, J. J., Colon, E. J., Stegeman, D. F., & Visco, Y. M. (1987b). The maturation of the central auditory conduction in preterm infants until three months post term. IV. Composite group averages of the cortical auditory evoked responses (ACRs). *Hearing Research*, *27*(1), 85–93.

Rotteveel, J. J., de Graaf, R., Colon, E. J., Stegeman, D. F., & Visco, Y. M. (1987). The maturation of the central auditory conduction in preterm infants until three months post term. II. The auditory brainstem responses (ABRs). *Hearing Research, 26*(1), 21–35.

Rotteveel, J. J., de Graaf, R., Stegeman, D. F., Colon, E. J., & Visco, Y. M. (1987). The maturation of the central auditory conduction in preterm infants until three months post term. V. The auditory cortical response (ACR). *Hearing Research, 27*(1), 95–110.

Rotteveel, J. J., Stegeman, D. F., de Graaf, R., Colon, E. J., & Visco, Y. M. (1987). The maturation of the central auditory conduction in preterm infants until three months post term. III. The middle latency auditory evoked response (MLR). *Hearing Research, 27*(3), 245–256.

Saito, Y., Fukuhara, R., Aoyama, S., & Toshima, T. (2009). Frontal brain activation in premature infants' response to auditory stimuli in neonatal intensive care unit. *Early Human Development, 85*(7), 471–474.

Salavitabar, A., Haidet, K. K., Adkins, C. S., Susman, E. J., Palmer, C., & Storm, H. (2010). Preterm infants' sympathetic arousal and associated behavioral responses to sound stimuli in the neonatal intensive care unit. *Advances in Neonatal Care, 10*(3), 158–166. doi:10.1097/ANC.0b013e3181dd6dea

Schneider, B. A., Trehub, S. E., Morrongiello, B. A., & Thorpe, L. A. (1989). Developmental changes in masked thresholds. *The Journal of the Acoustical Society of America, 86*(5), 1733–1742.

Sininger, Y. S., Abdala, C., & Cone-Wesson, B. (1997). Auditory threshold sensitivity of the human neonate as measured by the auditory brainstem response. *Hearing Research, 104*(1–2), 27–38.

Slater, R., Fitzgerald, M., & Meek, J. (2007). Can cortical responses following noxious stimulation inform us about pain processing in neonates? *Seminars in Perinatology, 31*(5), 298–302. doi:10.1053/j.semperi.2007.07.001

Slevin, M., Farrington, N., Duffy, G., Daly, L., & Murphy, J. F. (2000). Altering the NICU and measuring infants' responses. *Acta Paediatrica, 89*(5), 577–581.

Sokolov, E. N. (1963). Higher nervous functions; the orienting reflex. *Annual Review of Physiology, 25*, 545–580. doi:10.1146/annurev.ph.25.030163.002553

Sokolov, E. N. (1990). The orienting response, and future directions of its development. *The Pavlovian Journal of Biological Science, 25*(3), 142–150.

Therien, J. M., Worwa, C. T., Mattia, F. R., & deRegnier, R. A. (2004). Altered pathways for auditory discrimination and recognition memory in preterm infants. *Developmental Medicine and Child Neurology, 46*(12), 816–824.

Trapanotto, M., Benini, F., Farina, M., Gobber, D., Magnavita, V., & Zacchello, F. (2004). Behavioural and physiological reactivity to noise in the newborn. *Journal of Paediatrics and Child Health, 40*(5–6), 275–281. doi:10.1111/j.1440-1754.2004.00363.x

van Noort-van der Spek, I. L., Franken, M. C., & Weisglas-Kuperus, N. (2012). Language functions in preterm-born children: A systematic review and meta-analysis. *Pediatrics, 129*(4), 745–754. doi:10.1542/peds.2011-1728

Vila, J., Guerra, P., Munoz, M. A., Vico, C., Viedma-del Jesus, M. I., Delgado, L. C., … Rodriguez, S. (2007). Cardiac defense: From attention to action. *International Journal of Psychophysiology, 66*(3), 169–182.

Vranekovic, G., Hock, E., Isaac, P., & Cordero, L. (1974). Heart rate variability and cardiac response to an auditory stimulus. *Biology of the Neonate, 24*(1), 66–73.

Wachman, E. M., & Lahav, A. (2011). The effects of noise on preterm infants in the NICU. *Archives of Disease in Childhood. Fetal and Neonatal Edition, 96*(4), F305–F309. doi:10.1136/adc.2009.182014

Webb, A. R., Heller, H. T., Benson, C. B., & Lahav, A. (2015). Mother's voice and heartbeat sounds elicit auditory plasticity in the human brain before full gestation. *Proceedings of the National Academy of Sciences of the United States of America, 112*(10), 3152–3157. doi:10.1073/pnas.1414924112

Werner, L. A. (2004). Early development of the human auditory system. In R. A. Polin, W. W. Fox, & S. H. Abman (Eds.), *Fetal and neonatal physiology* (3rd ed., pp. 1803–1819). Philadelphia, PA: Saunders.

Wharrad, H. J., & Davis, A. C. (1997). Behavioural and autonomic responses to sound in pre-term and full-term babies. *British Journal of Audiology, 31*(5), 315–329.

White, R. D., Smith, J. A., Shepley, M. M., & Committee to Establish Recommended Standards for Newborn, I. C. U. D. (2013). Recommended standards for newborn ICU design, eighth edition. *Journal of Perinatology, 33*(Suppl 1), S2–16. doi:10.1038/jp.2013.10

Williams, A. L., Sanderson, M., Lai, D., Selwyn, B. J., & Lasky, R. E. (2009). Intensive care noise and mean arterial blood pressure in extremely low-birth-weight neonates. *American Journal of Perinatology, 26*(5), 323–329. doi:10.1055/s-0028-1104741

Zahr, L. K., & Balian, S. (1995). Responses of premature infants to routine nursing interventions and noise in the NICU. *Nursing Research, 44*(3), 179–185.

Zahr, L. K., & de Traversay, J. (1995). Premature infant responses to noise reduction by earmuffs: Effects on behavioral and physiologic measures. *Journal of Perinatology, 15*(6), 448–455.

Zaramella, P., Freato, F., Amigoni, A., Salvadori, S., Marangoni, P., Suppjei, A., … Chiandetti, L. (2001). Brain auditory activation measured by near-infrared spectroscopy (NIRS) in neonates. *Pediatric Research, 49*(2), 213–219.

Part III
The Early Vocal Contact in the NICU

Chapter 8
Early Vocal Contact: Direct Talking and Singing to Preterm Infants in the NICU

Manuela Filippa

Abstract *Introduction*: Early vocal contact aims to enhance closeness between preterm infants and their caregivers, principally through the medium of the voice. In this chapter we will refer, in particular, to the maternal voice, due to its special status for foetuses and newborn infants, but vocal contact should also be sustained between preterm infants and their fathers, siblings, nurses and caregivers.

Aim: the specific aims of this chapter are (1) to review the literature on maternal voice and preterm infants in the neonatal intensive care unit (NICU); (2) to identify and to describe the pathways through which early vocal contact acts as an early, family-based intervention for preterm infants in the NICU; and (3) to suggest some final recommendations.

Conclusions: Encouraging live vocal contact, with preterm infants, far from being only a sensory/acoustical stimulation, can activate a number of related and consequential actions (intuitive parenting, multimodal co-regulation, reciprocal synchronisation, unconscious mimicry). These normal actions in full-term birth are at the foundation of bonding and attachment processes and can lead to long-term and sustained positive effects on the development of preterm infants.

The Maternal Voice in the NICU: Current Practice

In recent years a number of studies of the effects of the maternal voice on preterm infants have been conducted (for a systematic review of the literature, see Filippa et al., 2017). One of the main findings of the review indicates that the maternal voice, either recorded or live, had beneficial effects on the stability of preterm infants: significant short-term effects on stability measures, both in the physiological and behavioural domains, were reported. In particular, the maternal voice seemed to support systemic oxygenation in preterm infants and in consequence

M. Filippa (✉)
Independent Researcher, Aosta, Italy
e-mail: manuela.filippa@gmail.com

© Springer International Publishing AG 2017
M. Filippa et al. (eds.), *Early Vocal Contact and Preterm Infant Brain Development*, DOI 10.1007/978-3-319-65077-7_8

reduce the frequency of critical respiratory events, such as episodes of bradycardia and apnoea.

Achieving stability is one of the major goals for hospitalised preterm infants during the first weeks of life in NICUs; however, the reasons why early closeness with parents, through the medium of the body, multimodal or vocal contact, enhances stability among preterm infants, are still under debate.

One of the more promising hypotheses links early parental closeness, especially through skin-to-skin contact (SSC), to the maturation of the autonomic nervous system (ANS) (Feldman & Eidelman, 2003). One clinically relevant index for the integrity and maturity of the nervous system in preterm infants, together with state regulation, is the cardiac vagal tone activity which, in turn, affects changes in heart rate variability (HRV): greater gains in vagal tone are fundamental indicators of an increase in autonomic maturation. When vagal tone is less active, preterm infant regulation relies on the sympathetic nervous system to increase heart rate in response to distress or to express mobilisation behaviours. Thus, HRV is a crucial measure for evaluating the maturation of ANS in preterm infants (Sahni et al., 2000): even in cases in which heart rate levels are similar, a healthy full-term neonate has much greater beat-to-beat variability compared to a high-risk preterm (Porges, 2011).

To summarise, ANS maturation plays a critical role in the infant's survival during the transition from prenatal to postnatal environments. It provides a neural platform from which to support the developing abilities of the infant to engage with caregivers and with objects in a social-interactive context with another person (Porges & Furman, 2011).

Early vocal contact, together with other programmes enhancing relationship-based care and multimodal contact during a preterm infant's hospitalisation in the NICU, acts as a tool for early stabilisation of the child and, as a consequence, supports the infant's development (Arnon et al., 2014).

Several different outcomes should be taken into account in future studies to evaluate the effects of the maternal voice on preterm hospitalised infants.

There is a lack of evidence on the effects of early vocal contact on an infant's long-term language and cognitive abilities, on parent-infant synchrony (physiological synchrony, HR synchrony), on the maturation of the ANS, on an infant's readiness and flexibility in responding to positive environmental stimuli (such as parental care behaviours) and on epigenetic processes empowering individual resilience to illness or pain-related stress.

The Pathways Through Which the Early Vocal Contact Acts

The specific aim of this paragraph is to underline the pathways through which early vocal contact can act, both in short- and long-term perspectives.

Early proximity and physical contact between parents and preterm infants are supported by years of research and positive practices, mainly linked to SSC. Early closeness and proximity in SSC bring into play a multimodal sensory experience which is primarily vibrotactile and olfactory. Breast feeding is supported both for its nutritional values and for the close proximity it implies. Practitioners and researchers can only provide transitory substitutes for early sensory experiences: the early multimodal closeness with his caregiver constitutes the best conditions for preterm infant development.

In these early experiences of closeness, the role of vocal contact has been underestimated; substitutes for early vocal contact (e.g. recorded maternal voice) have been accepted in current practice and are found far more frequently than live vocal contact in current scientific investigations (for a systematic review, see Filippa et al., 2017).

However, a number of perspectives support the vocal medium as fundamental for social experiences promoting bonding and attachment in the early phases of an infant's development. In the following paragraph, we demonstrate the pathways through which early vocal contact acts in the context of early intervention in the NICU (Fig. 8.1).

Early Vocal Contact Is a Family-Based Early Intervention

Early vocal contact is a special form of early intervention actively involving parents in a specifically meaningful and emotional contact with their infants.

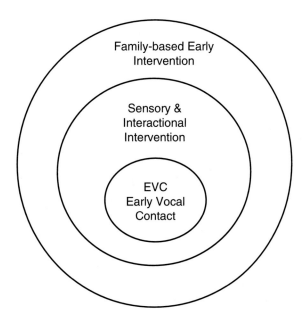

Fig. 8.1 Early vocal contact: a general framework

A chapter of this book has been dedicated to family-based interventions and developmental care programmes (see Roué, Rioualen, Sizun, Chap. 17) and the theoretical framework supporting their rationale, as well as a critical overview of the results, based on scientific evidence from different programmes.

Family-centred care strategies reported in systematic reviews and meta-analyses show the importance of early interventions involving parents, both actively in the intervention, and in teaching parents techniques for enhancing infant development (Vanderveen, Bassler, Robertson, & Kirpalani, 2009). In general, involving parents in the care of their preterm infants can decrease the risks linked to an early mother-infant separation which may lead to a wide array of adverse physiological, emotional and behavioural consequences persisting throughout life (Hofer, 1996). However, in early interventions for preterm infants, the outcomes for both mothers and preterm infants should be thoroughly assessed in order to better understand the underlying mechanisms for change (Benzies, Magill-Evans, Hayden, & Ballantyne, 2013).

Early vocal contact, as an early intervention actively involving parents in close contact with their preterm infants, can enhance not only individual but family resilience to adverse early experiences linked to prematurity.

Early Vocal Contact Is a Cross-Modal and Redundant Sensory Intervention

Defining the optimal sensory experience for preterm infants in the NICU is complex and challenging. However, some indications can be evinced by observing some particular characteristics of the infant's prenatal and postnatal sensory and brain development (Lagercrantz, 2016). For a detailed description of the foetal auditory environment, see Christine Moon's contribution, and for the postnatal environment in the NICU, see Pierre Kuhn and Kathleen Philbin's chapters in this book.

In the prenatal period, the environment provides the foetus with a variety of sensory information: among the most prominent are the auditory, tactile, vestibular, olfactory ones. However, the role of this prenatal intersensory experience in the development of sensory integration is far from well understood. During the early stages of infant development, senses work in concert, and the various sensory systems provide intermodal information regarding objects and events (Calvert, Spence, & Stein, 2004). Since birth, newborns are sensitive to audiovisual synchrony (Spelke, 1976) in particular for speech (Lewkowicz, 2010).

An "integrated" view of sensory organisation has been traced in the last decades. Voice, touch, sight and movement are linked in an infants' perception, and this is particularly true for very preterm infants who, in principle, "may see the thunder and hear the flash of lightning" (Lagercrantz, 2016). In fact, during early periods of brain development, there are redundant connections, for example, between the cochlea and the visual cortex, and the retina is connected to the auditory cortex. These links diminish during development, but multimodal perception still remains active during infancy. Due to this strong integration between different sensory systems, both in foetuses and in neonates, we can hypothesise that preterm infants also seek for intersensory experience during hospitalisation (Lickliter, 2011).

Preterm birth imposes significant modifications in the sensory experience reducing, for example, the amount of tactile and vestibular stimulation and increasing amounts of other types of stimulation not present in the uterine environment (unfiltered auditory stimulation and different visual stimulation). These alterations in light, sound and movement lead to perceptual and cognitive consequences with enduring effects on the developing premature brain (Als et al., 2003). In particular, preterm infants are exposed to a reduced availability of intersensory redundancy which, in turn, can be detrimental to the development of early sensory integration (Lickliter, 2000).

Bahrick and Lickliter define intersensory redundancy as "a particular type of multimodal stimulation in which the same information is presented simultaneously and in a spatially coordinated manner across two or more sensory modalities. For the auditory-visual domain, redundancy entails the temporally synchronous alignment of the information available to each modality" (Bahrick & Lickliter, 2000).

From the above-mentioned studies, we can hypothesise that a sensory intervention with preterm infants should be based on opportunities for intersensory redundant contact, especially that provided by social communication, in particular through audiovisual speech and songs.

Early vocal contact, communicating through the privileged medium of the voice, is not only an auditory experience for parents and preterm infants. Talking and singing face-to-face or in close proximity such as SSC involve sight, the olfactory system and the touch. For newborn infants the typical linguistic environment is inseparably linked with visual proximity, and the information comes from acoustical (voice) and visual (facial expression, eye contact) clues.

Adults, intuitively, speak to their babies, accompanying the vocal contact with synchronised and well-adapted gestures. For example, they intuitively soothe their babies with a descending vocal profile (diminishing the pitch or the intensity) and a descending gesture, from the top of the head to the neck, or, in the same way, they imitate an infant's rising vocal profile, both by gesture and with the voice.

Case Vignette 1: A Father and His Preterm Newborn Infant During SSC

Parents can do it intuitively in the NICU, when environmental conditions allow closeness and intimacy. In the following example, a father interacts vocally with his preterm baby during SSC. The baby vocalises, and they interact in a so-called protoconversation. The sensory information that is provided redundantly by the kinaesthetic stimulation (bouncing and rhythmically moving) and by the vocalisations occurs in response to the preterm infant's ones (see the Figs. 8.2 and 8.3).

Fig. 8.2 The father, during
SSC, interacts vocally with
his preterm baby.
Unpublished data

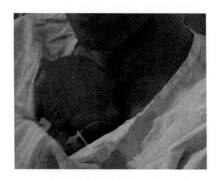

Fig. 8.3 Acoustical
analysis of the father and
infant's utterances with the
software Praat. The
analysis extracted the
variation of the pitch (Hz)
in time (seconds).

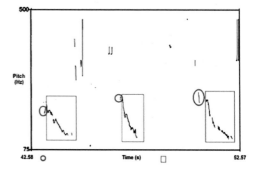

The father coordinates his vocal interventions (in blue) to the infant's one (in red circles), with a regular and descending vocal shape.

The father's three vocalisations are repeated at regular intervals of 4 s (the first starts at 43.06, the second at 47.10 and the third at 51.11); they share the same shape, starting with very close initial heights and concluding under 100 Hz. The second vocalisation has a shorter duration (0.75 s), than the first (1.12 s) and the third (1.38 s), but keeping the same shape, showing some variations in a repetitive vocal pattern. The analysis of the vocal pitch reveals a general tendency of the father's vocalisations to cope with the infant's pitch and to emit a descending intonation profile. The father's three vocalisations immediately follow the baby's "calls", producing a very regular and rhythmical temporal form (Fig. 8.4).

Case Vignette 2: Stefano and His Mother: An Intermodal Exchange. Unpublished Data The following description is taken from a research corpus of recordings and data collected between 2010 and 2013 in Aosta NICU (Italy). The main results of the research project are published in Acta Paediatrica (Filippa, Devouche, Arioni, Imberty, & Gratier, 2013), but some data are still unpublished. In the following paragraph, data on microanalysis of early interactions between a mother and her preterm infant are discussed.

Spontaneous exchanges between infant and caregiver are part of a dynamic process of continuous and bidirectional reciprocal adaptation. During their interactions,

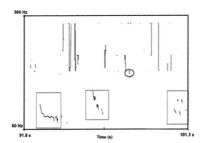

Fig. 8.4 Acoustical analysis of the father and infant's utterances (time in seconds and pitch in Hz) performed with the software Praat. The father continues vocalising for the following period, until the infant closes the eyes. Infant's arm and body movements gradually diminish in amplitude and he acquires a more stable state.

they dynamically modify their behaviour according to a precise sequential temporal organisation (Fogel, 1977).

Infants, far from being silent and receptive partner of maternal stimuli, are active constructors of the dyadic relationship (for details see Chap. 4 by Gratier and Devouche). The adult, in early communicative exchanges, is able to adjust her voice, gestures and proximity to the behavioural expressions of newborn infants: her "ID speech" varies greatly according to the infant's age and state and to the purposes of the communication (for detailed description see Chap. 3 by Trehub).

A similar process happens in preterm dyads during hospitalisation. In a preliminary study (Filippa et al., in press), we demonstrated that mothers of preterm infants are sensitive to their infant's positive behavioural displays in the first weeks of life in the NICU. More specifically, maternal infant-directed speech and song are significantly different during a baseline condition where infants are passive and expressionless, as opposed to a condition where infants display positive facial expression, opening the eyes or smiling: vocal pitch is higher on average, and maximum intensity level and standard deviation from standard are both higher in interactions when the infant is displaying positive response.

In this case vignette, the mother is encouraged to interact with her infant in a condition of proximity: the preterm infant moves his head with an ascending motor profile ╯. The mother imitates the same movement with the head and with the vocal profile ╯. The vocal profile, in the imitation process, has the same shape of her head movement and of the infant's head movement, describing an ascending profile that can be both seen and heard. This intermodal pattern, being both auditory, the mother's voice, and visual, the head movement, was used intuitively by the mother and precedes a shared smile, where she mirrored the infant's simultaneous lip corner raising. We can observe that, during early vocal contact, parents in the NICUs are intuitively able to use intersensory and redundant information to communicate with young infants when an opportunity for closeness and intimacy is offered (Figs. 8.5, 8.6, 8.7, 8.8, and 8.9).

The presence of a transfer of the imitation from one modality to another, and the correspondences between the two observable behaviours, that of the mother's voice/movement and that of the infant's, leads us to assume that the early forms of

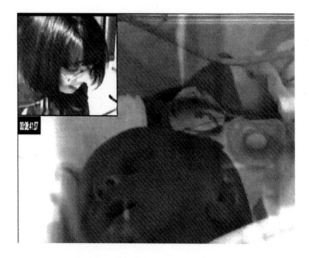

Fig. 8.5 (Timing 6.41.07) Initial condition: the mother is talking in an affective way to her infant Stefano (32 weeks post menstrual age). In the incubator, Stefano's head is turned to the mother and no movement is shown.

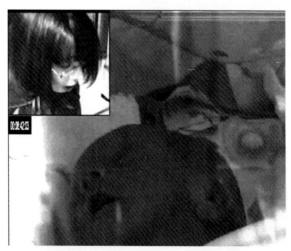

Fig. 8.6 (Timing: 6.42.03) Stefano's mouth and head movement and the beginning of the mother's imitation. Stefano closes the mouth corners and raises his head. The mother's imitation, rounding her mouth shape according to the infant's one, begins the imitation 0, 041 s after the baby's initial movement. The baby raises his head from the chin, and the mother follows the ascending line of his movement with her head (see transition between photos 2 and 3, kinetic-postural imitation, in the same sensory modality) and, especially, with her voice (intermodal imitation, the acoustical profile copies the motor head profile). This is a clear example of maternal intersensory redundant stimulation, in a condition of close imitation, which is crucial for infant's development of early sensory integration.

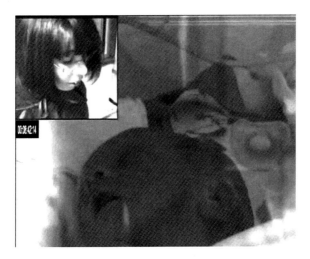

Fig. 8.7 (Timing: 06.42.14) Climax and intermodal imitation. Mother and infant raise their head in an ascending movement. A detail of the ascending movement of both mother and infant is shown in Fig. 8.8. The simultaneous raise stops at 06.42.14. The mother's imitation of Stefano's head movement is reinforced by her intonation profile (pitch raising ⬛) and intensity raising profile.

communication between the mother and her premature newborn in an incubator can constitute salient moments of intersubjective exchanges, laying the ground for infantile matching experiences (Stern, 1999).

In these conditions, where the mother tunes her affects with her newborn infant, the two partner's behaviours match with similar timing, intensity and shape characteristics of gestures, infant's head movement, and voice, mother's ascending voice profile and imitative gesture (Stern, 1998).

This analysis leads us to reflect on the potential clinical implications of the presence of such forms of intermodal imitation that would underlie emotional tuning in an at-risk dyad and the need to promote early interventions for supporting the emotional and affective connection between caregivers and newborns in the NICU.

Early Vocal Contact Sustains Synchrony and Facilitates Intuitive Parenting

Early vocal contact can represent a preferential tool for sustaining synchrony in early social interactions with preterm infants in the NICU.

Synchrony between human beings is based on a shared timing experience which coordinates the exchanges during social interactions that are fundamental for the infant's growth and development. The parental brain is endowed with the necessary abilities to regulate on his/her infant since early gestational phases of development,

Fig. 8.8 (Timing: 06.43.10) The beginning of the last phase of the sequence: a simultaneous smile. In order to analyse the last phase of the sequence, we placed two markers near the mother and infant's mouth corners. The preterm infant begins to open simultaneously the lip corners and is followed by the beginning of the mothers' smile 0.05 s later.

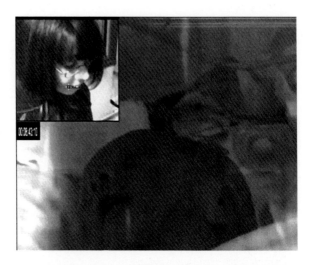

Fig. 8.9 (Timing: 06.44.02) Climax of a shared smile. The mother approaches her head to the incubator (as shown by the yellow marker) and smiles. The sequence ends with the mother's words: "You're so nice".

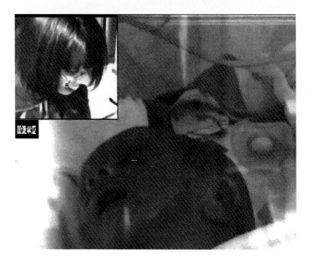

the parental brain shapes, and is shaped by infant physiology and behaviour (Feldman, 2015). The reciprocal exchanges regulated by synchrony are not only vocal and auditory in their character but concomitantly entails biological co-regulations in which hormones and physiological regulations play a fundamental role, while a lack of synchrony is hypothesised to have a detrimental role in communication disorders of preterm infants (Feldman, 2007). A detailed description of the role of synchrony in communication development is outlined in Chap. 10 by Filippa and Kuhn.

In typical conditions, vocal and multimodal communication between parents and infants functions as a didactic system to support the development of thought and speech.

During face-to-face vocal contact, in early exchanges, adult and infants are in the best condition for imitating and being imitated. Neonatal imitation is a process in which a newborn matches the gestures of an adult, even if the adult model is not his parent. In this process, neonates copy the gestures – tongue protrusion, mouth opening, eyes opening, finger movements and vocalisations – that are already within their behavioural repertoire (Kugiumutzakis, 1993, 1999; Meltzoff & Moore, 1977; Nagy & Molnar, 2004). The neonatal imitation, also known as unconscious mimicry, is present only in face-to-face conditions and is sustained by vocal calls. The question whether the mirror neuron system is involved in early forms of imitation in a face-to-face condition is still unanswered.

Newborns, during these episodes, copy the actions that are already within their behavioural repertoire. Newborns both imitate and provoke imitation from an adult, with different patterns of heart rate changes accompanying imitation, with a decreasing heart rate, and provocations, with an increasing heart rate (Nagy & Molnar, 2004).

It's arguable that neonatal imitation aims mainly to foster social interaction and communication between the young infant and his mother (Bjorklund, 1987).

According to some hypothesis (Rizzolatti, Fadiga, Fogassi, & Gallese, 2002) under the heading of imitation, fundamental and ancient mechanisms of resonance can be at the basis of interindividual relations: whether these mechanisms could involve also early interactions between infants and parents is still under debate.

Over the course of infancy, parents and infants continue this reciprocal imitative relationship. Episodes of mimicry are in fact very frequent, and infants are endowed with the necessary abilities to imitate since the first hours of life (for details, see Chap. 4 by Gratier and Devouche). The circle of reciprocal imitation is essential for newborns who can imitate by motor patterns what they have already experienced in utero and, through repetition and variation, they enlarge their "motor vocabulary"; in reverse, being imitative produces in infants a sudden increase in oxytocin (Delaveau, Arzounian, Rotgé, Nadel, & Fossati, 2015). This mechanism acts as a reward, with effects also in adults (Chartrand & Bargh, 1999), so that the proprioceptions match with sensorial audio/visual inputs. In the same way, infants begin imitating the vocal sounds they are exposed to, and by means of adaptations and variations, in mutual concert with the caregivers, they enlarge their vocabulary of vocal sounds. What the role of gestural and vocal mimicry may be in prematurity, and when/how it is displayed, is an interesting research topic but still needs to be explored.

Empirical evidence shows that the emotional dimensions of social bonds are controlled by highly conserved biological processes (Panksepp, 1998).

Other forms of support for communicative competence, biological rather than cultural, are defined as intuitive parental behaviours (Papoušek & Papoušek, 1986): they escape the parent's conscious awareness and are not intentional. In the vocal communication with newborns, parents unknowingly adjust the structure and dynamics of speech and songs to the infant's abilities and use it in expressive forms: in this and other similar ways, parents offer, through an abundance of learning situations, a platform for communicative development.

The adult voice changes strikingly when directed to infants (see Chap. 3 by Trehub), and interestingly it becomes more tied to interactional context and to the infant's behavioural-emotional state than to the lexical content. These observations confirm that it is not the lexical but the prosodic message, the musicality, that plays a crucial role (see Chap. 1 by Trevarthen).

Language and communication skills develop during social interchanges: especially the earliest phases of language acquisition – during the transition from an initial universal state of language processing to one that is language specific – it requires social interaction with caregivers (Kuhl, 2007), and it occurs subconsciously in parents, confirming the hypothesis that these complex didactic abilities have biological roots. However, it often happens that, in the context of hospitalisation, maternal care remains unexpressed, and therefore parents need specific conditions of closeness and intimacy in order to express their intuitive behaviours. If rational and didactic recommendations were to be prepared in support of preterm infants' language and communicative development in NICUs, they would hardly differ from these same intuitive didactic conditions and co-regulation patterns that parents already intuitively use in normal conditions. Therefore, considering the ecology of the NICU as a whole, the main aim of practitioners is to create an optimal environment in which intuitive parental competences may be expressed and supported.

This leads to a different paradigm of early intervention in the NICU, where clinicians do not interfere with the dyad but support and create the best environment for the promotion of intuitive parenting expression.

One of the best ways to allow intuitive non-verbal vocal communication is to encourage early forms of vocal and multimodal interactions in the ecology of the NICU.

Preterm Infant-Directed Songs During Early Vocal Contact

In its singing form, early vocal contact acts as a form of musical communication which is beneficial for both mothers and infants (see Chaps. 1 by Trevarthen and 3 by Trehub), based on the effects of music on active perception in infant brains (see Chap. 5 by Grandjean).

When comparing maternal speaking and singing directed to preterm infants, differences in vocal sensitivity to infants' behavioural displays have been demonstrated, between speech and songs, in a preliminary study (Filippa, Gratier, Devouche, & Grandjean, in press). Comparison between acoustic features in preterm infant-directed speaking or singing shows that pitch variability and range are greater in maternal speech than in singing during an infant's behavioural display. When preterm infants open the eyes or smile, in a face-to-face interaction, mothers tend to adapt their voices to these behavioural signals, becoming more emotional and more expressive. It is possible that mothers' speech and singing become more clearly infant-directed in the presence of a discernible potentially communicative display by the infant, by increasing the pitch variability and range. This finding strongly suggests that mothers intuitively interpret infant facial displays as potential acts of communication and intuitively respond.

When compared to singing, maternal speech affords greater acoustic variations, both in pitch and intensity, in the presence of an infant display. One explanation for this difference is that heightened emotion in speech is indexed by greater pitch variability (Scherer, 2003), whereas it is indexed by greater timing variation in song and music (Clarke, 1999). Another explanation for lower pitch variability in song is that it is constrained by musical structure. We can argue that maternal singing, as a form of musical code, is a special signal for preterm infants, for its particular structure. In her chapter Sandra Trehub describes the ubiquity of maternal singing to infants: in the course of caregiving, adults commonly use a specific musical repertoire fulfilling specific functions, including lullabies, play songs and songs adapted from the adult repertoire (Shenfield, Trehub, & Nakata, 2003).

Mothers in the NICU are no exception: in our previous research (Filippa et al., 2013), we observed that early vocal contact increased preterm infant wakefulness but only in the speaking condition. In the case of singing, they tended to maintain the initial state. Based on the existing literature, we can hypothesise that singing can facilitate coordinated and repetitive communicative patterns.

In the same cohort of mothers, we analysed the maternal repertoire in preterm infant-directed songs. We asked mothers to sing to their babies from their own repertoire of familiar songs: the protocol called for mothers to sing a meaningful, easy song, with which they felt at ease. As vocal communication covers all aspects of emotional and affective communication, the songs had to have relevance to mothers as special tools with which to enter into close emotional contact.

The choice of repertoire was very varied: 40% of the repertoire came from popular music but also traditional Italian and regional songs (32%), while lullabies and children's songs in general accounted for 17% and 11% of the total repertoire. Contrary to initial expectations, the specific repertoire for children – lullabies, nursery rhymes, play songs, etc. – did not achieve high percentages.

These preliminary findings confirm that play songs and happy songs in which infants are engaged in repetitive gestures are frequently used in the context of interaction during infant waking states and in face-to-face communication also involving body contact and that they sustain an increase in arousal and new learning activities. However, in the context of the NICU, during hospitalisation, play songs are not frequently used: we can argue that this is due to the difficulty premature infants have in sustaining a calm state of wakefulness sufficiently long to allow reciprocal interplay.

Finally, mothers were encouraged to sing and speak in the language of their culture: early vocal contact is not only an affective attunement but also a medium through which adults begin sharing cultural practices and meanings with their children.

The "mother tongue" is not only a specific language but a communication system used among kin; mother tongues store information and meaning accumulated by parents or other relatives, meaning that there is a continued impulse to transmit (Fitch, 2004).

During hospitalisation, where standards of care are central to infant survival, parents can represent the link with cultural practice and meaning. Preterm infants, after discharge, will find themselves in a broader sociocultural context, in which different styles of parenting influence infant care. Early engagement in social and cultural practices can be a special challenge for individualised care in the NICU and requires early engagement in social interaction through the medium of the voice, the mother tongue and culturally based play songs and lullabies. This early form of protoconversation (see the paragraph on intuitive parenting for a more detailed description) contains all the elements of cultural and linguistic heritage which the adult brings to bear on the process of infant development.

Final Recommendations and Conclusions

Empowering Parents to Begin Earlier What They Will Be Doing for the Rest of Their Lives

The first argument often reported against active parental involvement in early vocal contact is parental emotional unavailability during an infant's stay in the NICU. For these reasons, certain practitioners could suggest "surrogates" of parental vocal presence, such as the provision of maternal voice recordings.

However, a number of successful early parental intervention programmes demonstrate that the parents' early involvement in a preterm infant's care is not only appropriate but fundamental, not only for the well-being of infants and to enhance parent-infant interaction but also in the interests of improving parent mental health outcomes (Melnyk et al., 2006).

Parental so-called unavailability is often attributed to high levels of parental stress and instability, frequently linked to the particular infant's state of health (Eriksson & Pehrsson, 2002). However, with the exception of rare situations – such mothers too severely ill to be able to look after themselves or their infants or giving their babies up for adoption – the overall experience of skin-to-skin contact indicates that, especially in critical conditions, separation causes adverse effects and that early closeness is beneficial and should be encouraged, both for infant's and mother's well-being (Bergman, Linley, & Fawcus, 2004).

Limitations for the Early Vocal Contact

The effects of an enhanced vocal contact between parents and very preterm infants with severe health complications or with very immature brains are currently unknown.

Most of the studies on the maternal voice effects and, in general, on early multisensory contact are limited to stable preterm infants (see Filippa et al., 2017). When exactly the early vocal contact can begin must be judged individually, and full account should be taken of the condition and status of each baby and his mother or father.

Fully account should be taken also of the very preterm infant's reactions to the intervention: very preterm infants' delayed or unexpected physiological (bradycardia, apnoea) and behavioural (muscular flaccidity and state fluctuation) responses are often difficult to read, especially for parents, when the baby health conditions are unstable. As mothers and fathers will deliver the vocal contact, their conditions must be stable but not necessarily optimal. Both parents and infants can, in fact, benefit from this intervention, and they can improve their health condition thanks to this early practice.

Conclusions and Suggestions for Further Interventions and Research

> *Care and intervention based on the infant's own behavior makes good biological sense and is also ethically attractive* (Westrup, 2014).

The aim of this chapter was to clarify the main pathways through which early vocal contact acts in a family-centred neonatal care unit.

Based on the principles of early family-based interventions and on individualised care programmes, in particular on the evidence reported in the research and practice of the skin-to-skin contact, early vocal contact is suggested as an effective tool with which to enhance parent-infant early affective closeness, which is fundamental for an infant's adaptation to his environment and for the creation of optimal conditions in which to sustain synchrony, intermodal connection and infant learning processes.

To conclude, preterm infants, seeking for closeness and social "companionship" that preterm infants have experienced already in the mother's womb, may be regained by the experience of parental singing and speaking, which, in turn if delivered sensitively in a multimodal fashion (e.g. during the skin-to-skin contact), will enhance the sensory environment and social interaction necessary for a positive long-term development.

Future research, based on integrated outcome measurements, especially neurological ones with neuroimaging techniques, e.g. electroencephalography (EEG), magneto-encephalography (MEG), functional near-infrared spectroscopy (fNIRS) and functional magnetic resonance imaging (fMRI), is promising and strongly encouraged.

Key Messages
- The maternal voice, either recorded or live, had beneficial effects on the stability of preterm infants.
- Early vocal contact is a family-based, cross-modal and redundant sensory intervention.
- Early vocal contact can represent a preferential tool for sustaining synchrony in early social interactions with preterm infants in the NICU.
- The effects of an enhanced vocal contact between parents and very preterm infants with health complications are currently unknown: full account should be taken of the condition and status of each baby and his mother or father.

Key Messages
The optimal conditions and the limitations for sustaining the early vocal contact:

When preterm infants are *stable*.

If babies are *unstable*, pay extra attention to the infant physiological and behavioural responses (can she/he handle it? does it improve/worsen his/her stability?).

In a condition of *intimacy* with mothers/fathers or primary caregivers (i.e. in an enough quiet environment allowing auditory perception/extraction).

In a condition of *physical closeness* (when possible, during skin-to-skin contact).

Avoid *starting* the vocalisations when preterm infants are in deep sleep.

References

Als, H., Gilkerson, L., Duffy, F. H., Mcanulty, G. B., Buehler, D. M., Vandenberg, K., … Butler, S. C. (2003). A three-center, randomized, controlled trial of individualized developmental care for very low birth weight preterm infants: Medical, neurodevelopmental, parenting, and caregiving effects. *Journal of Developmental & Behavioral Pediatrics, 24*(6), 399–408.

Arnon, S., Diamant, C., Bauer, S., Regev, R., Sirota, G., & Litmanovitz, I. (2014). Maternal singing during kangaroo care led to autonomic stability in preterm infants and reduced maternal anxiety. *Acta Paediatrica, 103*(10), 1039–1044.

Bahrick, L. E., & Lickliter, R. (2000). Intersensory redundancy guides attentional selectivity and perceptual learning in infancy. *Developmental Psychology, 36*(2), 190.

Benzies, K. M., Magill-Evans, J. E., Hayden, K. A., & Ballantyne, M. (2013). Key components of early intervention programs for preterm infants and their parents: A systematic review and meta-analysis. *BMC Pregnancy Childbirth, 13 Suppl 1*:S10.

Bergman, N. J., Linley, L. L., & Fawcus, S. R. (2004). Randomized controlled trial of skin-to-skin contact from birth versus conventional incubator for physiological stabilization in 1200-to 2199-gram newborns. *Acta Paediatrica, 93*(6), 779–785.

Bjorklund, D. F. (1987). A note on neonatal imitation. *Developmental Review, 7*(1), 86–92.

Calvert, G., Spence, C., & Stein, B. (2004). *The handbook of multisensory processes.* Cambridge, MA: MIT Press.

Chartrand, T. L., & Bargh, J. A. (1999). The chameleon effect: The perception–behavior link and social interaction. *Journal of Personality and Social Psychology, 76*(6), 893.

Clarke, E. F. (1999). Rhythm and timing in music. *The Psychology of Music, 2*, 473–500.

Delaveau, P., Arzounian, D., Rotgé, J. Y., Nadel, J., & Fossati, P. (2015). Does imitation act as an oxytocin nebulizer in autism spectrum disorder? *Brain, 138*(7), e360–e360.

Eriksson, B. S., & Pehrsson, G. (2002). Evaluation of psycho-social support to parents with an infant born preterm. *Journal of Child Health Care, 6*, 19–33.

Feldman, R. (2007). Parent–infant synchrony biological foundations and developmental outcomes. *Current Directions in Psychological Science, 16*(6), 340–345.

Feldman, R. (2015). The adaptive human parental brain: Implications for children's social development. *Trends in Neurosciences, 38*(6), 387–399.

Feldman, R., & Eidelman, A. I. (2003). Skin-to-skin contact (Kangaroo Care) accelerates autonomic and neurobehavioural maturation in preterm infants. *Developmental Medicine and Child Neurology, 45*(4), 274–281.

Filippa, M., Devouche, E., Arioni, C., Imberty, M., & Gratier, M. (2013). Live maternal speech and singing have beneficial effects on hospitalized preterm infants. *Acta Paediatrica, 102*(10), 1017–1020.

Filippa, M., Gratier, M., Devouche, E., & Grandjean, D. (in press). Changes in infant-directed speech and song are related to preterm infant facial expression in the neonatal intensive care unit. *Interaction Studies.*

Filippa, M., Panza, C., Ferrari, F., Frassoldati, R., Kuhn, P., Balduzzi, S., & D'Amico, R. (2017). Systematic review of maternal voice interventions demonstrates increased stability in preterm infants. *Acta Paediatrica. 106*(8):1220–1229. doi: 10.1111/apa.13832.

Fitch, W. T. (2004). Kin selection and 'mother tongues': A neglected component in language evolution. In *Evolution of communication systems: A comparative approach* (pp. 275–296). Cambridge, MA/London, England: MIT Press.

Fogel, A. (1977). Temporal organisation in mother-infant face-to-face interaction. In H. R. Schaffer (Ed.), *Studies in mother-infant interaction* (pp. 119–151). New York, NY: Academic.

Hofer, M. A. (1996). On the nature and consequences of early loss. *Psychosomatic Medicine, 58*(6), 570–581.

Kugiumutzakis, G. (1993). Intersubjective vocal imitation in early mother–infant interaction. In J. Nadel & L. Camaioni (Eds.), *New perspectives in early communicative development* (pp. 23–47). London, England: Routledge.

Kugiumutzakis, G. (1999). Genesis and development of early infant mimesis to facial and vocal models.

Kuhl, P. K. (2007). Is speech learning 'gated' by the social brain? *Developmental Science, 10*(1), 110–120.

Lagercrantz, H. (2016). *Infant brain development. Formation of the mind and the emergence of consciousness.* Cham, Switzerland: Springer.

Lewkowicz, D. J. (2010). Infant perception of audio-visual speech synchrony. *Developmental Psychology, 46*(1), 66.

Lickliter, R. (2000). The role of sensory stimulation in perinatal development: Insights from comparative research for care of the high-risk infant. *Journal of Developmental & Behavioral Pediatrics, 21*(6), 437–447.

Lickliter, R. (2011). The integrated development of sensory organization. *Clinics in Perinatology, 38*(4), 591–603.

Melnyk, B. M., Feinstein, N. F., Alpert-Gillis, L., Fairbanks, E., Crean, H. F., Sinkin, R. A., … Gross, S. J. (2006). Reducing premature infants' length of stay and improving parents' mental health outcomes with the creating opportunities for parent empowerment (COPE) neonatal intensive care unit program: A randomized, controlled trial. *Pediatrics, 118*(5), e1414–e1427.

Meltzoff, A. N., & Moore, M. K. (1977). Imitation of facial and manual gestures by human neonates. *Science, 198*(4312), 75–78.

Nagy, E., & Molnar, P. (2004). Homo Imitans or homo provocans? Human imprinting model of neonatal imitation. *Infant Behavior & Development, 27*(1), 54–63.

Panksepp, J. (1998). The periconscious substrates of consciousness: Affective states and the evolutionary origins of the SELF. *Journal of Consciousness Studies, 5*(5–6), 566–582.

Papoušek, H., & Papoušek, M. (1986). Structure and dynamics of human communication at the beginning of life. *European Archives of Psychiatry and Clinical Neuroscience, 236*(1), 21–25.

Porges, S. W. (2011). *The polyvagal theory: Neurophysiological foundations of emotions, attachment, communication, and self-regulation (Norton series on interpersonal neurobiology).* New York: WW Norton & Company.

Porges, S. W., & Furman, S. A. (2011). The early development of the autonomic nervous system provides a neural platform for social behaviour: A polyvagal perspective. *Infant and Child Development, 20*(1), 106–118.

Rizzolatti, G., Fadiga, L., Fogassi, L., & Gallese, V. (2002). 14 from mirror neurons to imitation: Facts and speculations. *The Imitative Mind: Development, Evolution, and Brain Bases, 6*, 247–266.

Sahni, R., Schulze, K. F., Kashyap, S., Ohira-Kist, K., Fifer, W. P., & Myers, M. M. (2000). Maturational changes in heart rate variability in low birth weight infants. *Developmental Psychobiology, 37*, 73–81.

Scherer, K. (2003). Vocal communication of emotion: A review of research paradigms. *Speech Communication, 40*(1–2), 227–256.

Shenfield, T., Trehub, S. E., & Nakata, T. (2003). Maternal singing modulates infant arousal. *Psychology of Music, 31*(4), 365–375.

Spelke, E. (1976). Infants' intermodal perception of events. *Cognitive Psychology, 8*(4), 553–560.

Stern, D. N. (1998). Aspects temporels de l'expérience quotidienne d'un nouveau-né: quelques réflexions concernant la musique. In E. Darbellay (Ed.), *Le temps et la forme* (pp. 167–189). Genève, Droz: Pour une épistémologie de la connaissance musicale.

Stern, D. N. (1999). Vitality contours: The temporal contour of feelings as a basic unit for constructing the infant's social experience. In P. Rochat (Ed.), *Early social cognition: Understanding others in the first months of life* (pp. 67–90). Mahwah, NJ: Erlbaum.

Vanderveen, J. A., Bassler, D., Robertson, C. M. T., & Kirpalani, H. (2009). Early interventions involving parents to improve neurodevelopmental outcomes of premature infants: A meta-analysis. *Journal of Perinatology, 29*, 343–351.

Westrup, B. (2014). Family-centered developmentally supportive care. *NeoReviews, 15*(8), e325–e335.

Chapter 9
Maternal Voice and Its Influence on Stress and Sleep

Fabrizio Ferrari, Giovanna Talucci, Luca Ori, Natascia Bertoncelli, Manuela Filippa, and Laura Lucaccioni

Abstract *Introduction*: Several developmental care programmes in NICU have been created to minimize the consequences of prematurity and to promote preterm infant's neurobehavioral and brain development. The foetus in the womb relies on the organic structure of the rhythms of mother's heart, her breath patterns and over-tone vibrations of her "voice-supported" organizational development. Preterm birth interrupts the dialog between mother and foetus: changes of the sensory inputs and mother-driven environmental enrichment at this stage deeply affect the brain development and the stress regulation.

Main aims of the chapter: We wonder if vocal intervention is associated to increased neuro-vegetative stability. Birth and neonatal adaptation to the extrauterine environment is terribly stressful, and early interventions should aim to stabilize neuro-vegetative functions from the delivery room and later on during the hospitalization. Early vocal contact (EVC), a specific form of acoustical intervention, seems to be able to reassure and stabilize the autonomic function of the baby. EVC appears to facilitate sleep and organization of behavioural states and the maturation of the autonomic nervous system.

Conclusions: Intrauterine environment should be taken into account to tailor possible interventions for prematurity. Future work should aim to find simple and easy implement tools to assess and measure sleep and physiological stability (vagal tone) of the newborn. In this prospective, maternal vocal intervention may play a fundamental role in supporting and integrating neonatal clinical care.

F. Ferrari (✉) • G. Talucci • L. Ori • N. Bertoncelli • L. Lucaccioni
Neonatal Intensive Care Unit, Department of Medical and Surgical
Sciences of Mothers, Children and Adults, University of Modena & Reggio
Emilia, Modena, Italy
e-mail: fabrizio.ferrari@unimore.it

M. Filippa
Independent Researcher, Aosta, Italy

© Springer International Publishing AG 2017
M. Filippa et al. (eds.), *Early Vocal Contact and Preterm Infant Brain
Development*, DOI 10.1007/978-3-319-65077-7_9

Introduction

A drop in very low birth weight (VLBW) infant mortality has been observed in the last decades particularly for very (29–32 weeks of gestation) and extremely (≤28 weeks) preterm births, although continuing concerns about the quality of outcome of these infants persist in relation to the high rate of neuromotor, cognitive, learning and behavioural problems observed at preschool and school age. A number of intervention strategies on preterm infants and their families, aiming to reduce and possibly overcome the risks linked to premature births and to improve preterm infant development, have been proposed and tested in few studies (Als & McAnulty, 2011; Baley, J., & Committee in Fetus and Newborn, 2015; Ortenstrand et al., 2010; Peters, Rosychuk, Henderson, McPherson, & Tyebkhan, 2009; Westrup, 2015) that rose huge expectations among NICU professionals and families. One of these strategies is early vocal contact (EVC) that has been already described (see Filippa, Chap. 8). This chapter reviews the existing literature dedicated to the ontogeny of behavioural states, examines the influence of sleep on the stability of the preterm baby and investigates the possible effects of mother voice on early stabilization and behaviour of the preterm infants exposed to maternal voice after birth. EVC seems to positively influence the development of the central nervous system of preterm newborn infants in terms of ameliorating the stabilization of vital signs and, possibly, developing behavioural states and sleep and promoting body movements.

Risks Linked to the Preterm Birth and Aim of the Chapter

The aim of this chapter is to discuss EVC in relation to behavioural states and well-being of preterm infants. Before addressing EVC it is worth recalling briefly the main risk factors related to prematurity, seen that all of them may have a direct link with EVC and that EVC itself may positively impact them. Three different types of risk affect the preterm newborn infant: neurological, relational and stress in NICU.

The neurological risk is related to the brain lesions that may occur in preterm infants during the first days after birth: germinal matrix–intraventricular haemorrhage (GMH–IVH) and cerebellar haemorrhages (CH) are haemorrhagic lesions that usually occur during the first week of life, mostly often during the first 48–72 h; their pathogenesis is multifactorial, although the fragility of a transient fragile brain structure as germinal matrix and the absence of cerebral blood flow autoregulation system, along with the respiratory and blood pressure instability, play a basic role. Periventricular cystic and non-cystic leukomalacia, on converse, is a subacute/chronic ischaemic lesion that needs a much longer period to develop: it needs 3–5 weeks to manifest as white matter ultrasound abnormalities. Most frequently the ischaemia of the border zones (last fields) leads to a necrosis of all types of cerebral cells. Stress and pain may have a relevant pathogenetic role as cofactors in brain ischaemic-anoxic damage (Volpe, 2009).

The relational risk consists in being separated from the mother and other family members for weeks or months during the NICU-long stay with several possible implications in terms of stabilization of vital signs and influence on the psychological processes of bonding and attachment between parents and their newborn infant (Westrup, 2015).

The "NICU-long-staying-related risk" is the risk of stress due to NICU clinical practice and setting, leading to an excess of light and noises and a burden of continual or semi-continual painful procedures such as blood sampling, intravenous lines and ventilator support. Apparently innocent caregiving procedures such as cleaning, handling and monitoring of basic vital parameters, which are part of the daily routine NICU care, are themselves source of stress and pain.

These three different types of risk occur during the period of maximal brain spurt, corresponding to the extraordinary brain growth and development, dendritogenesis, synaptogenesis, selective elimination of neuronal processes and synapses, glial proliferation and differentiation, and myelination will never be so intense and complex at later ages. However, period of maximal brain spurt also corresponds to the period of maximal brain vulnerability, and each single moment and each single variation in the environment may affect brain development. Robert D. White (2011) defines NICU as follows "NICU […] is the environment in which brain growth and development proceed at a pace unmatched at any other time in life with millions of neurons firing and wiring, for better or worse, minute by minute".

Targets for the Developmental Care

Developmental care is defined as that newborn care that minimizes the *toxic* impact of the NICU environment and invasive care practices and encourages parental participation promoting more appropriate brain development (Peters et al., 2009). Developmental care is conceived to limit pain and stress and to optimize the developmental potentialities of the preterm infant. Among the various risks, peri- and postnatal stress has a major role: containment of stress in NICU, as pulling down lights and noises and promoting sleep, is aimed to help the preterm baby to stabilize physical conditions and consequently to promote his wellbeing and development.

Maternal Voice and Intrauterine Life

Maternal voice plays a crucial role for foetuses and possibly for newborn infants' development. In fact, it may contribute to the homeostasis and stability of the foetus.

Most frequently, preterm birth is an unexpected event that sharply interrupts the continuity and stability of foetal life. In utero *foetal homeostasis* is promoted by many factors such as quietness and semi-darkness of the womb environment, *external* light and noise filtered by the abdominal wall, provision of oxygen and nutrients from the placenta and diurnal and circadian rhythms driven by the mother rhythms (see Moon, Chap. 2).

Maternal Voice and Motility

Very little is known about maternal voice and motor behaviour. It is not known whether a sensory stimulation may influence quantity and quality of the single movement pattern: motility is produced by central pattern generators (CPG) placed in the brain and should not be influenced by any sensory feedbacks, although there is evidence that changing in sensory environment may affect quality of general movements (GMs) (Ferrari et al., 2007).

The stable posture of the foetus is supported by the limited room available inside the womb, and the walls of the uterus support the trunk and the head aligned. The adduction of shoulders and hips allows limb movement to reach the midline. Movements of the limbs and of the trunk are facilitated by the amniotic fluid and by the limited force of gravity; the different body parts are in contact with other parts, such as the chin with the trunk, limbs with the head and trunk and hands and fingers with the face and mouth. This extensive mutual contact of the body parts provides a continual sensory feedback, which informs the brain about the posture, the movements and the sensations of all the body parts. This continuous physical contact is source of rich sensory inputs that contribute to create the physical self. Oxygenation of the blood and energy supply are provided by the mother through the placenta; rest and activity states are driven by the behavioural states of the mother. Maternal voice and continual rhythmical sounds from the heart and guts accompany the foetus during day and night.

Recently Marx and Nagy (2015) evaluated which is the foetal behavioural responses to maternal voice (mother reading a story) and to maternal touch of the abdomen (usual touching of the mother) compared to a control condition (mother laying with hands beside the body), utilizing 3D real-time (4D) sonography. Behavioural responses of 23 foetuses (from the 21st to 33rd week of gestation) were frame by frame coded and analysed in the three conditions.

Overall results suggest that maternal touch of the abdomen is a powerful stimulus, producing a range of foetal behavioural responses: increase in arm, head, and mouth movements was seen when the mother touched her abdomen as compared to maternal voice.

On the contrary, the response to maternal voice showed a decrease in arm and head movements supporting previous studies reporting a decrease also in foetal heart rate (FHR) when direct maternal voice was used to stimulate the foetus (see below). The behavioural quieting to maternal voice corresponds to the physiological response of decreased FHR. Moreover, foetuses in the third trimester showed increased regulatory (yawning), resting (arms crossed) and self-touch (hands touching the body) responses to the stimuli when compared to foetuses in the second trimester.

The study underlines how foetuses selectively and differently answer to external stimulations and that foetal maturation influences these differential responses to the environment: maternal voice plays a key role in reducing movements and FHR (Marx & Nagy, 2015).

What is the role of EVC on influencing neonatal movements once the newborn leaves the womb is still unclear. It would be useful to distinguish an immediate effect after birth (increasing or reducing spontaneous movements) from a medium-term effect, focusing on the maturity of spontaneous movements at term and at 3 months of age. In fact, it was recently seen by Picciolini et al. that the quality of general movements in 71 VLBW preterm newborn infants early exposed to maternal voice was better at term-corrected age compared to controls (Picciolini et al., 2014).

Foetal Hearing and Foetal Response to Mother Voice

Hearing function begins at about 25–26 weeks of gestational age (GA) when cochlear hair cells first translate acoustic vibrations and then airborne sound stimulation into coded electrical signals that are sent to the brainstem for additional processing. Consistent responses to vibro-acoustic stimuli have been observed in the foetus from approximately 27–28 weeks, particularly in response to low-frequency sounds. These basic auditory skills are known to constitute the basis for subsequent processing of human speech sounds, beginning with mother's voice (see Moon, Chap. 2).

Whereas the newborn and foetal response to mother's voice has been well studied, the sustainability of this response following a premature birth is not fully understood (see Kuhn, Chap. 7). Chronologically, a typically developed foetus at 28 weeks of gestation and an infant born 12 weeks prematurely are exactly of the same age; however, developmentally, they may show very different HR responses when hearing their mother's voice. The ability of preterm newborns to show a preference for their mother's voice while still in the neonatal intensive care unit (NICU) may be constrained by several factors including their immature nervous system, their hypersensitivity to loud noise, the sudden demands for hearing through air (instead of amniotic fluid) and their limited capacity to hear human speech sounds clearly in the noisy NICU environment. The prenatal response to mother's voice continues postnatal. Term newborns show perceptual sensitivities in response to familiar speech stimuli. This preferential response has been demonstrated in full-term infants by several measurements, including increased nonnutritive sucking and reactive movement towards the sound source. Interestingly, newborn infants also show a preference to the type of language used (i.e. native vs. foreign) based on their individual language experience in utero. Partanen and colleagues demonstrated that term newborns react differentially to familiar vs. unfamiliar sounds they were exposed to as foetuses, revealing a direct correlation between the amount of prenatal exposure and brain activity. The above studies suggest that auditory attention, learning and memory originate before birth to allow proper priming of language centres of the brain

(Filippa et al., 2017; Kisilevsky et al., 2009; Kisilevsky, Chambers, Parker, & Davies, 2014; Krueger, 2010; Partanen et al., 2013; Rand & Lahav, 2014).

Ontogeny of Sleep

Neurophysiology of the newborn infant has shown that sleep is critical for development: a large percentage of time is spent on active sleep (AS), characterized by intense firing in most areas of the brain. Eye and body movements, breathing movements, sucking, swallowing, yawning and stretching are typical spontaneous movement patterns in AS, generated by central pattern generators (CPG), mainly located in the brainstem, providing an endogenous stimulation of the sensory processing areas (Roffwarg, Muzio, & Dement, 1966).

Proof of this endogenous firing is the increase of regional blood flow in the brain stem and other areas of the brain during AS in foetal sheep, especially in those areas involved in AS generation (Peirano, Algarín, & Uauy, 2003). In animals deprived of AS, behavioural problems (such as hyperactivity, anxiety, reduced sexual activity, disturbed sleep) have been seen in conjunction with reduction in the cerebral cortex, brainstem size and tissue protein content and, more in general, with reduction of induced synaptic plasticity.

Quiet sleep (QS) has a different task in development: its maturation coincides with the formation of thalamocortical and intracortical patterns of innervation, periods of heightened synaptogenesis and synaptic remodelling. During QS, waking patterns of neuronal activity are reactivated, suggesting that information acquired during wakefulness is further processed during sleep.

It is therefore possible that QS contributes to synaptic remodelling by providing an endogenous source of repetitive, synchronized activity within specific neuronal pathway (Frank, Issa, & Stryker, 2001).

How is sleep developing?

- 24–27 weeks of GA: at this age neither wakefulness can be distinguished from sleep nor a wakefulness state can be observed because the foetus is in an undifferentiated state with continual body movements, closed eyes, rare eye movements, clonic movements of chin and tongue, discontinuous EEG (or occasional periods of more continues activity) and regular breathing and heart rate.
- Dreyfus-Brisac (1979) states that during a polygraphic and behavioural recording of foetus at this age, elements that can demonstrate the presence of a brain rest–activity cycle cannot be found. The same was observed by Sterman and Hoppenbrouwers (1971) during the recording of the foetus movements in utero.
- 28–31 weeks of GA: wakefulness cannot be clearly identified because the EEG is similar in wakefulness and sleep. Most of the sleep cannot be classified, and it has been described as "transitional" or "undetermined" sleep.
- The behavioural features of AS and QS are partially recognizable, but the correlation between continuous EEG and AS and discontinuous EEG and QS is still very poor.

- 32–36 weeks GA: AS starts to be well developed from both the EEG (continuous activities) and behavioural perspective (REMs are present, irregular breathing, body movements), and QS periods start to be present with a reduction or disappearance of the body movements, regular breathing, discontinuous EEG and clonic movements of the chin.
- Short periods of wakefulness start to appear which correlate with a continuous EEG pattern. After 34 weeks, the periods of transitional or undetermined sleep diminish. In general, the periods of AS and QS are shorts and variable in duration (Hoppenbrouwers et al., 1978). At this age, the percentages of AS and QS are difficult to be accurately determined and depend on the variables used for their classification. The quantity and the quality of the body movements, i.e. chin myogram, are not yet well correlated with the sleep state.
- From 36 weeks of GA: wakefulness is well differentiated from sleep, and the three typical states of the full-term baby can be identified: wakefulness, active sleep and quite sleep. After a rapid increase of the duration of the sleep periods between 32 and 36 weeks (Stern, Parmelee, & Harris, 1973), the sleep cycles stay stable.
- From 38 weeks of GA: a low-voltage EEG pattern appears in AS, often together with superimposed slow waves (pattern Mixed or M according to Anders, 1974), while a high-voltage (or more simply H of Anders, 1974) EEG pattern can be observed in the QS beside the *tracé alternant* (André et al., 2010).

During the ontogeny, the percentage of QS increases compared to AS. In fact, from 30 to 32 weeks of GA up to term age, the AS is clearly predominant, while after 44–48 weeks of postmenstrual age (PMA), the percentage of QS increases quickly and becomes clearly predominant during the first 2 months of life. The trend finds its explanation in neurophysiologic and maturational aspects. In fact, QS is produced by subcortical structures of the brainstem, which connect each other by a complicated feedback network with ascending and afferent tracts to the thalamus, to the hypothalamus and then to the cortex. In animal models, removing such structures implies the disappearance of the behavioural features of QS; this is not the case of AS, which continues to be present in animals with decorticated brain (this is the reason why AS was also defined rhombencephalic sleep and QS the telencephalic sleep).

At birth, QS results to be less present than AS because it is deeply controlled by complex interactions between cortical and subcortical structures involving the cortex, which is less mature at birth compared to the brainstem structures. During ontogeny QS increases in percentage according to the development of the CNS and in particular of the cortical structures. The increasing of QS during the first months of life is considered a sign of CNS maturation.

The cyclic sleep state organization shows a gradual evolution during ontogeny which means that as the PMA increases, the state cycle seems to be more stable and more regular with a gradual decrease of the undetermined sleep state, a reduction of the AS phases and an increase of the duration of the QS phases. The duration of the sleep cycle remains stable around 40–60 min up to 8 months of life.

Ontogeny of Behavioural States

Recognition of the behavioural states in the newborn period goes back to the 1960s of the twentieth century with the fundamental contribution of the French Paris school of Dreyfus-Brisac and Monod (André et al., 2010; Dreyfus-Brisac, 1970; Dreyfus-Brisac & Minkowski, 1968). Their studies led to a great achievement in neonatal neurology: it is now universally accepted that the priority in neurological examination of the newborn infant is the recognition of the behavioural states. Heinz Precthl was the first who described in details, either starting from pure naturalistic observation with naked eyes or with polygraphic electrophysiological recording of multiple parameters, the criteria to recognize the states.

Precthl affirms that "the states represent specific and distinct modes of neural activity that are stable over time and change from one to the other during short transition, consisting of rapid changes in concert with the parameters from the various states variables. This latter aspect makes it clear that state classifications based on only one variable are not appropriate. [...] Only when a certain association between state criteria is reached during foetal life can we speak of behavioural states, but not before" [...]. "The connotation of the term state derived from the Latin "status" and means the "condition or manner of existence". For Prechtl the identification of the behavioural states was a prerequisite for a quantitative neurological assessment.

He summarized the five behavioural states of the newborn infant, from state 1 to state 5 (see Table 9.1), as distinct—and not continual—modes of the nervous system (Prechtl, 1974). He underlined that the distinction of behavioural states is essential for neonatal neurological examination: reactions to proprioceptive stimulations are exaggerated during state 1 (i.e. eyes closed, respiration regular, gross movements absent, vocalizations absent) but can hardly be elicited during state 2 (i.e. eyes closed, respiration irregular, gross movements from time to time present, vocalizations absent). On the contrary, reactions to exteroceptive stimulations cannot be seen during state 1, but typically occur during state 2 (Prechtl, Vlach, Lenard, & Grant, 1967).

Dealing with sleep ontogenesis, the state criteria proposed by Dreyfus-Brisac (1979) will be here followed; however, it has to be outlined that there is no agreement among authors on pointing the emergence and development of behavioural states in the preterm period, especially for the timing of appearance.

The definition of behavioural states mildly changes according to the authors: Brazelton, in addition to the five states of Prechtl, identifies an extra state, called

Table 9.1 Behavioural states in newborn infant (From Prechtl, 1974)

	Respiration	Eyes	Gross movements	Vocalization
State 1	Regular	Closed	Absent, some startles	Absent
State 2	Irregular	Closed	Incidental	Absent
State 3	Regular	Opened	Absent	Absent
State 4	Irregular	Opened	Continuous	Absent
State 5	Irregular	Opened or closed	Present	Present, crying, fussing

awake/transition state, corresponding to the so-called drowsy or semi-dozing state (Brazelton & Nugent, 2011).

Postnatal Environment and Stress Stimuli: The Role of Sleep Cycles and Behavioural States

After birth the maternal diurnal and circadian rhythms are interrupted; the acoustic environment provided by the continual and rhythmical heart beating, gut movements and the voice of the mother are also lost. How does the environment act on sleep?

A quite silent and dark environment promotes falling asleep and protects the temporal cyclic alternation of the two sleep states, AS and QS (i.e. sleep cycles); it reduces the arousals and promotes the solidity of both AS and QS. Moreover, the preterm baby experiments another painful experience: inside the incubator the newborn infant is alone, isolated from parents and from the warm and reassuring uterine environment. The neonate spends most of the day away from the mother, being handled by different caregivers who are not the mother. The baby suffers from this condition of isolation, and, equally, the mother feels stressed and sorry for being apart from her baby. The mother–infant interaction cycle is inevitably disrupted: the more immature the preterm, the more fragile and sensitive the preterm infant in the NICU is.

The process of *postnatal adaptation* varies from one individual to another, and the evolution of this complex process in each baby is unpredictable. According to our clinical experience, a sequence of different phases may develop: the first stage, usually covering the first few days, consists on mobilization of available energies. It corresponds to the acute stress response. The second stage is the progressive consumption and possible exhaustion of the energy patrimony: the need of increasing respiratory and cardiovascular support indicates that the stress reaction is close to be over; there is the need of waiting for a new balance. This phase may last for days or weeks. Eventually, in the last phase, the balance is temporarily or steadily reached: this point may be the beginning of real adaptation and possible stability. At this time, cycles of sleep and wakefulness states start to be seen. Sleep organization is, at the same time, a marker of wellbeing and a trigger for a new spurt in development.

During prematurity, stability and cyclicity of *behavioural states* are critical: the presence of different behavioural states is a marker of normal neurological conditions, and, on converse, their absence indicates a state of disease or of instability. Recognition of behavioural states is the starting point of daily assessment of the infant wellbeing. For the aforementioned reasons (disruption of the mother–infant closeness and relationship), the new NICUs have changed their architecture and organization, and nowadays there is the trend to build new units able to reconstruct

Table 9.2 The main
ontogenetic steps of sleep and
behavioural organization

21–27 weeks of GA	Rest–activity cycles
28–30 weeks of GA	Indeterminate sleep
30–32 weeks of GA	Emergence of AS and QS
32–34 weeks of GA	Consolidation of AS and QS
34–36 weeks of GA	Wakefulness
From term age	Increasing of QS, reducing AS

the family context around the preterm baby: in Sweden and in few other countries, the new units provide the so-called couplet care, comprehensive of the intensive care cot and the family members, i.e. parents (including mothers with medical needs) and siblings, in the same single room (Ortenstrand et al., 2010; Westrup, 2015).

The impact of the old and new NICUs on brain development is still a matter of discussion. Despite initial evidences of a better development in the couplet care units, there is one study indicating that infants left alone in single rooms actually might do worse in regard to brain growth and development compared to infants cared for the traditional NICU with more sensory stimuli, although Lester et al. have demonstrated in 2016 that whatever the architectural design of NICU is, the mother's presence is a determining factor for better cognitive and language development before 2 years of age (Lester et al., 2016; Pineda et al., 2014).

Despite the great effort of the NICU professionals to reduce the invasiveness of resuscitation manoeuvres in the delivery room, of cardiorespiratory support during transfer to the unit and soon later in NICU, little attention is usually given to recognize the behavioural states and sleep organization of the preterm baby. Conversely, the presence of robust sleep states, cyclic recurrence of sleep states (sleep cycles) and identification of QS have been recently correlated with better stability of the autonomic nervous system. It is now several decades that a good or fairly good sleep state organization is recognized as a sign of appropriate brain maturation (Lombroso & Matsumiya, 1985).

In other words, the identification of behavioural states and of the sleep/wakefulness cycles (see Table 9.2) is important for several reasons: first of all, sleep and distinct behavioural states indicate wellbeing and maturation of the brain of the newborn; second, sleep disruption is a sign of stress and/or brain dysfunction; and third, the sleep states and the single variables that are selected as state criteria and form the state constellation may be markers of the maturation and integrity of the autonomous nervous system.

Final Remarks

One of the most important limitations in the study of neurobehaviour and monitoring of physiological variables is the lack of a shared method of evaluation of the autonomic nervous system function and of the sleep states. Studies are differently focused on hearth rate variability or blood pressure variability, respiratory rate, blood oxygenation and so on: polygraphic multidimensional recordings could ideally overcome these limitations and detect behavioural states and changes in singles parameters, but they are invasive especially in the preterm infant, expensive in terms of technicians needed for the demo and time-consuming for data analysis. Therefore, they cannot be proposed as standard of care. Clinical practice in NICU should be focused on reducing stress manoeuvres soon after birth, in order to promote proper sleep and the development of behavioural states. In addition to that, as it has been shown in a systematic review (Filippa et al., 2017), the maternal voice intervention, both recorded and live, has important beneficial effects on preterm infants' behavioural and physiological stability, decreasing the cardiorespiratory events, such as apnoeas and bradycardia, and increasing oxygen saturation levels. This stability can be evidenced in an increase of calm alertness states, as a precious state in which preterm infants attend to environmental stimuli and can benefit from an audio-visual affective contact, such the maternal voice (Filippa, Devouche, Arioni, Imberty, & Gratier, 2013) or in better autonomic stability, when the maternal voice is delivered during skin-to-skin contact (Arnon et al., 2014), promoting all the beneficial affects previously discussed in terms of cerebral wellness central nervous system maturation.

Key Messages
- Preterm birth interrupts the symbiotic dialog between the dyad mother and foetus: the development of the different body systems, including the central nervous system, is strongly influenced by the gestational age when the delivery happens and by all the medical care procedures in NICU. Intrauterine environment should be taken into account to tailor possible interventions for prematurity, and, in this context, maternal vocal intervention may positively influence and improve medical practice, encouraging the clinical stabilization of the preterm infant.
- The development of sleep cycles and of behavioural states is a complex process starting from the womb and continuing during the postnatal life. They are considered a marker of normal neurological development. Maternal vocal intervention may positively influence and improve this complex process thanks to the positive effect on preterm infant's stability and subsequently to the autonomic functions.
- EVC has the potential to improve the quality of posture and movement of the preterm infant, although this hypothesis should be demonstrated in future research in preterm infants.

References

Als, H., & McAnulty, G. B. (2011). The Newborn Individualized Developmental Care and Assessment Program (NIDCAP) with Kangaroo Mother Care (KMC): Comprehensive care for preterm infants. *Current Women's Health Reviews, 7*(3), 288–301.

Anders, T. F. (1974). The infant sleep profile. *Neuropediatrie, 5*(4), 425–442.

André, M., Lamblin, M. D., d'Allest, A. M., Curzi-Dascalova, L., Moussalli-Salefranque, F., S Nguyen The, T., ... Plouin, P. (2010). Electroencephalography in premature and full-term infants. Developmental features and glossary. *Neurophysiologie Clinique, 40*(2), 59–124.

Arnon, S., Diamant, C., Bauer, S., Regev, R., Sirota, G., & Litmanovitz, I. (2014). Maternal singing during kangaroo care led to autonomic stability in preterm infants and reduced maternal anxiety. *Acta Paediatrica, 103*(10), 1039–1044.

Baley, J., & Committee on Fetus and Newborn. (2015). Skin-to-skin care for term and preterm infants in the neonatal ICU. *Pediatrics, 136*(3), 596–599.

Brazelton, T. B., & Nugent, J. K. (2011). *The neonatal behavioural assessment scale*. London, England: Mac Keith Press.

Dreyfus-Brisac, C. (1970). Ontogenesis of sleep in human prematures after 32 weeks of conceptional age. *Developmental Psychobiology, 3*(2), 91–121.

Dreyfus-Brisac C. (1979). Ontogenesis of brain bioelectrical activity and sleep organization in neonates and infants. In F. Falkner & J. M. Tanner (Eds.), *Human growth* (Vol. 3, pp. 157–182). New York, NY: Plenum.

Dreyfus-Brisac, C., & Minkowski, A. (1968). Electroencephalographic maturation and too low birth weight. *Revue Neurologique (Paris), 119*(3), 299–301.

Ferrari, F., Bertoncelli, N., Gallo, C., Roversi, M. F., Guerra, M. P., Ranzi, A., & Hadders-Algra, M. (2007). Posture and movement in healthy preterm infants in supine position in and outside the nest. *Archives of Disease in Childhood. Fetal and Neonatal Edition, 92*(5), F386–F390.

Filippa, M., Devouche, E., Arioni, C., Imberty, M., & Gratier, M. (2013). Live maternal speech and singing have beneficial effects on hospitalized preterm infants. *Acta Paediatrica, 102*(10), 1017–1020.

Filippa, M., Panza, C., Ferrari, F., Frassoldati, R., Kuhn, P., Balduzzi, S., & D'Amico, R. (2017). Systematic review of maternal voice interventions demonstrates increased stability in preterm infants. *Acta Paediatrica, 106*(8), 1220–1229.

Frank, M. G., Issa, N. P., & Stryker, M. P. (2001). Sleep enhances plasticity in the developing visual cortex. *Neuron, 30*, 275–287.

Hoppenbrouwers, T., Ugartechea, J. C., Combs, D., Hodgman, J. E., Harper, R. M., & Sterman, M. B. (1978). Studies of maternal-fetal interaction during the last trimester of pregnancy: Ontogenesis of the basic rest-activity cycle. *Experimental Neurology, 61*(1), 136–153.

Kisilevsky, B. S., Chambers, B., Parker, K., & Davies, G. (2014). Auditory processing in growth-restricted fetuses and newborns and later language development. *Clinical Psychological Science: A Journal of the Association for Psychological Science, 2*(4), 495–513.

Kisilevsky, B. S., Hains, S. M., Brown, C. A., Lee, C. T., Cowperthwaite, B., Stutzman, S. S., ... Wang, Z. (2009). Fetal sensitivity to properties of maternal speech and language. *Infant Behavior & Development, 32*(1), 59–71.

Krueger, C. (2010). Exposure to maternal voice in preterm infants: A review. *Advances in Neonatal Care, 10*(1), 13–18.

Lester, B. M., Salisbury, A. L., Hawes, K., Dansereau, L. M., Bigsby, R., Laptook, A., ... Padbury, J. F. (2016). 18-Month follow-up of infants cared for in a single-family room neonatal intensive care unit. *The Journal of Pediatrics, 177*, 84–89.

Lombroso, C. T., & Matsumiya, Y. (1985). Stability in waking-sleep states in neonates as a predictor of long-term neurologic outcome. *Pediatrics, 76*(1), 52–63.

Marx, V., & Nagy, E. (2015). Fetal behavioural responses to maternal voice and touch. *PLoS One, 10*(6), e0129118.

Ortenstrand, A., Westrup, B., Broström, E. B., Sarman, I., Akerström, S., Brune, T., … Waldenström, U. (2010). The Stockholm Neonatal Family Centered Care Study: Effects on length of stay and infant morbidity. *Pediatrics, 125*(2), e278–e285.

Partanen, E., Kujala, T., Naatanen, R., Liitola, A., Sambeth, A., & Huotilainen, M. (2013). Learning-induced neural plasticity of speech processing before birth. *Proceedings of the National Academy of Sciences of the United States of America, 110*(37), 15145–15150.

Peirano, P., Algarín, C., & Uauy, R. (2003). Sleep-wake states and their regulatory mechanisms throughout early human development. *The Journal of Pediatrics, 143*(4 Suppl), S70–S79.

Peters, K. L., Rosychuk, R. J., Henderson, L., McPherson, C., & Tyebkhan, J. M. (2009). Improvement of short- and long-term outcomes for very low birth weight infants: Edmonton NIDCAP trial. *Pediatrics, 124*(4), 1009–1020.

Picciolini, O., Porro, M., Meazza, A., Giannì, M. L., Rivoli, C., Lucco, G., … Mosca, F. (2014). Early exposure to maternal voice: Effects on preterm infants development. *Early Human Development, 90*(6), 287–292.

Pineda, R. G., Neil, J., Dierker, D., Smyser, C. D., Wallendorf, M., Kidokoro, H., … Inder, T. (2014). Alterations in brain structure and neurodevelopmental outcome in preterm infants hospitalized in different neonatal intensive care unit environments. *The Journal of Pediatrics, 164*(1), 52–60.e2.

Prechtl, H. F. (1974). The behavioural states of the newborn infant (a review). *Brain Research, 76*(2), 185–212.

Prechtl, H. F., Vlach, V., Lenard, H. G., & Grant, D. K. (1967). Exteroceptive and tendon reflexes in various behavioural states in the newborn infant. *Biologia Neonatorum, 11*(3), 159–175.

Rand, K., & Lahav, A. (2014). Maternal sounds elicit lower heart rate in preterm newborns in the first month of life. *Early Human Development, 90*(10), 679–683.

Roffwarg, H. P., Muzio, J. N., & Dement, W. C. (1966). Ontogenetic development of the human sleep-dream cycle. *Science, 152*(3722), 604–619.

Sterman, M. B., & Hoppenbrouwers, T. (1971). The development of sleep-waking and rest-activity patterns from fetus to adult in man. In *Brain development and behavior* (pp. 203–227). New York: Academic Press.

Stern, E., Parmelee, A. H., & Harris, M. A. (1973). Sleep state periodicity in prematures and young infants. *Developmental Psychobiology, 6*(4), 357–365.

Volpe, J. J. (2009). The encephalopathy of prematurity – Brain injury and impaired brain development inextricably intertwined. *Seminars in Pediatric Neurology, 16*(4), 167–178.

Westrup, B. (2015). Family-centered developmentally supportive care: The Swedish example. *Archives de Pédiatrie, 22*(10), 1086–1091.

White, R. D. (2011). The newborn intensive care unit environment of care: How we got here, where we're headed, and why. *Seminars in Perinatology, 35*(1), 2–7.

Chapter 10
Support of Language and Communication Development as a Rationale for Early Maternal Vocal Contact with Preterm Infants

Manuela Filippa and Pierre Kuhn

Abstract *Introduction.* Preterm infants have an increased risk of language and communication disorders, and these disorders can occur even in the absence of brain lesions or major disabilities. There is a linear relationship between gestational age at birth and language development. This suggests that alterations in the anatomical and functional development of the premature brain contribute to the delayed language development of preterm infants.

Aim. The main aims of this chapter are to summarize the mechanisms and factors that affect language and communication delays in preterm infants and to present the rationale and discuss the potential use of early maternal vocal contact to promote language development.

Conclusions. Multiple medical and environmental factors contribute to language and communicative delays in preterm infants. Early and prolonged exposure of preterm infants to adult talk improves their language development. Competences in communication are acquired in social contexts. Physical closeness and early vocal contact between parents and preterm infants have the potentiality to support their language and communicative development. We suggest that clinicians consider the benefits of these interventions and that researchers further examine their effects.

M. Filippa (✉)
Independent Researcher, Aosta, Italy
e-mail: manuela.filippa@gmail.com

P. Kuhn
Médecine et Réanimation du Nouveau-né Hôpital de Hautepierre,
CHU Strasbourg, Strasbourg, France

Laboratoire de Neurosciences Cognitives et Adaptatives,
CNRS-Université de Strasbourg, Strasbourg, France

© Springer International Publishing AG 2017
M. Filippa et al. (eds.), *Early Vocal Contact and Preterm Infant Brain Development*, DOI 10.1007/978-3-319-65077-7_10

Introduction

Despite improvements in perinatal care, preterm birth remains a significant risk factor for long-term neurodevelopmental problems. In particular, very preterm infants have a high risk of cerebral palsy and also of altered cognitive development, with several nationwide population-based follow-up studies reporting that such disorder occurs in nearly 40% of very or extremely preterm infants (Larroque et al., 2008, Marlow, Wolke, Bracewell, & Samara, 2005). Although survival of these infants without disability has improved in the past decade (Moore et al., 2012), a broader view of all the neurodevelopmental challenges these infants face is now available. Thus, many studies have highlighted the risk of psychiatric disorders in these infants, such as autism spectrum disorder, in which there are alterations of early communication skills, and learning disabilities. The seminal work of Limperopoulos et al. reported a high prevalence of a positive initial screening for autism spectrum disorders in survivors of extreme prematurity (Limperopoulos et al., 2008). Although the tools used to screen for these disorders have been discussed, other studies have confirmed the findings of Limperopoulos et al., especially in extremely preterm infants (Johnson et al., 2010).

The mechanism(s) responsible for psychiatric disorders in this population may include cognitive impairment and early traumatic experiences, events that impact children and parents. The risk for this condition appears to be specific to symptoms and disorders associated with inattention and social and communication problems, and manifests as a significantly higher prevalence of emotional disorders (Johnson & Wolke, 2013). In line with these neurodevelopmental morbidities, vulnerable preterm infants also have increased risk of disorders in speech and language development. A meta-analysis of large-scale follow-up studies reported these problems in more than one-quarter of such infants (Barre, Morgan, Doyle, & Anderson, 2011). Adequate early forms of communication and language competencies are essential for development of skills in interpersonal communication and social interaction. Language delay may also be associated with additional neurodevelopmental morbidities. Poor language skills negatively affect school success and long-term developmental progress and can also adversely affect the quality of social interactions (McCabe & Meller, 2004).

Although, there is a need to fully understand the nature of the specific language impairments in this population to improve detection of these disorders, it is also essential to implement early interventions for infants with language difficulties to improve their long-term outcomes.

Infants develop other forms of communication before language (see Gratier, Devouche, Chap. 4). Language can be divided into different categories and subdomains, and language development can be assessed by different tests (Barre et al., 2011). Infants begin early language development by listening to others, and then they begin to talk. Listening to voices is critical for the development of early forms of communication and speech. Here, we summarize the nature and factors associated with communication and language delays in preterm infants and then discuss the potential of early maternal vocal contact as a strategy to promote language development in very preterm infants.

Communication Disorders and Language Delays in Preterm Infants

The aim of this first section is to identify and discuss the factors related to communication and language delays in preterm infants. During the process of language acquisition, early markers of general communication disorders can appear during the first months of life.

Ontogeny of Communication and Preterm Birth

Several components define social or communicative behaviors, such as vocalizations, facial expressions, gaze direction, and the capacity to coordinate these expressive behaviors during interactions with others. An infant learns these precursors of language based on rules of communication, such as reciprocal turn taking and shared timing and synchrony, through early social exchanges, and these are indices of co-regulation between adults and infants (Brazelton, Tronick, Adamson, Als, & Wise, 1975). Young infants develop a complex communication system within the first months of life. During development, they learn to coordinate their expressive behaviors between different modalities, such as vocalizations with mutual gazes at caregivers, and into specific patterns and thereby develop interactive and expressive competencies before the onset of speech (Yale, Messinger, Cobo-Lewis, & Delgado, 2003).

Within the first months of life, infants begin to organize patterns of shared social and interactive rhythms with sensitive parents or caregivers (Stern, Beebe, Jaffe, & Bennett, 1977). This parent-infant synchrony is central for the development of an infant's socio-emotional and cognitive capacities (Feldman & Eidelman, 2004).

Typical Synchrony in Communication

Synchrony between parents and infants, defined as the temporal coordination of microlevel social behaviors, follows from shared and repetitive rhythmic sequences (Bernieri & Rosenthal, 1991). Precursors of synchrony are evident in the first hours after birth and consist of gestures, postures, gazes, and vocalizations (Trevarthen, Chap. 1; Gratier, Devouche, Chap. 4). This suggests that humans are "wired" to engage in coordinated interactions, presumably because these interactions are essential for survival.

The different parameters of synchrony are useful in predicting infant development, because they shape the child's social-emotional and cognitive development. Synchrony correlates with better attachment behavior in 1-year-olds, with lower levels of behavioral problems in 2-year-olds, and with infant-directed and symbolic expression and several indices of self-regulation (Feldman, 2007).

As thoroughly described in Chap. 1, parents and infants gradually learn to achieve synchrony in their mutual exchanges as the infant develops. However, certain high-risk events, such as preterm birth, can disrupt the normal development of these interactions.

Lack of Synchrony due to Prematurity: An Early Marker of Communicative Delays

Preterm infants typically have different forms of communication than infants born at full term. Dyads with full-term infants show higher coherence than those with preterm infants at 3 and 5 months of age, and full-term infants more often led these interactions at both ages (Lester, Hoffman, & Brazelton, 1985). Parents often have difficulty reading the behaviors and emotional signals of premature infants (Eckerman, Oehler, Medvin, & Hannan, 1994), and these infants have limited ability to tolerate face-to-face interactions during a calm and awake state (Eckerman, Hsu, Molitor, Leung, & Goldstein, 1999). The preterm infant's biological dysregulation affects parental behavior, and parents are less coherent with infant displays during their interactions. Early contact experiences, such skin-to-skin contact (SSC), can modify these patterns into more cohesive styles. This leads mothers and fathers to be more sensitive and less intrusive and infants to exhibit a less negative affect (Feldman, Weller, Sirota, & Eidelman, 2003).

Prematurity has a negative impact on the bonding and attachment process between parents and infants for multiple reasons (Welch & Ludwig, Chap. 15). Thus, via shared vocalizations, gazes, and touch contacts, mothers of premature infants tend to have decreased coordinated social contact with their infants (Lester et al., 1985).

In addition to the different behaviors of mothers of preterm infants, preterm neonates are also less competent at coordinating their social behaviors during their limited moments of calm alertness. Moreover, premature infants have lower synchrony when interacting with their mothers. In fact, both tend to engage in short and frequent mutual gazes that break off soon after initiation (Feldman, 2007). The temporal organization of social interactions is less synchronous and less mutually adaptive in dyads with a preterm infant than those with a full-term infant (Feldman, 2006), and there is debate regarding the etiology of these behaviors.

It is possible that the differences in synchrony of full-term and preterm infants with their parents may explain the subsequent differences in language ability. In other words, when the rhythms of social interaction are disorganized and lack coherence, as with preterm infants, this may disrupt the early steps of learning language.

Language Delays in Preterm Infants and Causal Medical Factors

Preterm infants commonly develop speech and language impairments as they mature (Barre et al., 2011). These impairments include problems with receptive language processing and expressive language production and deficits in phonological memory. These language or phonetic difficulties also indicate general difficulties in cognitive function (Wolke, 2008). Compared to children who were full term, children who were preterm have deficits in vocabulary, semantics, verbal processing, and memory. Premature birth is also associated with delays in receptive and expressive language (Böhm, Katz-Salamon, Smedler, Lagercrantz, & Forssberg, 2002; Vohr et al., 2000). A systematic review showed that preterm infants have lower scores on simple and complex language function tests throughout childhood. The differences in complex language functions of full-term and preterm infants persist during childhood and even increase from 3 to 12 years of age (van Noort-van der Spek, Franken, & Weisglas-Kuperus, 2012). In particular, preterm infants have more deficits in vocabulary, semantics (van Lierde, Roeyers, Boerjan, & De Groote, 2009), verbal processing, and memory (Lee, Yeatman, Luna, & Feldman, 2011) as compared to their peers born at term. Several previous neurophysiological studies have pointed to the possible mechanisms or characterized the problems associated with the difficulties in language function experienced by preterm infants. Thus, problems in auditory discrimination seem to be associated with difficulties in naming objects in 4-year-old children born preterm who had birth weights less than 1500 g (Jansson-Verkasalo et al., 2003, 2004). This decreased auditory discrimination seems linked to difficulties in maintaining active auditory attention, although passive auditory attention seems to be relatively preserved in 5-year-old children who were preterm infants (Dupin, Laurent, Stauder, & Saliba, 2000). In agreement, children who were born preterm also have greater difficulties in vocal perception tasks that require sustained efforts up to the age of 2 years (Bosch, 2011). Another hypothesis is that these infants cannot discriminate phonemes because of deficiencies in specialization for their mother's language. In other words, these infants may have a reduced "perceptual narrowing" for phonemes that are ecologically meaningful: increased discrimination for phonemes from the mother's language and diminished discrimination for phonemes from a foreign language (Jansson-Verkasalo et al., 2010).

Poor language outcomes of preterm infants occur even in the absence of major disabilities, leading to questions regarding their etiology. These could result from the "nosocomial" auditory environment preterm infants that are exposed in the neonatal intensive care unit (NICU) or from early alterations in the neuronal circuits responsible for voice perception and motor language skills.

Insults to the developing brain, such as intraventricular hemorrhage or periventricular leukomalacia, disrupt neural network development and obviously contribute to language deficits. Neurosensory impairment in auditory processing is a well-known cause of speech delay in infants, highlighting the importance of auditory inputs for normal language development. Researchers first assumed that poor language learning in preterm infants was primarily related to socioeconomic factors (Adams-Chapman et al., 2015). However, other research indicated that language difficulties in preterm infants were independent of socioeconomic status (Van Noort-Van der Spek et al., 2012), indicating that preterm birth by itself increases the risk of language deficits. Moreover, language deficits are greater in infants who are more premature. In particular, there is a clear linear relationship between gestational age at birth and subsequent language abilities, and this association persisted after statistical control for child and family factors (Foster-Cohen, Edgin, Champion, & Woodward, 2007). These researchers suggested that alterations in the anatomical and functional development of the premature brain contribute to the language difficulties of preterm infants. Medical factors affecting brain growth and development, such as white matter injuries, certainly have a role (Woodward, Clark, Bora, & Inder, 2012). However, different neonatal white matter abnormalities lead to different language disabilities (Reidy et al., 2013).

Broncho-pulmonary dysplasia (Singer et al., 2001) and severe jaundice with associated hearing disorders (Amin, Orlando, Monczynski, & Tillery, 2015) can disrupt language development. Data regarding the impact of perinatal inflammatory processes, as in chorioamnionitis, are conflicting. A recent meta-analysis (van Vliet, de Kieviet, Oosterlaan, & van Elburg, 2013) and a multicenter longitudinal study of 1194 extremely preterm infants (Pappas et al., 2014) found no relationship between chorioamnionitis and language delay after adjustment for confounding factors. Interestingly, certain therapies can modulate language outcomes in infants with chorioamnionitis. More specifically, the timing of caffeine therapy seems to alter outcome, in that infants given early caffeine therapy had better outcomes than those given later caffeine therapy and no caffeine therapy (Gupte et al., 2016).

Oral motor coordination is necessary for expressive language competencies and good feeding skills. Indeed, there is overlap of the neural pathways involved in eating and language. Previous research reported associations between feeding difficulties and language impairment (assessed using the 3rd edition of the Bayley Scales of Infant and Toddler Development [Bayley III]) in a cohort of 1477 extremely preterm infants (Adams-Chapman et al., 2013). This suggests that feeding difficulties during infancy could help to identify infants who will subsequently develop language difficulties during early childhood.

A recent review concluded that the etiology of language deficits in children who were preterm infants is multifactorial, and is related to "degree of prematurity, neonatal morbidities, illness severity, hearing status, gender, language environment in the neonatal intensive care unit and in the home, maternal education level, social and environmental status of the family, and access to early intervention" (Vohr, 2016). Thus, many factors contribute to the language deficits of extremely preterm infants, with and without hearing loss (Vohr, 2014). Although environmental factors are not the only one involved, the deprivation of biologically meaningful auditory stimuli in preterm infants seems especially important in leading to poor language development.

Hospitalization as a Cause of Distress and Speech Deprivation: Environmental Factors Leading to Language Delays

The environment of the NICU, which can include painful stimuli and high levels of light and noise, can cause distress in preterm infants. These factors may also adversely affect the development of a preterm infant via epigenetic mechanisms (see Montirosso & Provenzi, Chap. 16). Moreover, early experiences play a critical role in shaping the development of the brain and of behavior. There are several critical periods – windows of opportunity – during brain development in premature infants (Lagercrantz, 2016). During these periods, synaptogenesis alters neural connectivity patterns, according to an individual's experiences and responses to the environment (Knudsen, 2004). The brain of a preterm infant does not develop as in the womb, and there are subtle differences in cerebral growth and development relative to a full-term infant (Ment, Hirtz, & Hüppi, 2009). This is due to prematurity itself and to exposure to a different environment (Perlman, 2001).

Among the many environmental factors that can influence language development in hospitalized preterm infants, we focus on two specific components: auditory dys-stimulation in the NICUs (amount, duration, and type) and early maternal/paternal separation.

Auditory Dys-stimulation After Preterm Birth

It is still unknown whether a preterm infant is exposed to too much or too little auditory stimulation during hospitalization, and there are many additional unanswered questions. How much sound is best for promotion of infant language and communicative development? How long should these sounds last? What kinds of sounds are best, and who should deliver these sounds to hospitalized preterm infants? Do preterm infants in the NICU experience acoustical deprivation (Philbin, Chap. 6; Pineda et al., 2012)? Or are they specifically deprived from significant, caring, and contingent visual-tactile-acoustical stimuli?

The NICU has many loud and unpredictable sounds, and these can have detrimental effects on the physiological stability of preterm infants (Kuhn et al., 2012). Even moderate acoustic changes can disrupt the sleep of very preterm infants (Kuhn et al., 2013).

Several studies have evaluated the impact of noise on preterm newborns (Wachman & Lahav, 2011). Noise levels in NICUs are only rarely beneath the threshold set by the American Academy of Pediatrics (45 dBA) (Lasky & Williams, 2009). Moreover, NICUs also have greater levels of high-frequency sounds compared to the womb, and this can negatively impact the anatomical organization of auditory cortical circuits (Lahav & Skoe, 2014). More specifically, an auditory stimulus, such as alarm sound, negatively impacts other sensory functions in premature infants. These sounds may reduce the ability of premature infants to memorize tactile manual information and detect differences between shapes (Lejeune et al., 2016).

Thus, preterm infants in NICUs are simultaneously overexposed to certain sounds but underexposed to the maternal voice relative to the in utero experience. During hospitalization, the preterm infant's exposure to the mother's voice declines dramatically from the prenatal period to the postnatal period (Hofer, 2005). The deprivation of the mother's voice in the NICU during this important period of synaptogenesis and sensitive brain development can impact auditory maturation and potentially impact communicative and language skills (Fifer & Moon, 1994.). During hospitalization, preterm infants hear the talk of medical professionals, often during stressful or painful medical interventions. These preterm infants hear much less infant-directed speech (IDS) in relational-based contexts that focuses on sharing of emotions.

No studies have compared the effects of exposure to direct and indirect speech in the NICU. However, one study showed that exposure to maternal voice recordings with high-pitch modulation increased the rate of nonnutritive sucking in preterm infants (Butler, O'Sullivan, Shah, & Berthier, 2014). This suggests that emotional speaking, which is typical of IDS, can motivate infant responses.

Moreover, talking in a simulated face-to-face situation to very low-birth-weight preterm infants, as opposed to the mere presence of a social partner, can help infants achieve a quiet attentive state (Oehler, Eckerman, & Wilson, 1988) and lead to increased eye opening and more time in an attentive state (Eckerman et al., 1994). To summarize, previous studies that documented the negative impacts of unpredictable and loud noises reinforce the importance of developing environmental measures to lower the sound level in NICUs. On the other hand, preterm infants are sensitive to IDS, so caregivers should provide appropriate multisensory stimuli to these infants in a reciprocal affective co-regulation and active contact. Listening to the mother's voice and integration of vocal, verbal, and facial emotional information provide an optimal environment for emotional exchange with preterm infants (Brück, Kreifelts, & Wildgruber, 2011).

Early Mother-Infant Separation

Historical studies of infants deprived from their parents have documented the detrimental effect this has on their growth and development. Fortunately, there are now very few conditions in which mothers and infants are separated – even for a limited amount of time. However, this still occurs in many NICUs in cases of premature birth. The presence of parents and other family members in European NICUs has increased over the past 10 years, but several barriers remain, particularly in southern European countries (Greisen et al., 2009). Although the continuous presence of a primary caregiver with a preterm infant, from admission to discharge, appears to improve short-term outcome (Örtenstrand et al., 2010), uninterrupted parental presence (24/7) is still rarely implemented, and its long-term effects are not yet established. Prematurity often imposes long periods of separation of mothers and infants, and this early separation can lead to diverse physiological, emotional, and behavioral problems that can persist throughout life.

Exposure to elevated stressors early in life can increase subsequent reactivity to stress in mammals (Maestripieri & Mateo, 2009). In particular, infants with medical problems are more susceptible to elevated stress reactions in response to poor parenting. However, during early stressful experiences, such as pain, the primary caregiver is often absent. The presence of a parent could reinforce an infant's resilience. In the intrauterine life, fetuses experience total closeness with their mothers, and this interaction provides a basis for parent-infant synchrony (Feldman, 2007). This co-regulation is both driven and evidenced by similarities in physiology, such as heart rate and respiration synchrony, regulation of hormones (e.g., oxytocin), and behavioral coordination of communicative patterns.

Unique Effects of the Voices of the Mother and Other People on Development of Communication and Language Skills in Infants

Human Voices, Speech Processing, and Language in Preterm Infants: Neuroscientific and Medical Perspectives

Listening to voices is crucial for language development, as shown by the deleterious effect of hearing loss on language learning. The human voice is the most important sound in our auditory environment because it is a uniquely human signal. The development of language skills is supported by different theories and occurs in several steps early in the infant's life, but these steps are not fully understood (Kuhl, 2004; Gervain & Mehler, 2010). The unique and important role of exposure to voices – particularly the mother's voice – is crucial (Mayberry, Lock, & Kazmi, 2002; May et al., 2011).

Speech Processing and Language Development

Neural and behavioral research studies have shown that exposure to language influences the neural circuitry of infants, even before they can speak their first words (Kuhl, 2010). Other studies showed that language acquisition involves specific neural networks, in which there is a neural commitment early in development. In other words, the basic elements of language, learned initially, are pivotal during critical period for language development (Kuhl, 2004). Neonates can discriminate the sounds of different prosodies and between their own and foreign languages shortly after birth (Moon, Lagercrantz, & Kuhl, 2013). At birth, the newborn's brain can perceive human speech and has the basic ability to process auditory signals (Telkemeyer et al., 2009). In adults, spoken language activates a bilateral frontotemporal network, including the superior temporal sulcus, with a left hemispheric dominance. After initial processing in the auditory cortex, vocal information is processed in dorsal and ventral pathways that are partially dissociated (Belin, Fecteau, & Bedard, 2004).

A brain of a full-term newborn responds to spoken language shortly after birth and uses an auditory language network that is similar to that of adults (Perani et al., 2011), although there are conflicting results regarding hemispheric predominance.

Some studies reported a right predominance, but others reported a left predominance already in full-term newborns (as in adults) following exposure to native language (Sato et al., 2012; Vannasing et al., 2016), infant-directed speech (Peña et al., 2003), and the mother's voice rather than an unfamiliar voice (Beauchemin et al., 2010). Taken together, all these studies argue for an essential biological basis for language acquisition early in the postnatal life. Other research also confirmed left hemisphere dominance in 2-month-old healthy newborns (Dehaene-Lambertz, Dehaene, & Hertz-Pannier, 2002). Moreover, the mother's voice, but not unfamiliar voices, triggers activity in other emotion-processing areas and in the left posterior temporal areas (Dehaene-Lambertz et al., 2010). This finding strongly suggests the mother's voice plays a special role in infants of this age in that it shapes early posterior language areas, especially in the left hemispheric language network.

Many studies of preterm infants indicate they have perceptual abilities and are attracted to the mother's voice (see Kuhn et al., Chap. 7). Cortical responses in the temporal and frontal areas, similar to those noted above, recorded using functional near-infrared spectroscopy (fNIRS) in preterm infants at ~30 weeks post-menstrual age, indicate these infants can discriminate two syllables (/ba/ vs. /ga/). Responses to novel male and female voices were also present but were more limited (Mahmoudzadeh et al., 2013). Using the same paradigm and high-density event-related potentials, these authors recently confirmed that early language processing networks are functional in infants born 10 weeks before term (Mahmoudzadeh, Wallois, Kongolo, Goudjil, & Dehaene-Lambertz, 2016). However, in this study of 19 very preterm infants, mismatch responses were more present and were precisely time-locked to event onset for changes in syllables, rather than changes in voices. The authors concluded that "human infants possess a strong genetic endowment to process speech features" and that the presence of these early networks before term constitutes a "functional intrinsic envelope" that can be "refined by exposure to a specific linguistic environment or impaired in the case of deprivation or inappropriate stimulation such as incubator noise." Despite the immaturity of the auditory pathways, a daily 3 h exposure to maternal sounds during the first postnatal month increased the width of the auditory cortex of 20 very preterm infants relative to controls, suggesting that the mother's voice can elicit auditory plasticity in the human auditory brain (Webb, Heller, Benson, & Lahav, 2015). Although there is still limited knowledge on how genetic and environmental factors interact during language development, researchers now acknowledge that both of these factors are important (Gervain, 2015).

Exposure to Human Voices, NICU Design, and Language Development

Consideration of the sensory part of language development indicates that exposure to human voices is crucial, as confirmed by an elegant prospective follow-up study of very preterm infants starting in the NICU. In particular, researchers recorded spontaneous vocalizations, the amount of adult word exposure, and the extent of reciprocal conversational turns in 36 preterm infants (at 32 and 36 weeks of post-menstrual age) who had a mean gestational age of 27 weeks (range: 23–30) (Caskey, Stephens, Tucker, & Vohr, 2011). Greater exposure to adult talk correlated with more conversational turns, and this association was stronger for parental talk. At 7 and 18 months of age, language competencies and cognitive development (assessed using Bayley III) correlated positively with the adult word counts at 32 and 36 weeks, respectively. This supports the view that a preterm infant's exposure to adult words in the NICU before term equivalent age is associated with better cognitive, language, and communicative development during toddlerhood (Caskey, Stephens, Tucker, & Vohr, 2014). Studies evaluating the impact of NICU design (single family room, private room, or open-bay NICU) on the development of preterm infants support this view. In particular, private rooms in which there was very little parental presence and infant holding correlated with reduced hemispheric asymmetry at term in the language processing areas (temporal sulcus) and with worse language skills at 2 years of age (Pineda et al., 2014). This is presumably due to sensory deprivation and the lack of exposure to parents. However, other studies showed that single family rooms, rather than open-bay NICUs, were associated with greater maternal presence and involvement and with better neurobehavioral and medical outcomes in infants whose gestational ages were below 30 weeks (Lester et al., 2014). Whatever the NICU design, high maternal involvement with skin-to-skin contact correlated with improved 18-month neurodevelopmental outcome (higher language composite and better expressive and receptive communication scores on the Bayley III). This was especially the case for infants cared for in single family rooms that supported high maternal involvement (Lester et al., 2016).

To conclude, the preterm infant's brain, although immature, appears able to process speech. Exposure to adult talk, especially from the mother or father, has the potential to enhance their development of language and communication.

Psychosocial Arguments Supporting Early Vocal Contact to Improve Communication and Language in Preterm Infants

Early exposure to the mother's voice can improve a preterm infant's overall learning experience, including learning of language and cognitive development. Preterm infants are particularly sensitive to the sounds of language, such as adult talk and the sound of their mother's voice. They react to emotional voices, and the mother's voice can regulate the preterm infant's behavior by increasing its emotional and infant-directed features (Butler et al., 2014). The mother's live voice is emotional, and it regulates infant state changes and behavioral displays (Filippa, Gratier, Devouche, & Grandjean, 2017), and the emotional tone of maternal utterances can activate the neonate's brain.

Early forms of affective communication, which begin very early during extra-uterine life and continue after birth, are fundamental for the reciprocal regulation of human beings and are important early forms of learning.

Table 10.1 tentatively summarizes the typical psychosocial conditions in the NICU and in an optimal environment, in which a preterm infant can learn communicative and linguistic skills, with particular attention to the fundamental role of the mother's voice. This table summarizes our view that the environments of many NICUs can detrimentally affect language development in preterm infants.

Table 10.1 Psychosocial characteristics of preterm infants in a typical NICU compared with an optimal environment for acquiring language skills

	Typical NICU	Optimal environment
Exposure to infant-directed speech	Hearing sounds that are not meaningful and limited exposure to the voices of the mother and family	Hearing-sensitive infant-directed speech (IDS) and songs since birth improves language acquisition, word segmentation, vocalization, and social contact
Indirect exposure to voices of adults and siblings	Indirect exposure is often associated with painful/stressful medical procedures. Indirect conversations may be helpful if they are not too loud	Infants are inadvertent observers of adult voices, indicating the presence of social partners. Nearby adult and sibling voices, not specifically directed to infants, are common, potentially aiding language learning and more complex behavior
Social context	A fragmented social context due to the presence of strangers (medical and nursing staff) and limited presence of the mother	Early mastery of communication, prelinguistic, and linguistic skills, with learning in a social context
Multisensory experience of voices	Sources of sounds are often not evident. Few opportunities to match sounds with their visual and tactile referents	Auditory experiences typically lead to orienting responses and turning toward the sound source. Social events provide sensory redundancy (audiovisual speech). Parents and other caretakers provide a social context that contains amodal redundancy of the tactile, auditory, and visual sensory systems
Meaningful auditory experience	Repeated and continuous exposure to sounds that are not meaningful and possibly detrimental	Parents act as mediators between infants and the sound environment and provide biologically relevant sounds
Reciprocity and early co-regulation	Early separation and limited exposure to parents	Reciprocal early regulation, adjustment behaviors, responses and reciprocal adaptation, and progressive construction of a microhabitat. Key elements of a natural social and communicative intimate environment are present

Conclusion

Children born prematurely may have difficulty learning language because of difficulties in establishing early social interactions with their parents. Early contact with a caregiver's live voice is essential for normal communicative and language development, especially during this sensitive period of brain growth. There are complex relationships between early vocal contact, especially the mother's voice, with contingent social interactions that involve infant-directed speech, and early communicative competencies. Preterm infants have a biologic need for timed sensory exposures to speech. Genetic and environmental factors affect an infant's social and communicative abilities, and their inherited cognitive and behavioral abilities are affected by the environment. Appropriate multimodal experiences with a parent may be the best intervention to promote language development in preterm infants. Models of interventions that are based on the biology of mother-infant early interactions may help determine the appropriate amount and timing of interventions. Early interventions in infants with language difficulties can be beneficial (Law, Garrett, & Nye, 2008; Girolametto, Wiigs, Smyth, Weitzman, & Pearce, 2001). Early vocal contact with the mother or father appears to be essential for normal language development. However, scientific data that support this specific hypothesis are needed. Several studies that will directly test this hypothesis are currently being planned or in progress. Early interventions that may help sustain parent-infant synchronization include methods that employ face-to-face vocal and affective contact delivered in close proximity, as during skin-to-skin contact.

Key Messages
- Vulnerable preterm infants have increased risk of disorders in communicative and language development, mainly due to medical and environmental factors.
- Auditory dys-stimulation and mother-infant separation can have detrimental effects on preterm infants' communicative and language development.
- Better cognitive, language, and communicative development of preterm infants are linked to exposure to human voices.
- Appropriate multimodal experiences with a parent, including methods that employ face-to-face vocal and affective contact delivered in close proximity, may be the best early intervention to promote language development in preterm infants.

References

Adams-Chapman, I., Bann, C. M., Vaucher, Y. E., Stoll, B. J., & Eunice Kennedy Shriver National Institute of Child Health. (2013). Human Development (NICHD) Neonatal Research Network (NRN). Association between feeding difficulties and language delay in preterm infants using Bayley Scales of Infant Development. *The Journal of Pediatrics, 163*, 680–685.

Adams-Chapman, I., Bann, C., Carter, S. L., Stoll, B. J., & Neonatal Research Network, N. I. C. H. D. (2015). Language outcomes among ELBW infants in early childhood. *Early Human Development, 91*(6), 373–379.

Amin, S. B., Orlando, M., Monczynski, C., & Tillery, K. (2015). Central auditory processing disorder profile in premature and term infants. *American Journal of Perinatology, 32*(04), 399–404.

Barre, N., Morgan, A., Doyle, L. W., & Anderson, P. J. (2011). Language abilities in children who were very preterm and/or very low birth weight: A meta-analysis. *The Journal of Pediatrics, 158*(5), 766–774.

Beauchemin, M., González-Frankenberger, B., Tremblay, J., Vannasing, P., Martínez-Montes, E., Belin, P., ... & Lassonde, M. (2010). Mother and stranger: an electrophysiological study of voice processing in newborns. *Cerebral Cortex.*, bhq242.

Belin, P., Fecteau, S., & Bedard, C. (2004). Thinking the voice: Neural correlates of voice perception. *Trends in Cognitive Sciences, 8*(3), 129–135.

Bernieri, F., & Rosenthal, R. (1991). Interpersonal coordination: Behavior matching and interactional synchrony. In R. Feldman & B. Rime (Eds.), *Fundamentals of nonverbal behavior* (pp. 401–432). Cambridge, UK: Cambridge University press.

Böhm, B., Katz-Salamon, M., Smedler, A. C., Lagercrantz, H., & Forssberg, H. (2002). Developmental risks and protective factors for influencing cognitive outcome at 5½ years of age in very-low-birth-weight children. *Developmental Medicine and Child Neurology, 44*(08), 508–516.

Bosch, L. (2011). Precursors to language in preterm infants: Speech perception abilities in the first year of life. *Progress in Brain Research, 189*, 239–257.

Brazelton, T. B., Tronick, E., Adamson, L., Als, H., & Wise, S. (1975). Early mother-infant reciprocity. *Parent-Infant Interaction, 3*, 137.

Brück, C., Kreifelts, B., & Wildgruber, D. (2011). Emotional voices in context: A neurobiological model of multimodal affective information processing. *Physics of Life Reviews, 8*(4), 383–403.

Butler, S. C., O'Sullivan, L. P., Shah, B. L., & Berthier, N. E. (2014). Preference for infant-directed speech in preterm infants. *Infant Behavior & Development, 37*(4), 505–511.

Caskey, M., Stephens, B., Tucker, R., & Vohr, B. (2011). Importance of parent talk on the development of preterm infant vocalizations. *Pediatrics, 128*(5), 910–916.

Caskey, M., Stephens, B., Tucker, R., & Vohr, B. (2014). Adult talk in the NICU with preterm infants and developmental outcomes. *Pediatrics, 133*(3), e578–e584.

Dehaene-Lambertz, G., Dehaene, S., & Hertz-Pannier, L. (2002). Functional neuroimaging of speech perception in infants. *Science, 298*(5600), 2013–2015.

Dehaene-Lambertz, G., Montavont, A., Jobert, A., Allirol, L., Dubois, J., Hertz-Pannier, L., & Dehaene, S. (2010). Language or music, mother or Mozart? Structural and environmental influences on infants' language networks. *Brain and Language, 114*(2), 53–65.

Dupin, R., Laurent, J. P., Stauder, J. E., & Saliba, E. (2000). Auditory attention processing in 5-year-old children born preterm: Evidence from event-related potentials. *Developmental Medicine and Child Neurology, 42*(7), 476–480.

Eckerman, C. O., Hsu, H. C., Molitor, A., Leung, E. H., & Goldstein, R. F. (1999). Infant arousal in an en-face exchange with a new partner: Effects of prematurity and perinatal biological risk. *Developmental Psychology, 35*(1), 282.

Eckerman, C. O., Oehler, J. M., Medvin, M. B., & Hannan, T. E. (1994). Premature newborns as social partners before term age. *Infant Behavior & Development, 17*(1), 55–70.

Feldman, R. (2006). From biological rhythms to social rhythms: Physiological precursors of mother-infant synchrony. *Developmental Psychology, 42*(1), 175.

Feldman, R. (2007). Parent–infant synchrony and the construction of shared timing; physiological precursors, developmental outcomes, and risk conditions. *Journal of Child Psychology and Psychiatry, 48*(3–4), 329–354.

Feldman, R., & Eidelman, A. I. (2004). Parent–infant synchrony and the social – Emotional development of triplets. *Developmental Psychology, 40*, 1133–1147.

Feldman, R., Weller, A., Sirota, L., & Eidelman, A. I. (2003). Testing a family intervention hypothesis: The contribution of mother-infant skin-to-skin contact (kangaroo care) to family interaction, proximity, and touch. *Journal of Family Psychology, 17*(1), 94.

Fifer, W. P., & Moon, C. M. (1994). The role of mother's voice in the organization of brain function in the newborn. *Acta Paediatrica. Supplement, 397*, 86e93.

Filippa, M., Gratier, M., Devouche, E., Grandjean, D., (2017). *Changes in infant-directed speech and song are related to preterm infant facial expression in the neonatal intensive care unit.*

Foster-Cohen, S., Edgin, J. O., Champion, P. R., & Woodward, L. J. (2007). Early delayed language development in very preterm infants: Evidence from the MacArthur-Bates CDI. *Journal of Child Language, 34*(3), 655.

Gervain, J. (2015). Plasticity in early language acquisition: The effects of prenatal and early childhood experience. *Current Opinion in Neurobiology, 35*, 13–20.

Gervain, J., & Mehler, J. (2010). Speech perception and language acquisition in the first year of life. *Annual Review of Psychology, 61*, 191–218.

Girolametto, L., Wiigs, M., Smyth, R., Weitzman, E., & Pearce, P. S. (2001). Children with a history of expressive vocabulary delay outcomes at 5 years of age. *American Journal of Speech-Language Pathology, 10*(4), 358–369.

Greisen, G., Mirante, N., Haumont, D., Pierrat, V., Pallás-Alonso, C. R., Warren, I., ... Cuttini, M. (2009). Parents, siblings and grandparents in the Neonatal Intensive Care Unit A survey of policies in eight European countries. *Acta Paediatrica, 98*(11), 1744–1750.

Hofer, M. A. (2005). The psychobiology of early attachment. *Clinical Neuroscience Research, 4*(5-6 spec iss), 291–300.

Jansson-Verkasalo, E., Ceponiene, R., Kielinen, M., Suominen, K., Jäntti, V., Linna, S. L., ... Näätänen, R. (2003). Deficient auditory processing in children with Asperger syndrome, as indexed by event-related potentials. *Neuroscience Letters, 338*(3), 197–200.

Jansson-Verkasalo, E., Korpilahti, P., Jäntti, V., Valkama, M., Vainionpää, L., Alku, P., ... Näätänen, R. (2004). Neurophysiologic correlates of deficient phonological representations and object naming in prematurely born children. *Clinical Neurophysiology, 115*(1), 179–187.

Jansson-Verkasalo, E., Ruusuvirta, T., Huotilainen, M., Alku, P., Kushnerenko, E., Suominen, K., ... Hallman, M. (2010). Atypical perceptual narrowing in prematurely born infants is associated with compromised language acquisition at 2 years of age. *BMC Neuroscience, 11*(1), 88.

Johnson, S., Hollis, C., Kochhar, P., Hennessy, E., Wolke, D., & Marlow, N. (2010). Psychiatric disorders in extremely preterm children: Longitudinal finding at age 11 years in the EPICure study. *Journal of the American Academy of Child and Adolescent Psychiatry, 49*(5), 453–463.

Johnson, S., & Wolke, D. (2013). Behavioural outcomes and psychopathology during adolescence. *Early Human Development, 89*(4), 199–207.

Knudsen, E. I. (2004). Sensitive periods in the development of the brain and behavior. *Journal of Cognitive Neuroscience, 16*(8), 1412–1425.

Kuhl, P. K. (2004). Early language acquisition: Cracking the speech code. *Nature Reviews Neuroscience, 5*(11), 831–843.

Kuhl, P. K. (2010). Brain mechanisms in early language acquisition. *Neuron, 67*(5), 713–727.

Kuhn, P., Zores, C., Langlet, C., Escande, B., Astruc, D., & Dufour, A. (2013). Moderate acoustic changes can disrupt the sleep of very preterm infants in their incubators. *Acta Paediatrica, 102*(10), 949–954.

Kuhn, P., Zores, C., Pebayle, T., Hoeft, A., Langlet, C., Escande, B., ... Dufour, A. (2012). Infants born very preterm react to variations of the acoustic environment in their incubator from a minimum signal-to-noise ratio threshold of 5 to 10 dBA. *Pediatric Research, 71*(4–1), 386–392.

Lagercrantz, H. (2016). *Infant brain development: Formation of the mind and the emergence of consciousness.* Cham, Switzerland: Springer.

Lahav, A., & Skoe, E. (2014). An acoustic gap between the NICU and womb: A potential risk for compromised neuroplasticity of the auditory system in preterm infants. *Frontiers in Neuroscience, 8*, 381.

Larroque, B., Ancel, P. Y., Marret, S., Marchand, L., André, M., Arnaud, C., ... Burguet, A. (2008). Neurodevelopmental disabilities and special care of 5-year-old children born before 33 weeks of gestation (the EPIPAGE study): A longitudinal cohort study. *The Lancet, 371*(9615), 813–820.

Lasky, R. E., & Williams, A. L. (2009). Noise and light exposures for extremely low birth weight newborns during their stay in the neonatal intensive care unit. *Pediatrics, 123*(2), 540–546.

Law, J., Garrett, Z., & Nye, C. (2008). Speech and language therapy interventions for children with primary speech and language delay or disorder (review). *The Cochrane Collaboration, 1*, 1–62.

Lee, E. S., Yeatman, J. D., Luna, B., & Feldman, H. M. (2011). Specific language and reading skills in school-aged children and adolescents are associated with prematurity after controlling for IQ. *Neuropsychologia, 49*(5), 906–913.

Lejeune, F., Parra, J., Berne-Audéoud, F., Marcus, L., Barisnikov, K., Gentaz, E., & Debillon, T. (2016). Sound interferes with the early tactile manual abilities of preterm infants. *Scientific Reports, 6*.

Lester, B. M., Hawes, K., Abar, B., Sullivan, M., Miller, R., Bigsby, R., ... Padbury, J. F. (2014). Single-family room care and neurobehavioral and medical outcomes in preterm infants. *Pediatrics, 134*(4), 754–760.

Lester, B. M., Hoffman, J., & Brazelton, T. B. (1985). The rhythmic structure of mother-infant interaction in term and preterm infants. *Child Development, 56*, 15–27.

Lester, B. M., Salisbury, A. L., Hawes, K., Dansereau, L. M., Bigsby, R., Laptook, A., ... Padbury, J. F. (2016). 18-Month follow-up of infants cared for in a single-family room neonatal intensive care unit. *The Journal of Pediatrics, 177*, 84–89.

Limperopoulos, C., Bassan, H., Sullivan, N. R., Soul, J. S., Robertson, R. L., Moore, M., ... du Plessis, A. J. (2008). Positive screening for autism in ex-preterm infants: Prevalence and risk factors. *Pediatrics, 121*(4), 758–765.

Maestripieri, D., & Mateo, J. M. (Eds.). (2009). *Maternal effects in mammals*. Chicago, IL: University of Chicago Press.

Mahmoudzadeh, M., Dehaene-Lambertz, G., Fournier, M., Kongolo, G., Goudjil, S., Dubois, J., ... Wallois, F. (2013). Syllabic discrimination in premature human infants prior to complete formation of cortical layers. *Proceedings of the National Academy of Sciences, 110*(12), 4846–4851.

Mahmoudzadeh, M., Wallois, F., Kongolo, G., Goudjil, S., & Dehaene-Lambertz, G. (2016). Functional maps at the onset of auditory inputs in very early preterm human neonates. *Cerebral Cortex.*, bhw103.

Marlow, N., Wolke, D., Bracewell, M. A., & Samara, M. (2005). Neurologic and developmental disability at six years of age after extremely preterm birth. *New England Journal of Medicine, 352*(1), 9–19.

May, L., Byers-Heinlein, K., Gervain, J., & Werker, J. F. (2011). Language and the newborn brain: Does prenatal language experience shape the neonate neural response to speech? *Frontiers in Psychology, 2*, 222.

Mayberry, R. I., Lock, E., & Kazmi, H. (2002). Development: Linguistic ability and early language exposure. *Nature, 417*(6884), 38–38.

McCabe, P. C., & Meller, P. J. (2004). The relationship between language and social competence: How language impairment affects social growth. *Psychology in the Schools, 41*(3), 313–321.

Ment, L. R., Hirtz, D., & Hüppi, P. S. (2009). Imaging biomarkers of outcome in the developing preterm brain. *The Lancet Neurology, 8*(11), 1042–1055.

Moon, C., Lagercrantz, H., & Kuhl, P. K. (2013). Language experienced in utero affects vowel perception after birth: A two-country study. *Acta Paediatrica, 102*(2), 156–160.

Moore, T., Hennessy, E. M., Myles, J., Johnson, S. J., Draper, E. S., Costeloe, K. L., & Marlow, N. (2012). Neurological and developmental outcome in extremely preterm children born in England in 1995 and 2006: The EPICure studies. *BMJ, 345*, e7961.

Oehler, J. M., Eckerman, C. O., & Wilson, W. H. (1988). Social stimulation and the regulation of premature infants' state prior to term age. *Infant Behavior & Development, 11*(3), 333.

Örtenstrand, A., Westrup, B., Broström, E. B., Sarman, I., Åkerström, S., Brune, T., ... & Waldenström, U. (2010). The Stockholm Neonatal Family Centered Care Study: effects on length of stay and infant morbidity. *Pediatrics.*, peds-2009.

Pappas, A., Kendrick, D. E., Shankaran, S., Stoll, B. J., Bell, E. F., Laptook, A. R., ... Higgins, R. D. (2014). Chorioamnionitis and early childhood outcomes among extremely low-gestational-age neonates. *JAMA Pediatrics, 168*(2), 137–147.

Peña, M., Maki, A., Kovačić, D., Dehaene-Lambertz, G., Koizumi, H., Bouquet, F., & Mehler, J. (2003). Sounds and silence: An optical topography study of language recognition at birth. *Proceedings of the National Academy of Sciences, 100*(20), 11702–11705.

Perani, D., Saccuman, M. C., Scifo, P., Anwander, A., Spada, D., Baldoli, C., ... Friederici, A. D. (2011). Neural language networks at birth. *Proceedings of the National Academy of Sciences, 108*(38), 16056–16061.

Perlman, J. M. (2001). Neurobehavioral deficits in premature graduates of intensive care— Potential medical and neonatal environmental risk factors. *Pediatrics, 108*(6), 1339–1348.

Pineda, R. G., Stransky, K. E., Rogers, C., Duncan, M. H., Smith, G. C., Neil, J., et al. (2012). The single-patient room in the NICU: Maternal and family effects. *Journal of Perinatology, 32*, 545–551.

Pineda, R. G., Neil, J., Dierker, D., Smyser, C. D., Wallendorf, M., Kidokoro, H., ... Van Essen, D. C. (2014). Alterations in brain structure and neurodevelopmental outcome in preterm infants hospitalized in different neonatal intensive care unit environments. *The Journal of Pediatrics, 164*(1), 52–60.

Reidy, N., Morgan, A., Thompson, D. K., Inder, T. E., Doyle, L. W., & Anderson, P. J. (2013). Impaired language abilities and white matter abnormalities in children born very preterm and/ or very low birth weight. *The Journal of Pediatrics, 162*(4), 719–724.

Sato, H., Hirabayashi, Y., Tsubokura, H., Kanai, M., Ashida, T., Konishi, I., ... Maki, A. (2012). Cerebral hemodynamics in newborn infants exposed to speech sounds: A whole-head optical topography study. *Human Brain Mapping, 33*(9), 2092–2103.

Singer, L. T., Siegel, A. C., Lewis, B., Hawkins, S., Yamashita, T., & Baley, J. (2001). Preschool language outcomes of children with history of bronchopulmonary dysplasia and very low birth weight. *Journal of Developmental & Behavioral Pediatrics, 22*(1), 19–26.

Stern, D. N., Beebe, B., Jaffe, J., & Bennett, S. L. (1977). The infant's stimulus world during social interaction: A study of caregiver behaviors with particular reference to repetition and timing. *Studies in Mother-Infant Interaction*, 177–202.

Telkemeyer, S., Rossi, S., Koch, S. P., Nierhaus, T., Steinbrink, J., Poeppel, D., ... Wartenburger, I. (2009). Sensitivity of newborn auditory cortex to the temporal structure of sounds. *Journal of Neuroscience, 29*(47), 14726–14733.

van Lierde, K. M., Roeyers, H., Boerjan, S., & De Groote, I. (2009). Expressive and receptive language characteristics in three-year-old preterm children with extremely low birth weight. *Folia Phoniatrica et Logopaedica, 61*(5), 296–299.

van Noort-van der Spek, I. L., Franken, M. C., & Weisglas-Kuperus, N. (2012). Language functions in preterm-born children: A systematic review and meta-analysis. *Pediatrics, 129*, 745–754.

van Vliet, E. O., de Kieviet, J. F., Oosterlaan, J., & van Elburg, R. M. (2013). Perinatal infections and neurodevelopmental outcome in very preterm and very low-birth-weight infants: A meta-analysis. *JAMA Pediatrics, 167*(7), 662–668.

Vannasing, P., Florea, O., González-Frankenberger, B., Tremblay, J., Paquette, N., Safi, D., ... Gallagher, A. (2016). Distinct hemispheric specializations for native and non-native languages in one-day-old newborns identified by fNIRS. *Neuropsychologia, 84*, 63–69.

Vohr, B. (2014). Speech and language outcomes of very preterm infants. *Seminars in Fetal and Neonatal Medicine, 19*(2), 78–83.

Vohr, B. R. (2016). Language and hearing outcomes of preterm infants. *Seminars in Perinatology, 40*(8), 510–519.

Vohr, B. R., Wright, L. L., Dusick, A. M., Mele, L., Verter, J., Steichen, J. J., ... Delaney-Black, V. (2000). Neurodevelopmental and functional outcomes of extremely low birth weight infants in the National Institute of Child Health and Human Development Neonatal Research Network, 1993–1994. *Pediatrics, 105*(6), 1216–1226.

Wachman, E. M., & Lahav, A. (2011). The effects of noise on preterm infants in the NICU. *Archives of Disease in Childhood - Fetal and Neonatal Edition, 96*(4), F305–F309.

Webb, A. R., Heller, H. T., Benson, C. B., & Lahav, A. (2015). Mother's voice and heartbeat sounds elicit auditory plasticity in the human brain before full gestation. *Proceedings of the National Academy of Sciences, 112*(10), 3152–3157.

Wolke, D., Samara, M., Bracewell, M., Marlow, N., & EPICure Study Group. (2008). Specific language difficulties and school achievement in children born at 25 weeks of gestation or less. *The Journal of Pediatrics, 152*(2), 256–262.

Woodward, L. J., Clark, C. A., Bora, S., & Inder, T. E. (2012). Neonatal white matter abnormalities an important predictor of neurocognitive outcome for very preterm children. *PLoS One, 7*(12), e51879.

Yale, M. E., Messinger, D. S., Cobo-Lewis, A. B., & Delgado, C. F. (2003). The temporal coordination of early infant communication. *Developmental Psychology, 39*(5), 815.

Chapter 11
Recorded Maternal Voice, Recorded Music, or Live Intervention: A Bioecological Perspective

Joy V. Browne

Abstract *Introduction*: The human infant develops in his or her expected bioecological niche based on experience-dependent regulation of physiology, motor control, and arousal, typically provided by close contact with the mother. Synchrony, intensity, tempo, and rhythm of a mother's physical and vocal communication are embedded in what the infant experiences and lay the foundation for attachment relationships and optimal development. Infants who have significant medical issues or are early born experience a different developmental niche than would a typically developing infant. This chapter addresses the complexities of exposure of the newborn in intensive care to different models of intimate caregiving, including the mother's recorded or live voice and recorded or live music, in the context of current knowledge of necessary species-specific, co-regulatory synchronous interactions. Additionally, the chapter explores opportunities and barriers to the provision of optimal mother-infant communication in intensive care.

Aims: The aims of this chapter are to describe foundational developmental science that contributes to our understanding of the components of optimal bioecological niches for developing infants in the NICU and to provide a rationale for promoting optimal intersensory, redundant, synchronous, and rhythmic experiences for the developing infant through the mother's presence. Additionally, an aim of the chapter is to examine current intervention strategies that may or may not provide optimal bioecological niches for developing infants under intensive care.

Conclusions: Developmental science contributes to our emerging understanding of the optimal bioecological niche for the developing infant. Medically fragile and/ or early born infants are thought to have over or underexposure to sensory experiences prompting the addition of live and/or recorded inputs such as the mother's

J.V. Browne, PhD (✉)
University of Colorado, School of Medicine, Center for Family
& Infant Interaction, Aurora, CO, USA

Fielding Graduate University Santa Barbara, Santa Barbara, CA, USA
e-mail: joy.browne@childrenscolorado.org

© Springer International Publishing AG 2017   183
M. Filippa et al. (eds.), *Early Vocal Contact and Preterm Infant Brain Development*, DOI 10.1007/978-3-319-65077-7_11

voice or music and other multisensory stimulation approaches. Research on such interventions has begun to explore their benefits and/or challenges, but findings are not consistently conclusive. From a developmental science and clinical research perspective, the likely most optimal niche for the developing infant is the mother's body and voice. NICU practices that encourage mothers to be with and communicate with their baby need to be promoted.

Underpinnings of an Ecological Perspective

The Infant's Ecological Niche

All human infants are born within the context of his or her parents, the extended family and the culture in which they live. The "developmental niche" is a framework for understanding the cultural microenvironment of the baby. Three subsystems have been identified and are used to understand the child's functioning within his or her personal developmental niche: the physical and social setting, customs of child care, and psychology of the caregivers (Super & Harkness, 1994). Infants who have significant medical issues or are early born experience a different developmental niche than would a typically developing infant.

Physical and social settings refer to interactions with people who determine the kind of environments infants are exposed to, as well as provision of nurturing social relationships that are elicited by the infant. Infants who experience a newborn intensive care unit (NICU) stay have a vastly different physical environment and social interactions due to medical interventions and specialized hospital care from that of infants who are born to and live in their family home (e.g., lighting, bedding, medical rounds, parental "visiting" restrictions).

Customs of child care are sequences of behavior common to members of the community and so embedded in the larger community that they need no particular rationale or conscious thought. NICU and hospital caregiving is often challenging for the newborn; however, routines and caregiving rituals of the NICU have become regimented and customary (e.g., the "ritual" of bathing infants in the middle of the night, the routine of blood drawn in the early morning hours, or diaper change and vital signs before being fed).

Psychology of the caregivers includes beliefs concerning the nature and needs of children, and the organizing parenting strategies of child rearing. Caregiver psychology provides an immediate structure to the children's development through the meaning it invests in universal behaviors and processes. In the NICU, caregiving may be influenced by different philosophies of care for infants (e.g., the perspective that infants do not perceive pain or infants do not have the capacity for emotions) and the lack of parental presence to guide their own child's caregiving.

The developmental niche of the newborn is embedded in and influenced by both the altered environment in which they live and the customs, rituals, and psychology of their various caregivers.

Gottfried and Gaiter, in their seminal book *Infant Stress Under Intensive Care*, coined the term "environmental neonatology" and stressed the importance of attending to the ecology of the NICU (Gottfried & Gaiter, 1985). In their description of the NICU environment in the 1980s, Linn et al. (Linn, Horowitz, Buddin, Leake, & Fox, 1985) described typical interactions, contingent responses during interactions, and state availability of the infant for communication that constitute the ecology of the newborn in the NICU. These initial studies focused on an aspect of the ecology of the newborn that had not been emphasized previously and began a larger view of the experience of the newborn in the NICU in terms of the impact of the physical and social environment, as well as the caregiving on infant development.

The Bioecological Perspective of Infant Development

Bronfenbrenner is known best for the development of the ecological theory of development that focuses primarily on the context in which a child develops. These include microsystems or the most proximal setting where the child develops; mesosystems, which are made up of two or more microsystems; exosystems which involve the politics and society's social policies; and macrosystems which are composed of economic, social, education, legal, and political systems (Rosa & Tudge, 2013). His shift from the term "ecology" to "bioecology" was to emphasize the participation of the individual in his or her own development (Bronfenbrenner & Ceci, 1994). The central aspect of his theoretical perspective is that of "proximal processes" which are considered the primary driving force in development (Rosa & Tudge, 2013). Proximal processes have four components, those of process, person, context, and time, which work interdependently.

Bronfenbrenner's bioecological framework serves to explain the integration of interactions of infants in the context of his or her personal characteristics, environment in which they develop, their family interactions, and the larger family culture. The newborn in the NICU can be seen to develop within his or her bioecological context that includes not only their own personal makeup (e.g., temperament, resilience) but also an altered physiological status (e.g., preterm birth, medical complications, reliance on technology). They also are born into a family that is also in an altered psychological state in addition to being in a very unexpected environment and NICU culture. Proximal processes are thus different from what might be expected had the infant been born into a more typical family, environment, and culture.

Experience Expectance and Dependence as a Foundation of Bioecology of the Newborn

Infant development is organized around neurodevelopmental expectations and changes that are either "experience expected" or "experience dependent." Greenough and colleagues (Greenough, Black, & Wallace, 1987) defined "experience expectant" brain development as common to all species, which is organized for expected environmental input. It can be viewed as neural preparation for incorporating specific information, for example, fetal to newborn maternal voice recognition. "Experience-dependent" brain development is when active formation of new synaptic connections is made in response to events that an infant experiences that provide information to be stored, for example, the physical sound environment or the specific vocabulary that a mother uses when she talks to the infant. These constructs are used to further explain the underlying mechanisms for how the infant's brain development has "plasticity" as in the definition of "critical" or "sensitive" periods during which they are sensitive to specific environmental input or lack thereof.

Sensory development of the preterm infant proceeds in a stepwise fashion and, depending on the stage of development they are in, may be impacted by inappropriate, mistimed, or overwhelming sensory inputs. Developing in a cacophonous NICU environment presents challenges to experience-dependent sensory integration (Lickliter, 2011).

Hidden Regulators as the Bioecological Underpinnings of Early Interactions and Attachment

Bioecology of the newborn can serve to explain the context in which infant development occurs. Infant development is most impacted by the microsystem where interactions with parents and caregivers provide physiological, sensory, social, psychological, and cultural foundations for growth. The developmental niche or bioecology of the newborn in the NICU is altered from what might be expected, as their micro- and mesosystems are significantly different from those experienced by the nonhospitalized newborn. One microsystem is that of the physical or "distal" environment such as sound, light, activity, drafts, odors, and visual array. Another is the interactional or "proximal" environment of movement when cared for, tactile sensations of bedding and touch, verbal communication, odor within the bed space, taste of food or medications, and visual opportunities during interaction. Within the proximal microsystem are the more qualitative interactions or proximal processes of nurturing, caring, and emotional and verbal exchange. All microsystems impact the development of the newborn in the NICU, but likely the most essential for their experience expectant brain is the intimate proximal interactions that are offered by the infant's mother and primary caregivers. These interactions can be seen as providing regulation of physiology, state, and movement to the infant and as assuring a sound foundation for later attachment relationships that are essential for optimal development (Bowlby, 1954, 1958, 1968; Hofer, 1994).

Mothers, as the most intimate and important microsystem for the developing infant, provide regulatory mechanisms for infant stability. Hofer (Hofer, 1994) has proposed that many of these regulators are hidden to view and are provided in typical interactions during feeding, play, and caregiving. Hidden regulators control the behavioral, autonomic, endocrine, and sleep-wake states of the infant and thus control the parts of the early emotion states associated with attachment, separation, and loss first described by Bowlby (Bowlby, 1982; Hofer, 1994). Interactions between the mother and infant regulate the infant's behavior and physiology and acts to insure physiological homeostasis and on the neuronal systems underlying behavior. Additionally, as the mother and infant are intimately together, they link their homeostatic systems into even more optimal organization called symbiosis. Symbiosis describes the mutual benefits during close proximity to each other. Loss of these regulatory functions results in changes in function and stability demonstrated through changes in the infant's and/or mother's behavior.

The Sensory Bioecology of the Newborn

During pregnancy, fetuses are developing in the ecological niche of the mother's body, and their sensory systems are primed for experience-dependent learning afforded by the mother's voice, body sounds, movement, day/night cycling, and other physiological exchanges. Sensory developmental preparation of the fetus results in physiological exchange in the newborn that is both familiar to and dependent on the mother's physical closeness. The infant born prior to term typically is separated from the familiarity of the mother's body yet is sensitive and responsive to the sensory environment of the NICU, even though they may not have sensory systems that are as developmentally mature.

Sensory systems do not develop in isolation, but are integrated with other sensory systems. Lickliter (Lickliter, 2011) in his studies of sensory development in avian and human infants proposed that infants utilize information derived from all sensory systems and then use this sensory information to increase the likelihood that events in their environmental niche can be detected, identified, and responded to. Infants, even at a young age, are able to integrate these multisensory inputs in order to make sense of their world, impacting how their brains detect, integrate, and use sensory information. He further describes how infants use amodal information that is not specific to a particular sensory modality but can be detected and used redundantly across multiple senses. These amodal characteristics are evident in most sensory experiences and include rhythm, tempo, synchrony, and prosody. Infants thus use redundancy across sensory systems to further understand their sensory environment.

Bahrick and Lickliter (Bahrick & Lickliter, 2014) proposed that intersensory redundancy is essential during infant development to describe how selective attention is allocated to properties of objects and events. The redundancy hypothesis further describes how the detection of information not specific to any one sense guides selective attention. In this way, infants learn to selectively attend to a vast array of environmental stimulation and multimodal input. The fetus receives multimodal input in utero appropriate to their sensory developmental phase. The infant in the NICU may not receive sensory input appropriate for their developmental stage and in contrast may be either bombarded with unisensory input or multisensory input that is not multimodal or salient, but is a part of their bioecological niche. Additionally, the delivery of the stimulation that preterm infants may experience in the NICU may reduce the amount or availability of intersensory redundancy and thus have repercussions for early sensory integration (Lickliter, 2011). Regardless of the environment in which the infant develops, they are sensitive to and dependent on the salience of the intersensory redundancy and amodal features of the input. As neuronal plasticity is significant in early development, sensory experiences during early development may leave lasting functional and structural brain changes that can influence long-term intersensory interactions.

The bioecology of the NICU lays the groundwork for understanding appropriate and expected sensory experiences within the infant's developmental niche. The experiences are best integrated by interactions afforded by both the physical and cultural and the proximal and relationship environment in which they grow and develop. Thus, the bioecology of the infant within an NICU setting must provide opportunities for the infant to attend to a sensory environment that has both redundancy across sensory modalities and also amodal aspects to their presentation. This means that the infant can benefit best from an environment that has not only auditory, but optimally has visual, kinesthetic, and tactile modalities. Additionally, the infant should be provided an auditory environment that has rhythm, prosody, and tempo, typical during verbal exchanges. Multisensory inputs should also be presented when the infant is able (from an arousal perspective) to manage all of these modalities at the same time without state or physiological decompensation. The optimal provision of sensory redundancy and amodal characteristics is when the mother is holding, touching, moving, talking, and looking at the baby so that the baby can experience redundancy across sensory modalities and experience the feeling of having a "conversation."

The Social Bioecology of the Infant

Proximal interactions between parent and their infant are widely acknowledged to play a central role in influencing a wide array of developmental outcomes. Social competence and emotional regulation emerge from early relationships and provide significant foundational elements for optimal development. Early relationships are enhanced by interactions that are bidirectional between the parent and child and are characterized by verbal and nonverbal communicative and emotional behaviors (such as postures, facial displays, vocalizations, and eye contact). They have the quality of coordination between the members of the dyad, and they share modalities during exchanges (Leclere et al., 2014). Thus, proximal environments such as those that support early interactions and positive relationships between mothers and their infants result in a supportive bioecology for the newborn and, in turn, optimize development.

Synchronous interactions between the mother and their infant provide the most important foundation for early relationship development. Synchrony occurs when the mother's and the child's responses and emotional capacity to respond to each other are maximized. It is a matching of behavior, emotional states, and biological rhythms that forms a single relational unit (Feldman, 2016; Leclere et al., 2014). Synchrony involves mutuality in regulation, reciprocal, flexible exchanges, rhythmicity in interactions, shared behavioral states and affect, and maintained engagement. Interaction synchrony addresses the matching of behavior, affective states, and biological rhythms between the members of the dyad to form a single relational unit. The familiarity of the partner's biobehavioral interaction and rhythms is exquisitely timed for highly aroused as well as comforting moments of interpersonal exchange (Feldman, 2015, 2016; Feldman & Eidelman, 2007; Leclere et al., 2014) which results from consistent and predictable caregiving.

Better mother child synchrony is associated with more positive cognitive and behavioral outcomes. Among preterm infants, opportunities for this shared synchrony are often limited, as studies have shown lower coherence during interactions, less mother and infant responsivity, and shorter episodes of gaze synchrony (Censullo, Lester, & Hoffman, 1985; Karger, 1979; Lester, Hoffman, & Brazelton, 1985; Lester et al., 2011). Main causes for the disruption in parent-infant synchrony among prematurely born infants relate to the baby's difficulties with physiological regulation and scant attention availability.

Imbedded in synchronous interactions is emotional exchange between mother and baby. The integration of vocal, verbal, and facial emotional information in a given situation provides the infant a context for emotional exchange (Bruck, Kreifelts, & Wildgruber, 2011). Processing of emotional exchanges associated with the perception of auditory and visual emotional signals includes extraction and integration of auditory and visual information into a single perception in the brain. Nonverbal vocal emotional signals such as the amodal components of sensory inputs are closely intertwined with verbal affective cues such as expressive words. In order to lay a foundation for social and emotional understanding and expressiveness during synchronous interactions, the infant needs both the verbal and the visual and the redundant and amodal characteristics inherent in emotional exchanges with a caregiver (Bruck et al., 2011).

Human mothers typically engage in complex, emotion-laden synchronous face-to-face exchanges with their newborns which include both gaze and physical contact (Brazelton, Tronick, Adamson, Als, & Wise, 1975; Cohn & Tronick, 1989; Lester et al., 1985; Tronick, 1989). These complex interactions imply that there is a motivation on the part of both members of the dyad to engage in social exchanges. Behaviors help caregivers understand the nature of what the infant needs (Simpson, Murray, Paukner, & Ferrari, 2014). Mothers are typically sensitive to the infant's alertness and initiate engagements with social expressiveness and imitation of the infant's facial expressions. Current research attributes these behavioral interactions to a shared neural basis of empathy that highlights the value of neonatal imitation and shared emotional exchange as a behavioral measure of infant perception and action underlying early attachment behavior (Braadbaart, de Grauw, Perrett, Waiter, & Williams, 2014; Gonzalez-Liencres, Shamay-Tsoory, & Brune, 2013; Simpson et al., 2014).

The Distal and Proximal Bioecology of the NICU

The Distal Bioecology of the Infant in the NICU

Neonates in the NICU, by necessity, experience a bioecosystem with a history of revolving around the needs of medical and nursing staff in order to provide efficient and timely interventions (Philbin, Lickliter, & Graven, 2000). In the 1970s, there was an emphasis on reducing ambient sound in the NICU, largely because loud sound measured in the NICU was attributable to possible physiological changes and infant hearing loss and found to be common in preterm infants (Long, Lucey, & Phillips, 1980; Philbin et al., 2000). Early recognition of the impact of the sound environment of the NICU led to a series of recommendations and criteria for ambient sound reduction (Gray & Philbin, 2000; American Academy of Pediatrics, 1976).

Until recently, careful study of the benefits of sound reduction has reportedly not been well designed and carried out (Almadhoob & Ohlsson, 2015; Lasky & Williams, 2009). There has been a resurgence in the recognition of the impact of sound on the behavioral and state organization as well as neurodevelopmental outcomes of babies in NICUs (e.g., Kuhn et al., 2013; Morris, Philbin, & Bose, 2000) leading to acoustical and architectural design recommendations for NICU environments. Numerous attempts to modify the NICU environment and caregiving practices to be less invasive have been advocated by organizations such as the American Academy of Pediatrics, the Gravens NICU Design Consensus Panel recommendations, and the NIDCAP Federation International (White, Smith, Shepley,, & Committee to Establish Recommended Standards for Newborn, 2013).

The Proximal Bioecology of the Infant in the NICU

In the last decades, there has been an emphasis on not only reducing the distal sound environment of the NICU but also supplementing the infant's sensory proximal environment with music, mother's heartbeat sounds, and mother's recorded voice. These studies have focused primarily on the physiological responsiveness of the infant, both during painful procedures and during routine care, with purported benefits such as weight gain, enhancement of physiologic parameters, and shorter hospital stays.

Provision of Music in the Infant's Proximal Environment

Research on music therapy in the NICU has been initiated by a number of scientists in the past few decades. A review in 2013 (Allen, 2013) found music therapy, as an emerging intervention in the NICU, to lack consistency in research methodology and findings of reduction of hypoxia during stressful events. Allen's review of the then current literature indicated that additional research would be necessary before utilizing music as an intervention for sick preterm infants. It is noteworthy that the provision of music to infants was at a decibel level that was higher than the recommended standards for sound exposure in an NICU.

More recently, several studies have emerged that have used recorded music to focus less on physiological responses of the infant, and more on support infant arousal and neurodevelopment, in hopes of supporting the attachment relationship between mothers and their infants. Shoemark and associates (Dearn & Shoemark, 2014; Shoemark, Hanson-Abromeit, & Stewart, 2015) recognized that infants may be exposed to an unpredictable auditory background as well as the need for individualized approaches and parent presence in providing music to infants. Their research design included the playing of recorded lullabies with the parent present compared with when the parent was not present. However, the results showed no discernable impact of the mother's presence compared to when she was not present. Current contributions by Shoemark emphasize the music therapists' partnership with parents as they support the parents with "containment and soothing, enticement into interplay…," emphasizing that the work is essential to support the parent's interaction with their infant (Shoemark, Chap. 12, this volume).

Other research that included the exposure of infants to recorded lullabies and maternal voice have indicated that neither cortisol concentrations nor activity/rest patterns were influenced by music interventions (Dorn et al., 2014). More recently, Loewy and colleagues published a study of the effects of live music therapy on vital signs, feeding, and sleep in premature infants (Loewy et al., 2016) in a randomized sequence design. Their approach was to provide parent-preferred lullabies, sung live by the music therapist over a 2-week period. Their intent was to enhance bonding and decrease stress parents find with NICU infant care. In addition to short-term heart rate, sucking rhythm, and sleep pattern changes, they found decreased parental stress perception.

The provision of recorded music in the proximal environment of the infant in the NICU does not appear to have yielded consistent beneficial outcomes either from a physiologic or a behavioral perspective. The recordings may have not been individualized to the availability of the infant and not provided by a familiar caregiver. Although there was a beginning shift to having parents present in the NICU to observe the administration of "music therapy," even if the therapists used parent-preferred lullabies, parents have largely been excluded from singing the live lullabies themselves. The most recent study emphasized the provision of live music with some enticing findings of better physiologic organization in the infants and lowered perceptions of parental stress. More studies of live music presentations are necessary and hopefully will include the provision of music by familiar parents and caregivers.

Provision of Recorded Mother's Voice and Heartbeat in the Infant's Proximal Environment

Continuity between fetal and newborn exposure to the mother's voice indicates that the fetus is not only able to detect the mother's voice but also responds after birth to familiar verbalizations and narratives that the mother had provided during pregnancy. Moon has published a comprehensive review auditory development in the fetus and newborn (Moon, 2011). The continuity of auditory experiences from fetal to infancy lays the groundwork for attachment, language, and cognition. However, infants who are born early or spend time in the NICU environment are not afforded the benefit of continuity of their mother's auditory interactions. Understanding the benefits of maternal voice and heartbeat sounds on the developing fetus, studies have emerged to augment the auditory environment with recorded maternal heartbeats and voice for the preterm infant.

Krueger (Krueger, 2010) reviewed studies conducted over the years of 1972 to 2007 of exposure to maternal voice and found little research that addressed the preterm infant's loss of maternal voice continuity. She found that maternal voice recordings in those studies presented recordings above the recommendations for sound levels in an NICU. Additionally, the findings did not indicate significant beneficial outcomes on infant responsiveness. Her study emphasized the need for more research, particularly in the area of developmental outcomes that are a result of interventions that encourage parents to interact with their preterm infants.

More recent studies of maternal recorded voice and heartbeat effects on preterm infants sucking have noted that exposure to pitch modulation of the mother's voice yielded an increase in sucking (Butler, O'Sullivan, Shah, & Berthier, 2014). Other studies of maternal voice provided through bone conduction showed autonomic changes, visual attention performance, and general movements at 3 months, but not at 6 months of corrected age (Picciolini et al., 2014). Others have used similar administration of mother's voice and heartbeat sounds and have concluded that there is evidence for experience-dependent plasticity in preterm infants' auditory cortex (Webb, Heller, Benson, & Lahav, 2015), comparing their results with those found in term newborns' language-related cortical regions. In response to Webb et al., El-Dib and Glass (El-Dib & Glass, 2015) raise the question of whether brain acceleration in one area due to repetitive recordings is, in the long term, beneficial to the infant's outcome. These comments add to the cumulative calls for additional research on not only the appropriateness of recorded maternal voice and heartbeat but also on the potential long-term benefits for the development of the infant.

These studies raise important questions about the impact of recorded maternal voice and heartbeat on the experience-dependent newborn brain but may lead to understanding the effect of the mother's voice and heartbeat on infant short- and long-term outcomes. Currently the literature is sparce and limited in comprehensive longitudinal studies of infant developmental outcomes.

Recorded maternal voice and heartbeat has also been used to help reduce stress during the invasive procedures experienced in their proximal environments.

Although the literature is limited, there are a few studies indicating that infant expo-sure to recordings of maternal voice during adverse interventions such as arterial blood stick showed reduced pain-related behavior (Azarmnejad, Sarhangi, Javadi, & Rejeh, 2015). More recently Morelius and colleagues (Morelius, He, & Shorey, 2016) in their review of salivary cortisol reactivity in preterm infants during routine NICU care discussed "pleasant interventions" which included music, acoustic stim-ulation, maternal voice, and skin-to-skin care. They concluded that the literature on cortisol reactivity was inconsistent and needed further study for a variety of inter-ventions including those defined as pleasant and which included music and moth-er's voice and heartbeat.

Other interventions for painful procedures that provide multisensory interven-tion include the provision of spoken vocalization. Initially Bellieni et al. and then Gitto and colleagues (Bellieni et al., 2007; Gitto et al., 2012) referred to non-pharmacological treatments such as "sensorial saturation" which included touch and olfactory and human auditory input during heel lancing. Bellieni found no dif-ference in pain responses between mothers and nurses when sensorial saturation was provided. Gitto included parent's presence during the procedure, but parents themselves were not active in providing multisensorial input or vocalization. Both Bellieni and Gitto concluded that sensorial saturation was an effective non-pharma-cological alternative treatment to relieve pain in neonates in the NICU.

Provision of Human Voice in Proximal Interaction in the NICU

The optimal proximal bioecology of the fetus is the uterine environment. Infants born early are typically devoid of the continuity of the consistent, predictable, orchestrated sensory experiences that were to be experience expected and are instead dependent on the NICU environment to provide coordinated sensory input. In contrast to the previously reviewed studies of the bioecological environment of infants in the NICU provided by recorded music and mother's voice and heartbeat, there are few studies that examine the benefits and/or difficulties of human live verbal exchanges between the mother and her infant in the NICU. One exception is the study by Filippa (Filippa, Devouche, Arioni, Imberty, & Gratier, 2013) and col-leagues where the infant's mother was supported to speak and sing directly to her incubator-bedded infant. Significantly greater oxygen saturation and heart rate and fewer negative critical events resulted, and the infants came to alertness as if to interact with their mothers.

Other approaches that incorporate mothers and primary caregivers in verbaliza-tion with their infants are multimodal and multisensory in nature. White-Traut and colleagues (White-Traut et al., 2013) supported mothers to provide twice-daily auditory, tactile visual, and vestibular/rocking stimulation to their infants while in the NICU and as they transitioned home. The social interaction patterns of the experimental infants and mothers showed significant increases in responsiveness at 6 weeks corrected age.

Similarly, Welch and colleagues (Welch et al., 2012; Welch et al., 2014) supported mothers of preterm-born infants to engage in maternally and infant-mediated multisensory experiences by utilizing skin-to-skin opportunities, repeated "calming cycles," and speaking with their baby in their original language with emotion-laden content. Babies had significant optimal brain and behavior changes, and mothers had less anxiety and symptoms of depression.

Evidence points to the responsiveness of newborn preterm infants to proximal human voice interactions. Neurobehavioral assessments such as the Brazelton Newborn Behavioral Assessment Scale, the NICU Neonatal Network Scale, and the Assessment of Preterm Infant Behavior (Als, Butler, Kosta, & McAnulty, 2005; Als, Tronick, Lester, & Brazelton, 1977; Lester, Andreozzi-Fontaine, Tronick, & Bigsby, 2014) all support the baby to come to an alert state and respond effectively to a human face and voice. The responsivity of the infant can be optimized in a microsystem that allows for them to hear and see the examiner's face and voice and to make efforts to locate and interact with the examiner (Als, 1998).

Infants are exposed to a variety of distal and proximal sound environments that may have an impact on later receptive and expressive communication. Some of these environmental aspects are related to their exposure to live verbal exchanges in the NICU. Caskey and her group examined exposure to words and conversations during NICU stays for preterm infants (Caskey, Stephens, Tucker, & Vohr, 2011). Their remarkable finding that preterm infants make vocalizations as early as 32 weeks post-conceptional age and increase vocalizations over time contributes to our understanding of the bioecology of the infant in the NICU. They found that adult language was but a fraction of the sound that the infants were exposed to during their NICU stay and that parental verbal communication, especially during feeding at 36 weeks, predicted increases in infant vocalization. Additionally, their subsequent findings (Caskey, Stephens, Tucker, & Vohr, 2014) associated parent talk with their infants with higher 7- and 18-month language and cognitive scores on the Bayley III. These findings highlight the necessity of parental presence in proximal interactions with their preterm infants while in the NICU and beyond.

Skin-to-skin contact (SSC) has a growing research base in support of early physiological and neurobehavioral organization for prematurely born infants in the NICU, leading to the conclusion that provision of supports for STS care is a neurophysiologic imperative for both the mothers and their infants (Browne, 2004). In one unique study, mothers who engaged in singing to their preterm infant during STS care had reductions in anxiety and more physiologic stability in their infants (Arnon et al., 2014).

During STS care, the proximal environment for infants is their mother's or father's body. Their body provides the continuity of familiar, consistent, and predictable physiologic, vocal, and movement multisensory input that was initiated in utero. Infants in STS care are exposed to the human sound of the mother's heartbeat, body sounds, and vocalization, and the mother is additionally provided with coregulatory processes including vocal exchanges with the infant. These multisensory inputs are the best example of the developmental niche—the bioecological proximal interactions—that are experience expectant and that set the stage for experience-dependent brain organization. Furthermore, they provide redundant learning across all sensory inputs—the sound of the mother's voice, her body movement and breathing, her familiar odor, and the physiologic organization provided by "hidden regulators." The amodal properties imbedded in these organized and intimate multisensory inputs provide the infant with an array of experiences that support their alertness and attention, their orientation to salient elements of their mother's location, and emotional detection and exchange. These building blocks are essential for social and emotional, language, and cognitive development (Feldman, Rosenthal, & Eidelman, 2014).

The Bioecology of NICU Design

With the recent advent of single family rooms within NICUs, where infants are cared for in separate rooms rather than one or two large multibed rooms or "pods," the bioecology of the newborn has evolved from the more historic infant grouping to individual or family unit design (White, 2003). Although there are data available on sound reduction in single family rooms as opposed to multibed units which were traditionally noisy (Philbin & Gray, 2002), research into the benefits of the single family room on infant developmental outcomes are emerging. Conflicting outcomes in the few current studies may be related to lack of sound input, isolation from sound experiences, or lack of opportunities for parents (White, 2003; Jobe, 2014; Lester et al., 2014; Pineda et al., 2014; Pineda et al., 2012; Rand & Lahav, 2014) to be interactive with their infant. Without opportunities for consistent interactions between infants and their mothers and other consistent caregivers, it appears that little vocal interaction and intimate exchanges are possible and could potentially have detrimental effects on infant development. Implications for assuring that parents are supported to be with their infants as primary caregivers and not "visitors" are apparent.

Initiated in Europe, "couplet care" focuses on never separating the preterm infant from his or her parents throughout the entire hospitalization (Ortenstrand et al., 2010; Westrup, 2015) and includes significant time for the parents to engage in skin-to-skin experiences. These experiences result in more optimal medical and developmental outcomes for the preterm-born infant. Thus, the infant is exposed to ongoing, consistent, familiar, and predictable verbal and other multisensory communication with parents.

Summary and Conclusions

Historically, the NICU has attended to the medical and caregiving needs of the preterm-born infant that included support for technology and personnel. Along with lifesaving interventions were an ambient environment that was technology based and largely excluded parent participation in their infant's care. More recent recognition of the impact of the environment on the infant's organization and the benefits of parental care has provided an evolution in NICU caregiving and environmental design.

Understanding that the environment in which the infant grows impacts their experience-dependent brain organization and realizing that the NICU environment is not conducive to helping the infant transition from the "expected" environment of parental interactions and culture, professionals have developed strategies thought to enhance the infant's organization and neurodevelopment. Some of these strategies have included the provision of music in the form of lullabies, the mother's recorded voice and heartbeat, and, more recently, live singing of lullabies. As with the introduction of any new technology and/or innovative intervention for immature infants, questions arise as to the reproducibility of positive physiologic findings. Other questions include whether physiologic changes are the desired or appropriate measures to be investigated and if there are benefits to short and/or long term outcomes.

The fetus is already familiar with his mother's voice and body sounds and is expecting continuity when born into his human ecological niche. The mother's body provides regulation of her baby's physiology, arousal, and behavior, many of which are hidden to observation, yet are essential for survival. Unless there are significant opportunities for mother/infant closeness, an infant who spends time in the NICU may not benefit from these hidden regulators and alternatively is regulated by technology.

The human infant is dependent on experience within his or her proximal environment, largely through interaction with his or her parents and primary care providers. The sensory inputs that the infant is expecting are across systems, in fact, redundant and amodal so that the infant experiences the richness of the interactions with his mother. The best example of redundant, amodal sensory integration is provided by the proximal interaction when hearing the mother's voice, perceiving the emotionality of the interaction, seeing her face, smelling her particular odor, and moving in concert with her body such as when the dyad engage in skin-to-skin care. Efforts to reproduce these interactive components with technology cannot match the opportunities that infants are expecting of their developmental niche.

Synchronous interactions between the infant and his or her parents or consistent caregivers are now thought to lay a foundation for social and emotional development, which in turn results in more optimal cognitive, motor, and speech outcomes. Recorded administration of music or mother's voice and heartbeat represents a "one-way street," where the infant does not have a chance to reciprocally and synchronously develop social or emotional exchange, nor do they elicit emotional exchange between the members of the dyad. Further, parents often perceive that technology is an obstacle to interacting freely with their infant and may present unintended and ethically laden consequences (Lantz & Ottosson, 2013; van Manen, 2015).

Efforts by professionals to provide aspects of the mother's familiar voice, heartbeat, and preferred music reflect that the infant many times does not have parents available to provide their personal sensory experiences. Might NICUs, hospitals, and indeed the social and economic fabric of our countries work hard to remove obstacles and promote families to be together during this critical developmental phase? Approaches in support of parental participation in the care of their infants where families are encouraged to be together and to sing, laugh, play, hold, and interact with their infants should become the optimal bioecology for developing infants. What is needed is NICU design that encourages family presence 24 h a day, 7 days a week; a culture change that incorporates strategies for integrating families into the caregiving fabric of the NICU; and abolishment of the viewing of families as "visitors." Strategies such as these will go far in assuring that the new bioecology of both distal and proximal environments of the preterm newborn will encourage synchronous verbal, physical, and emotional interactions and optimize infant neurodevelopmental outcomes.

Key Messages
- Developmental science has provided a foundation for understanding the need for appropriately timed and redundant intersensory experiences in order to optimize neurodevelopmental outcomes.
- The optimal bioecological niche of the infant in the NICU is the mother's body, voice, and movement where sensory familiarity, rhythmicity, and synchrony contribute not only to the emerging attachment relationship but also to later cognitive, neurophysiological, and socioemotional development.
- To enhance the bioecological niche of the infant in the NICU, obstacles should be removed, and opportunities should be promoted for families, and, in particular, mothers, to interact with their infants in intimate physical and vocal exchanges as frequently as possible.

References

Allen, K. A. (2013). Music therapy in the NICU: Is there evidence to support integration for procedural support? *Advances in Neonatal Care, 13*(5), 349–352. doi:10.1097/ANC.0b013e3182a0278b

Almadhoob, A., & Ohlsson, A. (2015). Sound reduction management in the neonatal intensive care unit for preterm or very low birth weight infants. *Cochrane Database of Systematic Reviews, 1*, CD010333. doi:10.1002/14651858.CD010333.pub2

Als, H. (1998). Developmental care in the newborn intensive care unit. *Current Opinion in Pediatrics, 10*(2), 138–142.

Als, H., Butler, S., Kosta, S., & McAnulty, G. (2005). The Assessment of Preterm Infants' Behavior (APIB): Furthering the understanding and measurement of neurodevelopmental competence in preterm and full-term infants. *Mental Retardation and Developmental Disabilities Research Reviews, 11*(1), 94–102. doi:10.1002/mrdd.20053

Als, H., Tronick, E., Lester, B. M., & Brazelton, T. B. (1977). The Brazelton Neonatal Behavioral Assessment Scale (BNBAS). *Journal of Abnormal Child Psychology, 5*(3), 215–231.

American Academy of Pediatrics, C. o. E. H. (1976). Noise pollution: Neonatal aspects. *Pediatrics*, *54*(4), 476–479.

Arnon, S., Diamant, C., Bauer, S., Regev, R., Sirota, G., & Litmanovitz, I. (2014). Maternal singing during kangaroo care led to autonomic stability in preterm infants and reduced maternal anxiety. *Acta Paediatrica*, *103*(10), 1039–1044. doi:10.1111/apa.12744

Azarmnejad, E., Sarhangi, F., Javadi, M., & Rejeh, N. (2015). The effect of mother's voice on arterial blood sampling induced pain in neonates hospitalized in neonate intensive care unit. *Global Journal of Health Science*, *7*(6), 198–204. doi:10.5539/gjhs.v7n6p198

Bahrick, L. E., & Lickliter, R. (2014). Learning to attend selectively: The dual role of intersensory redundancy. *Current Directions in Psychological Science*, *23*(6), 414–420. doi:10.1177/0963721414549187

Bellieni, C. V., Cordelli, D. M., Marchi, S., Ceccarelli, S., Perrone, S., Maffei, M., and Buonocore, G. (2007, March/April). Sensorial saturation for neonatal analgesia, *The Clinical Journal of Pain* 23 3, 219-221.

Bowlby, J. (1954). The effect of separation from the mother in early life. *Irish Journal of Medical Science*, *339*, 121–126.

Bowlby, J. (1958). The nature of the child's tie to his mother. *The International Journal of Psycho-Analysis*, *39*(5), 350–373.

Bowlby, J. (1968). Effects on behaviour of disruption of an affectional bond. *Eugenics Society Symposia*, *4*, 94–108.

Bowlby, J. (1982). Attachment and loss: Retrospect and prospect. *The American Journal of Orthopsychiatry*, *52*(4), 664–678.

Braadbaart, L., de Grauw, H., Perrett, D. I., Waiter, G. D., & Williams, J. H. (2014). The shared neural basis of empathy and facial imitation accuracy. *NeuroImage*, *84*, 367–375. doi:10.1016/j.neuroimage.2013.08.061

Brazelton, T. B., Tronick, E., Adamson, L., Als, H., & Wise, S. (1975). Early mother-infant reciprocity. *Ciba Foundation Symposium*, *33*, 137–154.

Bronfenbrenner, U. U., & Ceci, S. J. (1994). Nature-nurture reconceptualized in developmental perspective: A bioecological model. *Psychological Review*, *101*(4), 568–586.

Browne, J. V. (2004). Early relationship environments: Physiology of skin-to-skin contact for parents and their preterm infants. *Clinics in Perinatology*, *31*(2), 287–298., vii. doi:10.1016/j.clp.2004.04.004

Bruck, C., Kreifelts, B., & Wildgruber, D. (2011). Emotional voices in context: A neurobiological model of multimodal affective information processing. *Physics of Life Reviews*, *8*(4), 383–403. doi:10.1016/j.plrev.2011.10.002

Butler, S. C., O'Sullivan, L. P., Shah, B. L., & Berthier, N. E. (2014). Preference for infant-directed speech in preterm infants. *Infant Behavior & Development*, *37*(4), 505–511. doi:10.1016/j.infbeh.2014.06.007

Caskey, M., Stephens, B., Tucker, R., & Vohr, B. (2011). Importance of parent talk on the development of preterm infant vocalizations. *Pediatrics*, *128*(5), 910–916. doi:10.1542/peds.2011-0609

Caskey, M., Stephens, B., Tucker, R., & Vohr, B. (2014). Adult talk in the NICU with preterm infants and developmental outcomes. *Pediatrics*, *133*(3), e578–e584. doi:10.1542/peds.2013-0104

Censullo, M., Lester, B., & Hoffman, J. (1985). Rhythmic patterning in mother-newborn interaction. *Nursing Research*, *34*(6), 342–346.

Cohn, J. F., & Tronick, E. (1989). Specificity of infants' response to mothers' affective behavior. *Journal of the American Academy of Child and Adolescent Psychiatry*, *28*(2), 242–248. doi:10.1097/00004583-198903000-00016

Dearn, T., & Shoemark, H. (2014). The effect of maternal presence on premature infant response to recorded music. *Journal of Obstetric, Gynecologic, and Neonatal Nursing*, *43*(3), 341–350. doi:10.1111/1552-6909.12303

Dorn, F., Wirth, L., Gorbey, S., Wege, M., Zemlin, M., Maier, R. F., & Lemmer, B. (2014). Influence of acoustic stimulation on the circadian and ultradian rhythm of premature infants. *Chronobiology International*, *31*(9), 1062–1074. doi:10.3109/07420528.2014.948183

El-Dib, M., & Glass, P. (2015). Does exposure of premature infants to repetitive recorded mother sounds improve neurodevelopmental outcome? *Proceedings of the National Academy of Sciences of the United States of America, 112*(31), E4166. doi:10.1073/pnas.1507315112

Feldman, R. (2015). The adaptive human parental brain: Implications for children's social development. *Trends in Neurosciences, 38*(6), 387–399. doi:10.1016/j.tins.2015.04.004

Feldman, R. (2016). The neurobiology of mammalian parenting and the biosocial context of human caregiving. *Hormones and Behavior, 77*, 3–17. doi:10.1016/j.yhbeh.2015.10.001

Feldman, R., & Eidelman, A. I. (2007). Maternal postpartum behavior and the emergence of infant-mother and infant-father synchrony in preterm and full-term infants: The role of neonatal vagal tone. *Developmental Psychobiology, 49*(3), 290–302. doi:10.1002/dev.20220

Feldman, R., Rosenthal, Z., & Eidelman, A. I. (2014). Maternal-preterm skin-to-skin contact enhances child physiologic organization and cognitive control across the first 10 years of life. *Biological Psychiatry, 75*(1), 56–64. doi:10.1016/j.biopsych.2013.08.012

Filippa, M., Devouche, E., Arioni, C., Imberty, M., & Gratier, M. (2013). Live maternal speech and singing have beneficial effects on hospitalized preterm infants. *Acta Paediatrica, 102*(10), 1017–1020. doi:10.1111/apa.12356

Gitto, E., Pellegrino, S., Manfrida, M., Aversa, S., Trimarchi, G., Barberi, I., & Reiter, R. J. (2012). Stress response and procedural pain in the preterm newborn: The role of pharmacological and non-pharmacological treatments. *European Journal of Pediatrics, 171*(6), 927–933. doi:10.1007/s00431-011-1655-7

Gonzalez-Liencres, C., Shamay-Tsoory, S. G., & Brune, M. (2013). Towards a neuroscience of empathy: Ontogeny, phylogeny, brain mechanisms, context and psychopathology. *Neuroscience and Biobehavioral Reviews, 37*(8), 1537–1548. doi:10.1016/j.neubiorev.2013.05.001

Gottfried, A. W., & Gaiter, J. L. (1985). *Infant stress under intensive care*. Baltimore, MD: University Park Press.

Gray, L., & Philbin, M. K. (2000). Measuring sound in hospital nurseries. *Journal of Perinatology, 20*(8 Pt 2), S100–S104.

Greenough, W. T., Black, J. E., & Wallace, C. S. (1987). Experience and brain development. *Child Development, 58*, 539–559.

Hofer, M. (1994). Hidden regulators in attachment separation and loss. *Monographs of the Society for Research in Child Development, 59*(2/3), 192–207.

Jobe, A. H. (2014). A risk of sensory deprivation in the neonatal intensive care unit. *The Journal of Pediatrics, 164*(6), 1265–1267. doi:10.1016/j.jpeds.2014.01.072

Karger, R. H. (1979). Synchrony in mother-infant interactions. *Child Development, 50*(3), 882–885.

Krueger, C. (2010). Exposure to maternal voice in preterm infants: A review. *Advances in Neonatal Care, 10*(1), 13–18.; quiz 19–20. doi:10.1097/ANC.0b013e3181cc3c69

Kuhn, P., Zores, C., Langlet, C., Escande, B., Astruc, D., & Dufour, A. (2013). Moderate acoustic changes can disrupt the sleep of very preterm infants in their incubators. *Acta Paediatrica, 102*(10), 949–954. doi:10.1111/apa.12330

Lantz, B., & Ottosson, C. (2013). Parental interaction with infants treated with medical technology. *Scandinavian Journal of Caring Sciences, 27*(3), 597–607. doi:10.1111/j.1471-6712.2012.01061.x

Lasky, R. E., & Williams, A. L. (2009). Noise and light exposures for extremely low birth weight newborns during their stay in the neonatal intensive care unit. *Pediatrics, 123*(2), 540–546. doi:10.1542/peds.2007-3418

Leclere, C., Viaux, S., Avril, M., Achard, C., Chetouani, M., Missonnier, S., & Cohen, D. (2014). Why synchrony matters during mother-child interactions: A systematic review. *PLoS One, 9*(12), e113571. doi:10.1371/journal.pone.0113571

Lester, B. M., Andreozzi-Fontaine, L., Tronick, E., & Bigsby, R. (2014). Assessment and evaluation of the high risk neonate: The NICU Network Neurobehavioral Scale. *Journal of Visualized Experiments, 90*. doi:10.3791/3368

Lester, B. M., Hawes, K., Abar, B., Sullivan, M., Miller, R., Bigsby, R., ... Padbury, J. F. (2014). Single-family room care and neurobehavioral and medical outcomes in preterm infants. *Pediatrics, 134*(4), 754–760. doi:10.1542/peds.2013-4252

Lester, B. M., Hoffman, J., & Brazelton, T. B. (1985). The rhythmic structure of mother-infant interaction in term and preterm infants. *Child Development*, *56*(1), 15–27.

Lester, B. M., Miller, R. J., Hawes, K., Salisbury, A., Bigsby, R., Sullivan, M. C., & Padbury, J. F. (2011). Infant neurobehavioral development. *Seminars in Perinatology*, *35*(1), 8–19. doi:10.1053/j.semperi.2010.10.003

Lickliter, R. (2011). The integrated development of sensory organization. *Clinics in Perinatology*, *38*(4), 591–603. doi:10.1016/j.clp.2011.08.007

Linn, P. L., Horowitz, F. D., Buddin, B. J., Leake, J., & Fox, H. A. (1985). An ecological description of a neonatal intensive care unit. In *Infant stress under intensive care* (pp. 83–112). Baltimore, MD: University Park Press.

Loewy, R., Fisher, M., Schlosser, D. A., Biagianti, B., Stuart, B., Mathalon, D. H., & Vinogradov, S. (2016). Intensive auditory cognitive training improves verbal memory in adolescents and young adults at clinical high risk for psychosis. *Schizophrenia Bulletin*. doi:10.1093/schbul/sbw009

Long, J. G., Lucey, J. F., & Phillips, A. C. (1980). Noise and hypoxemia in the neonatal intensive care unit. *Pediatrics*, *65*(1), 143–145.

Moon, C. (2011). The role of early auditory development in attachment and communication. *Clinics in Perinatology*, *38*(4), 657–669. doi:10.1016/j.clp.2011.08.009

Morelius, E., He, H. G., & Shorey, S. (2016). Salivary cortisol reactivity in preterm infants in neonatal intensive care: An integrative review. *International Journal of Environmental Research and Public Health*, *13*(3). doi:10.3390/ijerph13030337

Morris, B. H., Philbin, M. K., & Bose, C. (2000). Physiological effects of sound on the newborn. *Journal of Perinatology*, *20*(8 Pt 2), S55–S60.

Ortenstrand, A., Westrup, B., Brostrom, E. B., Sarman, I., Akerstrom, S., Brune, T., … Waldenstrom, U. (2010). The Stockholm Neonatal Family Centered Care Study: Effects on length of stay and infant morbidity. *Pediatrics*, *125*(2), e278–e285. doi:10.1542/peds.2009-1511

Philbin, M. K., & Gray, L. (2002). Changing levels of quiet in an intensive care nursery. *Journal of Perinatology*, *22*(6), 455–460. doi:10.1038/sj.jp.7210756

Philbin, M. K., Lickliter, R., & Graven, S. N. (2000). Sensory experience and the developing organism: A history of ideas and view to the future. *Journal of Perinatology*, *20*(8 Pt 2), S2–S5.

Picciolini, O., Porro, M., Meazza, A., Gianni, M. L., Rivoli, C., Lucco, G., … Mosca, F. (2014). Early exposure to maternal voice: Effects on preterm infants development. *Early Human Development*, *90*(6), 287–292. doi:10.1016/j.earlhumdev.2014.03.003

Pineda, R. G., Neil, J., Dierker, D., Smyser, C. D., Wallendorf, M., Kidokoro, H., … Inder, T. (2014). Alterations in brain structure and neurodevelopmental outcome in preterm infants hospitalized in different neonatal intensive care unit environments. *The Journal of Pediatrics*, *164*(1), 52–60. e52. doi:10.1016/j.jpeds.2013.08.047

Pineda, R. G., Stransky, K. E., Rogers, C., Duncan, M. H., Smith, G. C., Neil, J., & Inder, T. (2012). The single-patient room in the NICU: Maternal and family effects. *Journal of Perinatology*, *32*(7), 545–551. doi:10.1038/jp.2011.144

Rand, K., & Lahav, A. (2014). Impact of the NICU environment on language deprivation in preterm infants. *Acta Paediatrica*, *103*(3), 243–248. doi:10.1111/apa.12481

Rosa, E. M., & Tudge, J. (2013). Urie Bronfenbrenner's theory of human development: Its evolution from ecology to bioecology. *Journal of Family Theory & Review*, *5*(4), 243–258. doi:10.1111/jftr.12022

Shoemark, H., Hanson-Abromeit, D., & Stewart, L. (2015). Constructing optimal experience for the hospitalized newborn through neuro-based music therapy. *Frontiers in Human Neuroscience*, *9*, 487. doi:10.3389/fnhum.2015.00487

Simpson, E. A., Murray, L., Paukner, A., & Ferrari, P. F. (2014). The mirror neuron system as revealed through neonatal imitation: Presence from birth, predictive power and evidence of plasticity. *Philosophical Transactions of the Royal Society of London. Series B, Biological Sciences*, *369*(1644), 20130289. doi:10.1098/rstb.2013.0289

Super, C. M., & Harkness, S. (1994). The developmental niche: A theoretical framework for analyzing the household production of health. *Social Science & Medicine, 38*(2), 217–226. doi:10.1016/0277-9536(94)90391-3

Tronick, E. Z. (1989). Emotions and emotional communication in infants. *The American Psychologist, 44*(2), 112–119.

van Manen, M. A. (2015). The ethics of an ordinary medical technology. *Qualitative Health Research, 25*(7), 996–1004. doi:10.1177/1049732314554101

Webb, A. R., Heller, H. T., Benson, C. B., & Lahav, A. (2015). Mother's voice and heartbeat sounds elicit auditory plasticity in the human brain before full gestation. *Proceedings of the National Academy of Sciences of the United States of America, 112*(10), 3152–3157. doi:10.1073/pnas.1414924112

Welch, M. G., Hofer, M. A., Brunelli, S. A., Stark, R. I., Andrews, H. F., Austin, J., ... Family Nurture Intervention Trial, G. (2012). Family nurture intervention (FNI): Methods and treatment protocol of a randomized controlled trial in the NICU. *BMC Pediatrics, 12*, 14. doi:10.1186/1471-2431-12-14

Welch, M. G., Myers, M. M., Grieve, P. G., Isler, J. R., Fifer, W. P., Sahni, R., ... Group, F. N. I. T, Group, F. N. I. T. (2014). Electroencephalographic activity of preterm infants is increased by Family Nurture Intervention: A randomized controlled trial in the NICU. *Clinical Neurophysiology, 125*(4), 675–684. doi:10.1016/j.clinph.2013.08.021

Westrup, B. (2015). Family-centered developmentally supportive care: The Swedish example. *Archives de Pédiatrie, 22*(10), 1086–1091. doi:10.1016/j.arcped.2015.07.005

White, R. D. (2003). Individual rooms in the NICU – An evolving concept. *Journal of Perinatology, 23*(Suppl 1), S22–S24. doi:10.1038/sj.jp.7210840

White, R. D., Smith, J. A., Shepley, M. M., & Committee to Establish Recommended Standards for Newborn, I. C. U. D. (2013). Recommended standards for newborn ICU design, eighth edition. *Journal of Perinatology, 33*(Suppl 1), S2–16. doi:10.1038/jp.2013.10

White-Traut, R., Norr, K. F., Fabiyi, C., Rankin, K. M., Li, Z., & Liu, L. (2013). Mother-infant interaction improves with a developmental intervention for mother-preterm infant dyads. *Infant Behavior & Development, 36*(4), 694–706. doi:10.1016/j.infbeh.2013.07.004

Part IV
Family-Centered Music Therapy Experiences in the NICU

Chapter 12
Empowering Parents in Singing to Hospitalized Infants: The Role of the Music Therapist

Helen Shoemark

Abstract *Introduction*: While we understand the potential benefits of mothers and fathers singing to their infants in the Neonatal Intensive Care Unit (NICU), the process is not simple. The challenges can be personal, contextual, and temporal. Singing is not a natural action for everyone. With rapidly increasing individualized music listening technology and decreasing opportunities for active music making in many countries, people have less experience and awareness of their own musicality. This can hinder their capacity to use music as part of nurturing their infant. Additionally, across their time in the NICU, parents can feel concerned about singing in a "public" place.

Main aims: This chapter outlines how the music therapist works in the real-world lived experience with parents. Three phases – anticipatory, cautious interplay, and active parenting – offer parents a different range of potential for their voice and the unfolding relationship with their infant.

Conclusion: The music therapist works with mothers and fathers to reconnect them to their own vocal potential and to normalize the sound of singing in the NICU. These processes are underpinned by theories of attachment and infant neurodevelopment and are responsive to the evolving needs of the mother and infant.

The everyday lived experience of people is never as tidy as the findings of research studies convey. Even in experience-near qualitative research (Frogget & Briggs, 2012) which allows the reader to share in the experience of the participant, the descriptions are still orchestrated by the researcher to illustrate a predetermined point. Real life in the NICU is not so linear, but a "roller coaster" (Layne, 1996),

H. Shoemark (✉)
Temple University, Philadelphia, PA, USA
e-mail: helen.shoemark@temple.edu

© Springer International Publishing AG 2017   205
M. Filippa et al. (eds.), *Early Vocal Contact and Preterm Infant Brain Development*, DOI 10.1007/978-3-319-65077-7_12

during which families treasure the "normal" things like touching, holding, feeding, and washing.

While singing may not always be on that list of normal things, using the voice is. Families talk to their infants, regardless of whether they know their infant is aware or not (Shoemark & Arnup, 2014). This vocal potential is a simple but vital indication of parent role and status in their infant's well-being. We are familiar with the portrayal of families in the Neonatal Intensive Care Unit (NICU) feeling that they are both figuratively and literally without a voice. They are characterized as displaced, powerless, and without a voice in their infant's life. In reality, the scope of parenting experience also includes those parents who demand a pivotal role as advocate and voice for their infant, creating partnerships with nursing and medical teams to promote their infant's care and experience. The therapist in the clinical context must hold this scope in mind so no assumptions are made about the inner or outward expressions of the family's experience.

It is important to note that the role of the music therapist will depend on the culture of the country, the region, the hospital, the ward, and the music therapist (Shoemark, 2015). Each influences the acceptable theoretical premise and implementation of the actual intervention. This chapter is provided by an Australian music therapist with 20 years' experience in a pediatric NICU, informed by a preceding practice in special education and early intervention. The writing will reflect that experience, while also drawing in other known perspectives. There is also a movement to acknowledge fathers in the NICU, and the lived experience of singing in the clinical context pertains equally to fathers as mothers. Therefore, the term "parent" is used instead of mother to build the precedent for the inclusion of fathers.

Most music therapists working in the NICU take referrals from other NICU team members. For some staff, peer-reviewed evidence of the effect of singing may be needed before they will refer, but when parents and bedside nurses clinically observe change in the infant or parent to music therapy, this will usually provide sufficient evidence of effect to engender referrals. The team will be willing to refer infants and families for music therapy even when their understanding of the process is quite limited. Beyond individual team members, embedding music therapy in the standard clinical pathway for infants and families is reliant on the individual music therapist's capacity to articulate the mediating pathway in a manner which is congruent with the culture of the NICU.

Depending on the music therapist's training and theoretical framework, singing becomes an intervention or a strategy, when it is brought into the parent's consciousness within the therapeutic relationship. In a family-centered model, the music therapist creates a partnership with the parent by first understanding the parent's status in their life trajectory (Perry Black, Holditch-Davis, & Miles, 2009), alongside their evolving experience of parenting and their own musical self (Shoemark & Arnup, 2014). By first calling to consciousness the parents' own capacities to generate an optimal presence, parents can begin to find a comfortable use of their voice and singing and integrate it into their day with their infant. In other

NICU cultures where the NICU team member is still considered to be the expert, the family might be able to put aside their own uncertainties to follow the stipulated intervention.

Parents Actually Singing in the NICU

The modest research about parents singing live in the NICU has identified the primacy of the mother's voice for NICU infants. Dearn and Shoemark (2014) identified the significance of maternal presence in the NICU even when they were very passive, and recent research has begun to report the significance of the primacy of parental voices as optimal stimulus (Filippa, Devouche, Arioni, Imberty, & Gratier, 2013; Loewy, Stewart, Dassler, et al., 2013).

Before singing might be considered as a viable experience for families, availability and use of voice serves as a starting point. We understand that parents who believe that singing is useful or can think of a reason for singing in the NICU are likely to go on and use their voices to sing to their baby (Shoemark & Arnup, 2014). So the music therapist can first gently inquire about the parent's beliefs and knowledge, to ascertain the probability of singing. While the person introducing the idea of singing obviously has a belief in the usefulness of such action, there should be no assumption that any parent shares this belief. On this basis, the discussion about singing should never actually begin with singing. The discussion should begin with the most likely existing use of voice, talking. If the music therapist has observed the parent talking to their infant, then affirmation is the starting point, "I can see you are already talking to your baby, that's lovely." Where there is no possibility of observing the parent talking to their infant, then the music therapist asks, with an expectation that the parent has been talking (Shoemark & Arnup, 2014). This question affords the therapist the opportunity to bring to the parent's consciousness their experiences of talking to their baby. Where a parent reveals they are not talking, the music therapist understands that there is a rupture to the parent's sense of self and the program must proceed cautiously to reconstruct that parent's sense of self in relation to their infant while also referring back to a mental health team if there is one.

The act of singing is revealing and potentially embarrassing, and without understanding the parent's proclivity for singing, it is not likely that a parent will actually sing (Blumenfeld & Eisenfeld, 2006). The capacity to sing may be moderated by a lack of musical heritage. Singing in the NICU is possible for parents who can think of a reason or imagine singing but is also made possible by their own experience of being sung to as a child and their own experiences of playing/learning an instrument or playing and singing in an ensemble (Shoemark & Arnup, 2014). The music therapist accounts for these factors, when initiating contact with parents.

The everyday lived experience of music is rapidly changing. Like others, parents perceive that music making is something undertaken by recording artists. As active music education is discarded from the education systems, the opportunities for becoming musical are also diminishing in high-income countries. It is not unusual for parents to report that they cannot sing. The music therapist reframes this perception by inquiring gently about everyday singing experiences, most commonly *singing along* to a recorded music source while in the car or shower or while doing house work. This often allows parents to realize that they actually do sing and thereby overcoming their reluctance.

When introducing singing as an intervention, it is important to consider that the experience of singing is not a singular phenomenon but occurs in and across time. Singing is a temporal process which both takes time and creates time for "being" together (Shoemark, 2017). It takes time to sing the chorus of a song, to hum a verse, and to recite a nursery rhyme. Within that bounded time of a song, there is opportunity. A song creates a time in which parent and infant can be engaged in the same experience of contingency or reciprocity (Trevarthen & Malloch, 2000; Trehub, Plantinga, & Russo, 2015) and potentially a significant moment of meeting (Tronick, 1998) or synchrony (Feldman, Magori-Cohenc, Galili, Singerb, & Louzounc, 2011). Song is a time-bound pattern of replicable expectation, joy, and memory building:

> Everything gets interrupted by medical ... there's always someone at the door. Having a program like this [music therapy] that everyone understands could help parents to make that time happen...."[1] *Kyra*

Across the time of the NICU admission, a parent's opportunities for singing can be organized loosely into three time frames. The first phase is *anticipatory,* when the infant is not available for interplay because of medical instability or sedation and the role of the parent is constrained to a simple presence and limited sensory support. Once the infant has stabilized and is socially available but restricted by their condition or complex care regimes, the parents enter a phase of *cautious interplay,* in which they are unsure about what they can do. Finally is the phase of *active parenting,* in which the infant may have periods of medical stability and social availability and parents focus on opportunities for development.

Anticipatory

The early days of NICU admission are usually marked by functional and technical medical care serving to stabilize or maintain stability of the infant's physical status. During this time, neurological immaturity, sedation, intubation, and analgesia may prevent the infant from being available to his parents in ways they might have expected or hoped for. The loss of role is profound. This can immediately undermine a parent's identity as primary nurturer, knowing simply how to be with their

---

[1] All names are changed. All quotes are drawn from the study reported in Shoemark, H. (2017).

infant, while for some, it inflames a fierce determination to protect and advocate for their infant as a baby:

> I know. I've seen, I've had Liam on machines breathing for him… when they're not available, all you might get is the occasional eye open and that always caught me because that's something the machines can't do, that's him…Which is why I read to him. That's what I did, that's all I had. In the end I had hope and to let him know that I'm here. Just keep going…. It was hard, but I just had go 'Alright, regardless, I'm just going to be there'. He needs to know I'm going to be there for him. *Jo*

During this time, the music therapist may partner with the parents to be witness to the baby's simplest capacities and to help parent understand their baby's behavioral cues and the potential of their own expression:

> If we'd known how important our voices were, and she's still going to love us and know who we are by our voices rather than touch, it would have made me feel a lot better. *Ann*

Knowledge is often key at this point, giving parents enough reason to continue their presence and actions even when there is no obvious response. As needed, the music therapist introduces key information about what is known about infant auditory processing, the difference between ambient sound and the detectable stimulus of voice, recognition of parental voice, and answering all and any questions parents ask. A further strand of the discussion acknowledges the infant's inability to obviously respond at this time. For some parents, a discussion about how their infant's heart rate and oxygen saturation can indicate their response to stimulation is an accessible pathway to understanding their baby's experience. However, as far as possible, the purpose of family-centered practice is to humanize and maintain a meaningful connection between parent and infant, so singing is a human act of nurturing care, not medical care. The focus remains on the parent's direct experience of their baby's response or complete lack of response to their presence and action.

Where an infant is unable to respond at all, the music therapist can work with parents to help them hold the potential of their baby in mind. This can be achieved by encouraging parents to see their efforts as storing experience in their baby's brain and "heart." The prospect that their loving care and interaction might be processed by their infant in a way which we do not yet understand is usually enough to sustain a parent when there is no obvious response from their infant.

In the *anticipatory* phase, the parents may note that they would use their voice, but because their infant is unavailable, they have not talked at all or much. The music therapist can introduce the possibility that the sound of the parent's voice is at least useful and at best critical for their infant's ongoing brain development which will usually override any sense that it serves no purpose.

Once the usefulness of voice is established, many parents will spontaneously discuss other voices use such as reading, humming, singing, or prayer. This opens the discussion about acceptable voice use and promotes the potential for leading the parent toward the idea of singing or patterned voice use. Patterned voice use is any kind of speech in which a replicable pattern may be developed. This most commonly includes (a) little rhymes which may be a familiar part of the family heritage shared with other siblings or in own childhood and (b) chants which are little phrases of comfort such as "there, there, there" or "sh-sh-sh" repeated for soothing the infant.

The music therapist may demonstrate any and all possibilities to the parents, to confirm they have understood the action as intended but also to give labels to new actions as actual supportive strategies. Mothers often note that they use chant but do not necessarily think of this as a conscious action, despite it being the most common way in which any adult soothes an infant. The categorization of this little action as a strategy helps parents claim their role as the pivotal person who knows intimate details about their infant and enables them to inform other carers such as nurses about this action as a successful strategy.

Because of the acute environment, many parents do not want to make any more noise, and most will whisper to their infant (Shoemark & Arnup, 2014). Whispering does not contain a melodic contour, and therefore the intention of the message is lost to the infant (Spence & Freeman 1996). The music therapist will demonstrate whispering and quiet talking, and parents almost always detect the loss of the melodic content in the whispering. The parent immediately understands that voiced sound is needed to make their intention clear to their baby.

In some music therapy practice, it might also be that the music therapist first creates musical sound in that anticipatory phase so that parents can experience the sound without being responsible for it. The song of kin (Loewy et al., 2013), which is a song selected by the parent for its familiarity and comforting, is adapted to a closely contained form of lullaby (3/4 or 6/8 time, slow repetitious, breathy) to create a supportive auditory experience which is shared by all within hearing. Where opening their mouth to sing might feel too revealing, the parent might be able to hum. The creation of such moments of intimacy can provide pivotal support for parent as nurturer.

Cautious Interplay

Infants with complex medical needs can provide the greatest challenge for their parents. Conditions which cause ongoing pain or discomfort, treatments which limit positioning or scope of movement, and regimes which include nasogastric, naso-pharyngeal, or orogastric tubes can all compromise or distort infant's capacities to achieve regulation and interact with their parent or carer. The capacity of the infant to respond may vary greatly both in actual behavior and in the time it takes (see below in *Active Parenting* for more discussion on this). The infant's windows of availability may be brief and infrequent, and the cues they give may be idiosyncratic to their medical condition or their emerging personality. Despite perplexing responses, parents are eager to maximize the window of availability and can unwittingly be overwhelming to hospitalized infants. They can be very anxious about every nuance of behavior or seemingly oblivious to significant cues. At either extreme, their infant can withdraw, complain, or outright protest. In units where a family-centered approach is lacking, less than optimal parental interaction may cause the parents to feel judged:

> "We were told not to over-stimulate her and then when she woke up we were like"ooh-ooh Taylor.....'[demonstrates very excited, big smiling face] and the nurses were like "leave her alone"!" *Tyra*

The music therapist works in partnership with parents to understand their baby's thresholds for stimulation and the behaviors that indicate tolerance, acceptance, and engagement:

> *Vignette*: As Shelley approaches Tyron's bed, she is already talking to him brightly, "good morning bubba, your Mama is here". She touches his cheek, strokes his head, runs her hand down his torso, and pats his tummy. Tyron looks at her brightly and stretches his legs and arms out tight, then turns away, taking several minutes before he returns. Shelley is disappointed, "don't you wanna talk to me today?"

Shelley interprets Tyron's response as disinterest or, worse, rejection; when in most cases, this response is more likely to be a disengagement from the overwhelming variety of stimuli Shelley offered. The therapist can help Shelley to be aware that she brings sight, sound, smell, touch, and sometimes vestibular action, without necessarily thinking about how overwhelming that presence might be. The music therapist helps her to identify that this disengagement is about Tyron's tolerance for stimulation and not an indication of his interest in her. On arrival, Tyron recognizes her voice, so while she washes her hands, she can talk to him to give him an opportunity to gently alert to her presence and prepare for when he subsequently sees her. This sort of incremental transition will also allow the parent's space to observe their baby's availability for interaction allowing both parties a gentler and often more successful start to interplay.

The infant's capacity to be engaged may be short-lived, and the change from engaged to disengaged can come without obvious warning. Pain, discomfort, hunger, or physical restriction (intravenous drips, mittens, tubes, etc.) can impinge on the infant. Also, for some infants, conditions such as Pierre Robin syndrome are associated with frequent periods of protracted irritability. The "zero to ten" shift into distress or seeming anger can leave parents confused, powerless, and feeling betrayed. The music therapist can demonstrate and work with parents to help them understand the power of their voice in that moment to preempt or even momentarily override escalating distress. By understanding and controlling the pitch, timbre, and tempo of their voice, parents can create a low, steady, flat intonation to reassure their infant that escalating distress is not needed (Shoemark & Grocke, 2010).

It is important to help parents understand that meaningful sound and interaction are about taking turns or an even more rudimentary balance of sound and silence. Without silence, sound becomes noise. For the anxious or intrusive parent, a problem can arise when they think that if they're not making a sound, they're not doing something:

> My husband and I are do-ers.... so we find it very hard not to do something. It's hard to get your head around [giving space] because we feel as though we're not helping or we're not being worthwhile... *Ann*

To sit quietly during the sought-after periods of infant availability can be counterintuitive. So rather than telling parents to stop or wait for a response, it can be more helpful to encourage them to *create a space* for their infant. To create a quiet space in which their infant can answer them makes sense to the active parent:

> I think she's missing out on because she's asleep so much, that I might actually need to just give her space in that awake time and if I am being too intense with her then she might just go back to sleep rather than stay awake." *Karla*

Voice use and singing in this phase can still emulate the sounds and singing for soothing (as offered in the *anticipatory* phase) to encourage transition to sleep or a quiet awake state for other interactions. Understanding the characteristics of a lullaby is not difficult for parents. They can readily imagine that a lullaby is quiet, slow, and gentle. The value added at this point is helping parents see the impact of changing any and all of the elements of music one at a time. For parents with musical heritage (instrument learned, choir experience), this can be readily achieved, using musical terminology drawing on mastery in other parts of life. For the parent without musical heritage, this is introduced through demonstration and shared experience. The music therapist helps parents to hear and sing a little quieter, a little breathier, a little slower, etc. By singing a song over and over, the parent will also embed this song in the memory of the nurse caring for their infant, and on departure it might just be that the nurse will return to that song if the baby stirs.

Alongside this, playsongs can now be added to promote more active interplay in the available infant. These are discussed in the next section where they are even more pertinent.

Active Parenting

During the NICU admission, the infant may be medically stable and developmentally more available for interplay. Such opportunities might occur while infants await surgery or diagnosis or toward the end of the admission. The purpose of singing now becomes to acknowledge the "good enough" baby (Winnicott, 1971) whose potential as a developing baby now comes into focus.

Parents, now mindful of scaffolding their baby's experiences so they do not overwhelm, can add the bright and joyful playsong during active interplay. Playsongs are identifiable by their bright and clipped timbre, their faster tempo, regular pulse (4/4 time), and the introduction of rhythmic interest. These are the songs that parents imagined singing at home. They create experiences of tangible happiness. The parent's fatigue and ongoing stress often impinge on their capacity to remember even the best known songs of their own childhood. The music therapist helps a parent to recall a selection of songs and, where appropriate, calls on extended family for suggestions which in turn creates a wider context for songs to be shared. Because playsongs are more characterful and expressive, this can be a time when a parent's embarrassment or lack of confidence may override their inclination to sing:

I'll do it when I get home. I just feel stupid doing it in a hospital. *Hailey*

If we were in a room by ourselves it would be a lot better. If I had my earphones or I knew some nursery rhymes or something I might. *Sandra*

The music therapist may resource the family with simple playlists of constructed renditions of songs that provide a "soundtrack" to which they can sing along. Singing along with a recording is a familiar, everyday experience which also provides some masking for their shared experience.

Song becomes a vehicle by which parents can shape the day. This is drawing them toward the regular everyday use of music at home (Ansdell & DeNora, 2016), casually singing a familiar song, while drying their toes, and humming a little tune while settling into feeding or to sleep. The music therapist helps parents to find their creativity, making up songs to label their experiences:

We just make up random stuff [laughs]. I must say my husband sings more than I do. He's sung a few songs. I think it was quite funny; he started off with nursery rhymes and then made up bits at the end. I don't know if he couldn't remember the words or just put his own spin on it. He actually tends to do more of the singing and the reading than I do. *Ann*

During the song, parents can also construct opportunities for the rehearsal of motor and communication skills. A parent's song creates an unspoken but predictable duration to any task, whether it is bathing or physical therapy. For communication, the music therapist helps parents to understand turn-taking through musical games and a repertoire of songs which promotes vocalization, protoconversation, and joyful creative expression.

It is worth noting that singing in the NICU is not always about the infant and parents' emerging life together. When an infant has a life-limiting condition, families can be eager to create memories with their baby. The music therapist may use singing and a song to create shared experiences to be treasured. Amidst anticipatory grief, songs can serve as an accessible and recognizable experience, providing a legacy that is easily recalled. It is unlikely that the parent will be able to sing through the emotion of this moment, so the music therapist metaphorically holds infant and parents together, singing for them all in the moment of the song.

Singing to create a legacy might occur in the days or weeks leading up to an infant's death, but the music therapist can also create a warmer auditory context via songs and other music during final extubation from ventilator support and even in the hours after death. For the infant's funeral, the music therapist may record or actually play requested songs to celebrate the joyful moments of the baby's life. The experience of singing together and the song serve as symbols of the baby as baby, leaving behind the complexities of their medical condition.

Conclusion

The music therapist works in partnership with parents to understand their preexisting relationship with music and their current capacities to utilize singing to nurture and support their baby. The music therapist facilitates the parent's psychological access to their voice, as a tool for infant containment and soothing, as an enticement into interplay, as a vehicle for development, and as a meaningful memento when needed.

> **Key Messages**
> - The usefulness of singing in the NICU can be conceptualized in three phases: anticipatory, cautious interplay, and active parenting.
> - There should be no assumption that singing is a viable action for parents in the NICU.
> - The music therapist brings to consciousness in the parent their own current use of voice and supports ways in which that action can be extended.
> - To actually sing in the NICU, a parent must first be able to think of a reason or imagine singing to their infant in hospital.

References

Ansdell, G., & DeNora, T. (2016). *Music and change: Ecological perspectives: How music helps in music therapy and everyday life*. London, UK: Routledge.

Blumenfeld, H., & Eisenfeld, L. (2006). Does a mother singing to her premature baby affect feeding in the neonatal intensive care unit? *Clinica Pediatricas, 45*, 65–70.

Dearn, T., & Shoemark, H. (2014). The effect of maternal presence on premature infant response to recorded music. *JOGNN, 43*, 341–350.

Feldman, R., Magori-Cohenc, R., Galili, G., Singerb, M., & Louzounc, Y. (2011). Mother and infant coordinate heart rhythms through episodes of interaction synchrony. *Infant Behavior & Development, 34*, 569–577.

Filippa, M., Devouche, E., Arioni, C., Imberty, M., & Gratier, M. (2013). Live maternal speech and singing have beneficial effects on hospitalized preterm infants. *Acta Paediatrica, 102*(10), 1017–1020. doi:10.1111/apa.2013.102.issue-10

Frogget, L., & Briggs, S. (2012). Practice-near and practice-distant methods in human services research. *Journal of Research Practice, 8*(2.) Retrieved from http://jrp.icaap.org/index.php/jrp/article/view/318/276

Layne, L. (1996). "How's the baby doing?" Struggling with narratives of progress in a neonatal intensive care unit. *Medical Anthropology Quarterly, 10*, 624–656.

Loewy, J., Stewart, K., Dassler, A.-M., et al. (2013). The effects of music therapy on vital signs, feeding, and sleep in premature infants. *Pediatrics, 131*, 902–918.

Perry Black, B., Holditch-Davis, D., & Miles, M. (2009). Life course theory as a framework to examine becoming a mother of a medically fragile preterm infant. *Research in Nursing & Health, 32*, 38–49.

Shoemark, H. (e-pub 2017). Time Together: A feasible program to promote parent-infant interaction in the NICU. *Music Therapy Perspectives*. https://doi.org/10.1093/mtp/mix004

Shoemark, H. (2015). Culturally transformed music therapy in the perinatal and paediatric neonatal intensive care unit: An international report. *Music and Medicine, 7*(2), 34–36.

Shoemark, H., & Arnup, S. (2014). A survey of how mothers think about and use voice with their hospitalized newborn infant. *Journal of Neonatal Nursing, 20*, 115–121.

Shoemark, H., & Grocke, D. (2010). The markers of interplay between the music therapist and the medically fragile newborn infant. *Journal of Music Therapy, 47*, 306–334.

Spence, M., & Freeman, M. (1996). Newborn infants prefer the maternal low-pass filtered voice, but not the maternal whispered voice. *Infant Behavior and Development, 19*, 199–212.

Trehub, S., Plantinga, J., & Russo, F. (2015). Maternal vocal interactions with infants: Reciprocal visual influences. *Social Development*. doi:10.1111/sode.12164

Trevarthen, C., & Malloch, S. (2000). The dance of wellbeing: Defining the musical therapeutic effect. *Nordic Journal of Music Therapy*, *9*(2), 3–17.

Tronick, E. (1998). Dyadically expanded states of consciousness and the process of therapeutic change. *Infant Mental Health Journal*, *19*, 290–299.

Winnicott, D. (1971). *Playing and reality*. London, England: Tavistock.

Chapter 13
Sounding Together: Family-Centered Music Therapy as Facilitator for Parental Singing During Skin-to-Skin Contact

Friederike Haslbeck and Pernilla Hugoson

Abstract *Introduction*: When it comes to the delicate relationship between a baby and its parents, the voices of the parents have a significant role in communicating love, tenderness, and closeness as well as in supporting self-regulation as necessary for secure attachment. Under suboptimal experiences, such as premature birth, infant-directed singing takes on an even more important and therapeutic role since preterm infants miss the finely attuned auditory stimulation of the womb and the mother-infant dyad is disrupted too early.

Main aims of the chapter: In this chapter, we will draw from theory foundation, research, and clinical experience to explore the role of the parents' voices in early family-centered interventions in the NICU. Topics will include how infant-directed singing may create meaningful interaction, mutual co-regulation, emotional synchronization, and finely attuned stimulation for vulnerable preterm infants at risk of neurodevelopmental alterations. We will describe how singing for and with parents can motivate and empower parents in using their own voice for their baby. We will introduce how working with parents facilitates sensitivity to infant cues, thus enhancing the quality of parent-infant interactions and ultimately promoting paternal self-efficacy. We will discuss it in the light of the importance of early close relationship building between baby and parent, a base for further development of cognition, language, and emotions.

Conclusions: When we support parents to sing and/or use their voice in an infant-directed and responsive way, e.g., during skin-to-skin contact, we can facilitate self-regulation and nurture multimodal stimulation in a perfectly natural way for both, the baby and the parents. It contains the baby's need for closeness and safety and the parents' need of taking care and connecting emotionally.

F. Haslbeck, PhD (✉)
Clinic of Neonatology at University Hospital Zurich and University Hospital Bern,
Zurich & Bern, Switzerland
e-mail: friederike.haslbeck@usz.ch

P. Hugoson, PhD student
University of Jyväskylä, Finland and Karolinska Institute, Solna, Sweden
e-mail: pernilla.hugoson@ki.se

© Springer International Publishing AG 2017
M. Filippa et al. (eds.), *Early Vocal Contact and Preterm Infant Brain Development*, DOI 10.1007/978-3-319-65077-7_13

Introduction

From the very first moment in life, we are depending on our senses. Through our senses we embrace our environment, and they give us all the important information that we need when we slowly assimilate to the world. Already in the womb, we are being rocked by the movements of our mother, we taste her amniotic fluid, we feel her heartbeat, and we "hear" her voice through viscous sounds in utero and bone conduction. We experience with all our senses in an already-interactive and multisensory manner which is essential for further neurobehavioral development and bonding (Als, 1983; Lopez-Teijon, Garcia-Faura, & Prats-Galino, 2015; Moon & Fifer, 2000; Moon, 2011).

Our human brain is highly dependent upon this multisensory stimulation and is built out of the relation with a loving caregiver that can stimulate and regulate the baby's feelings and emotions (Hart, 2011). The neurosensory system needs an appropriate context to get the organization of neural networks in place, and the ultimate environment for the prenatal brain to develop is, of course, the womb of the mother (Lickliter, 2000). When born preterm, the baby is exposed for incoming sensory stimulation that it is yet not prepared to handle and can lead to many stressful and painful experiences (Mörelius, 2006). They must cope with the potential sensory tensions of overstimulation and deprivation at a time when their brains conventionally grow more rapidly than during any other period in their lives (Als, 2009). They are at the risk for neurodevelopmental deficits and language delays (Aarnoudse-Moens, Weisglas-Kuperus, van Goudoever, & Oosterlaan, 2009; Serenius et al., 2013; Adams-Chapman, 2015).

Also, the environment in the NICU can be stressful for the parents (Thomas & Martin, 2000). The sudden end of pregnancy, separation from the infant, trauma of premature birth, and uncertainty of the infant's survival can evoke feelings of fear, guilt, loss, grief, and confusion (Bruns-Neumann, 2006; Jotzo & Poets, 2005). These reactions increase parental stress and can have a negative impact upon the attachment process between infants and parents. Early separation and the parents' lack of self-confidence and autonomy as primary caregivers in the unfamiliar environment of an intensive care unit may compromise bonding between the mother and infant (Bialoskurski, Cox, & Hayes, 1999; Brisch, Bechinger, Betzler, & Heinemann, 2003).

The importance of constructing a properly suited environment for ultimate development, emotional closeness, bonding, and attachment cannot be overestimated. In the light of this knowledge, one can see the importance of parents being involved in the care of their prematurely born baby as necessary both for the baby's development and for the emotional attachment and bonding between baby and parents. Who can better shape an ultimate environment of love, tenderness, and gentle sensory input that is so essential for the development of a human being than the parents.

The Lullaby: An Emotional Bridge Between Baby and Parents

For thousands of years, in every human culture, parents have been singing to their babies. It is a most natural and genuine way to create security and comfort and to share love and tenderness. In the high-tech environment of the NICU, where both baby and parents are in a vulnerable situation, the humming of a lullaby can be the bridge they need to come in tune and reconnect (Stern, 1985). A humming human voice and the melody of a well-known lullaby can facilitate an emotionally sound environment that is familiar both for the baby and the parents and may lead to reciprocal interaction (Haslbeck, 2013b; de l'Étoile, 2006; O'Gorman, 2006).

Singing lullabies has cross-cultural features: slow tempo, a simple and repetitive melody hummed without words and simple pitch contours, and it is sung in a smooth, breathy, and loving voice timbre often accompanied with gentle touch (Trehub & Trainor, 1998; Unyk, Trehub, Trainor, & Schellenberg, 1992). Lullabies that are sung in an infant-directed style are further characterized by higher pitch, loving tone, more lively variables in tempo and dynamics, and longer pauses between the phrases and repetitiveness (de l'Étoile, 2006; Trainor, Clark, Huntley, & Adams, 1997; Rock, Trainor, & Addison, 1999).

These specific features of responsive singing to infants have been shown to modify infant state and to help regulate infant arousal as to strengthen and build the bond between a baby and its parents (de l'Étoile, 2006; Trainor et al., 1997; Rock et al., 1999). Under suboptimal experiences, such as premature birth, infant-directed singing takes on an even more important and therapeutic role since preterm infants miss the finely attuned auditory stimulation of the womb and the mother-infant dyad is disrupted too early (O'Gorman, 2005; Philbin, 2000; Graven, 2000).

Kangaroo Care: A Multimodal Sensory Intervention

The history of how kangaroo mother care (KMC) became a standard care practice in many NICUs worldwide started in Colombia in 1978. Dr. Rey and Dr. Martinez at the Instituto Materno Infantil proposed KMC as an alternative way of caring for preterm-born infants. Due to a lack of incubators, they started to place all preterm infants with a birthweight lower than 2000 g on the bare chest of their mothers around the clock. The three main components in the original KMC intervention were (1) kangaroo position i.e., skin-to-skin contact in a strict upright position; (2) kangaroo nutrition, i.e., exclusive or nearly exclusive breast-feeding; and (3) kangaroo discharge policies, i.e., early discharge in kangaroo position regardless of weight or gestational age (Charpak, Ruiz-Palaez, & de Calume, 1996). During the following years, up-to-date KMC or skin-to-skin contact (SSC) has developed to become standard care in many NICUs worldwide, and there have been outlined evidence-based guidelines to support establishment (Ruiz and Charpak, 2007).

SSC has been associated with stabilizing effects on (preterm) infants regarding respiratory rate, oxygenation, and temperature but also improved breastfeeding, bonding, and reduced paternal stress (Cho et al., 2016) Boundy, Dastjerdi, Spiegelman, et al., 2016; Moore, Anderson, Bergman, & Dowswell, 2014). In supporting the self-regulatory skills in preterm infants, SSC promotes more organized sleep-wake cyclicity and adaptation to regulating negative emotions, modulating arousal, sharing engagement, and sustaining effortful exploration (Feldman, Weller, Sirota, & Eidelman, 2002) with also long-lasting effects on executive functions and enhanced cognitive development at 10 years of age (Feldman, Rosenthal, & Eidelman, 2014). As SSC is a highly multimodal intervention with direct access to the parents' skin, heartbeat, vibrations through the bone, smell, and loving voice, one can assume that adding lullabies in this context may support even furthermore the fragile dyad of parents and preterm infants.

Music Therapy in Neonatal Care: Development Toward Multimodal Family-Centered Approaches

In the last few decades, there has been growing awareness that many of the health conditions of preterm infants, as well as the problems of parents and challenges in the parent-child relationship, may be prevented through improved therapeutic and preventative care initiated in the very beginning (EFCNI, 2011). There is a general shift from standardized treatment toward individualized relationship-based approaches including parental support, which is recognized within the discipline of music therapy as well (Haslbeck, 2012a). In the twentieth century, receptive, stimulatory types of recording were predominantly played only for infants (e.g., recordings of the mother's voice, womb sounds, and lullabies). Over the past decades, more and more (inter)active approaches with live music/singing have been implemented, also taking into account the complex triad of infant, parent(s)/families, and the NICU environment (e.g., engaging and encouraging parents to sing for their infants to support the infant-parent attachment process) (Haslbeck, 2013a, 2013b; Loewy, 2015; Shoemark, 2011; Teckenberg-Jansson, Huotilainen, Pölkki, Lipsanen, & Järvenpää, 2011; Whipple, 2000).

Even though music therapy in NICUs is a young field of practice and research, an astonishing quantity of evidence already exists. For instance, a systematic integrative review (Haslbeck, 2012a) illustrates with 43 included studies that music therapy particularly supports pacification and stabilization in preterm infants, e.g., more stable measures of heart rate and oxygen saturation and more beneficial behavioral states. This is in line with the results of the meta-analysis of Standley (2012) and the systematic review of Hartling et al. (2009). It also emphasizes that the preterm infants' perceptive faculties and capabilities are actively engaged in music therapy to a greater extent than had been previously recognized in the literature and that benefits were greatest from live music therapy (Haslbeck, 2012; Standley, 2012).

Current studies focus more on including parental support, e.g., by combining music with skin-to-skin contact (SSC). For instance, in the study of Lai et al. (2006), the dyad of mothers and their preterm infants listened to recorded lullabies of their own choice for 60 min/day for 3 days during SSC. The study showed lower maternal anxiety and an occurrence of more quiet sleep states and less crying among the preterm infants in the treatment group. Schlez et al. (2011) evaluated active live harp music therapy versus SSC and demonstrated that active music therapy reduces maternal anxiety more than SSC alone. Similarly, Teckenberg-Jansson et al. (2011) have suggested that live harp music and humming are better than SSC alone in terms of the preterm infant's physiological parameters and parental well-being. In another study on maternal singing and SSC, it was shown that singing improved the autonomic stability in preterm infants and reduced maternal anxiety compared to silent SSC (Arnon et al., 2014). In a small pilot study, reported in a master thesis, four mothers of premature-born babies report that singing during SSC got them to feel more relaxed, helped them to be in the moment, and gave them something to do (Tuomi, 2014).

An updated world perspective on NICU music therapy shows that live music and parental integration currently dominate music therapy practice in neonatal care, with singing being the central and most important modality in all regions (Shoemark & Group, 2014). For instance, in their multicentered RCT, Loewy, Stewart, Dassler, Telsey, and Homel (2013) demonstrated that interactive live music therapy can increase cardiac and respiratory function in the preterm infant, decrease parental stress, and potentially enhance bonding. Shoemark and Arnup (2014) surveyed 60 mothers of babies in the NICU about their beliefs, thoughts, and actions regarding using their voice in the NICU. Sixty percent of these Australian mothers reported that they sang spontaneously, irrespective of maternal age, education, and parenting experience. All these results call for providing more family-centered models of live music therapy with parental singing in the NICU.

Creative Music Therapy in Neonatal Care

One of these more interactive and family-centered music therapy approaches that incorporate parental involvement is called "creative music therapy with preterm infants and their parents" (CMT). The approach was introduced initially as a single case study (Haslbeck, 2004) and evaluated in greater detail in a qualitative study (Haslbeck, 2013a, 2013b).

CMT with preterm infants and their parents is an individualized, resource- and needs-oriented music therapy approach that is based upon "creative music therapy" (Nordoff & Robbins, 1977). It has been adapted to address the specific needs of that particularly vulnerable group of preterm infants and their parents within a NICU setting (Haslbeck, 2013b) combined with principles of CMT used on comatose patients (Aldridge, Gustorff, & Hannich, 1990). With this approach, the music therapist establishes human contact with the preterm infant through improvised, entrained infant-directed humming. CMT with preterm infants is based upon the premise that infants should be neither overwhelmed nor overstimulated. The parents, if available and willing, are involved individually in the therapeutic process, e.g., by supporting them in singing to their infant and fostering an intuitive parent-infant interaction, so as to strengthen the bonding process. CMT involves the model of psychological traumatization, incorporating specific aspects to facilitate relaxation, stabilization, and the healthy development of parent-infant relationships (Fischer & Riedesser, 2009).

In creative music therapy, we believe that everyone can respond to music, no matter how ill or disabled or even premature an infant is (Nordoff & Robbins, 1977). The Nordoff-Robbins approach implies the unique qualities of music as therapy: enhancing communication, supporting change, and enabling people to live more resourcefully and creatively (Nordoff & Robbins, 1977). If we accept that everyone is sensitive to music, which can be utilized for personal growth, health, and development, then we can accept that, through interactions with music, therapists can support and enhance the clients' expressive skills and their ability to relate to others. The noninvasive potential of creative music therapy for prelinguistic communication allows even vulnerable, severely affected individuals like preterm infants to become "active" rather than being given a solely receptive and passive role. Moreover, the focus of creative music therapy with preterm infants and their parents is on creating an individual relationship with the infant. This takes place through music, as well as by facilitating his or her relationship with parents to support the infant "coming into being," (Aldridge, 1996) the parents into parenthood, and the triad into bonding.

The preterm infant is seen as a social being (Buber, 1958; Malloch & Trevarthen, 2009a) since the newborn (including those who are premature) depends on others to construct his/her own structure and requires "regulatory input from others to sustain even basic homeostatic and physiological processes" (Ham & Tronick, 2009, p. 621) and to develop himself/herself through the reciprocal affect attunement that evolves between human beings (Papousek, 2012; Schore, 2003; Stern, 2010a). Stern's theory of *affect attunement* (Stern, 2010b), as well as the theory of *communicative musicality* by Malloch and Trevarthen (Malloch & Trevarthen, 2009b), emerged in the qualitative study of CMT (2013b) as sensitizing concept. The study results demonstrate that preterm infants are already capable of sharing subtle vitality forms in improvised live music, acting like the intuitive affect attunement of a healthy parent-infant performance, since this communicative event is highly musical and improvisational in nature (Lenz & von Moreau, 2004; Malloch & Trevarthen, 2009a; Papousek & Papousek, 1991; Trondalen & Skarderud, 2007).

As evident in the qualitative study, the finely attuned and entrained infant-directed singing of CMT offers the potential for preterm infants to engage in communicative

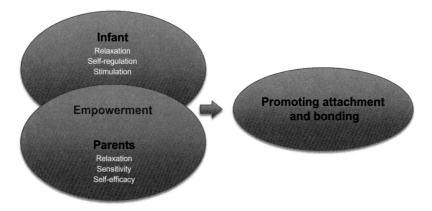

Fig. 13.1 The interactive potential of family-centered creative music therapy

musicality that can help them to get back in tune, in rhythm, in mutual co-regulation, in self-synchrony, and in interactional synchrony, even in an overwhelmingly arrhythmic intensive care environment (Haslbeck, 2013a, 2013b). The microanalysis suggests that CMT may be particularly effective at pacifying, engaging, and empowering pre-term infants without being overwhelming. Furthermore, the results demonstrate that CMT may empower parents, by enhancing their well-being, self-confidence, and quality of interactions with their infant through music. By integrating parents in the therapeutic process and by supporting them in singing, they are empowered in the quality of their interactions with their infants and, thus, in their attachment process, as well as their self-confidence (Fig. 13.1) (Haslbeck, 2015b).

CMT in neonatal care is a true family-centered music therapy approach in which each family is encouraged to find their innate way of relating through singing and music (Haslbeck, 2016). With this approach, health is promoted by integrating fam-ilies into the therapeutic process by providing emotional, social, and developmental support as warranted in family-centered care (Gooding et al., 2011) and highlighted in the literature of music therapy (Hanson-Abromeit, 2003; Haslbeck, 2015a; Loewy, 2015; Shoemark, 2014). This approach can also be linked to the tradition of Swedish pediatricians and nurses interested in parental singing and its impact on infant development and attachment between the baby and parents (Eulau, 2007; Lagercrantz, 2012; Lind, 1980; Ådén, 2014).

Clinical Approach

The main goals of working with preterm infants and their parents are to reduce stress and anxiety, to stabilize and empower both infants and parents, and to support parent-infant bonding. Neonatal music therapy is mostly part of a complementary psychosocial support in neonatal care.

Starting Up

Prior to initiating music therapy, an in-depth assessment of the current state and needs of the infant and its family must be conducted with the NICU team (primary nurse and/or physician/psychologist); it also must be well documented, as described in more detail in Haslbeck (2013a) and Hanson-Abromeit, Shoemark, and Loewy (2008). By identifying the needs of the infants and parents, specific short- and long-term goals can be created and adapted individually over time to the therapeutic process, in accordance with the principles of the individualized, relationship-based care model NIDCAP (Newborn Individualized Developmental Care and Assessment Program) and family-centered care approach (Craig et al., 2015; Als, 2009; American Academy of Pediatrics, 2003). Music therapy can only be offered when the infant is medically stable enough, as determined by leading members of the NICU team. Before conducting each music therapy session, again detailed information and permission must be obtained from the neonatal team. As soon as possible, we meet with parents to introduce ourselves, to personally assess their needs, to introduce the benefits of singing for their infant and themselves, and to assess their musical heritage, culture, context, and wishes. In other words, we ask a lot of questions over the whole course of the therapeutic process to guarantee individualized, resource- and need-based strategies.

The Role of the Music Therapist

In the neonatal environment, we must subordinate our therapeutic services to the priority of medical treatment and intensive care. We have to be flexible, creative, adaptive, and therapeutically responsive. By using this responsiveness, we see our role as a facilitator for meaningful interactions, which take place in the therapeutic moment with the infant and also between parents and infants by promoting the parents' sensitivity during interactions with their infants through music. Also, when music therapy only takes place between the therapist and the infant, the role of the therapist is to support the social development of the infant, not by being a surrogate for the parents but rather by functioning as an additional source of shared communicative musicality (Shoemark, 2011).

In the vulnerable situation of premature birth, a contact with a professional that is not part of the medical team may give parents a somehow broader space to share their situation and experiences on a deeper emotional level (O'Gorman, 2005; Shoemark & Dearn, 2008). Therefore, our role is also to give parents space for sharing emotions, feelings, and thoughts concerning their situation and life in general. We share our knowledge and act as a role model, when needed, in mediating the preferred way to sing to a premature-born baby and/or mediating knowledge about signs of overstimulation and signs of the baby's intentions to interact (Als, 2009). However, when working with parents, our role is not to educate them but rather to lure out endogenous capabilities of parenting and caring that are often hidden by stress, anxiety, and trauma (Boukydis, 2012). We understand our role within the purpose of family-centered principles as coach and collaborator (American Academy of Pediatrics, 2003).

This is of great value, considering their curtailed parental role and autonomy. In this context, the task of the music therapist is to respect, integrate, and attune to the individual cultural backgrounds of families. Moreover, our role is to facilitate empowerment – empowering both the infant (e.g., by facilitating self-regulation and engagement) and the parents (e.g., by supporting their well-being, self-confidence, autonomy, and quality of interactions with their infant through music) (American Academy of Pediatrics, 2003; Haslbeck, 2013b).

Methods and Techniques

While working only with the infant, the infant is placed in the incubator or warming bed. Mostly, the music therapist starts with initial touch (touch at the infant's head and feet) that transforms into therapeutic touch to offer contact as well as to feel and stimulate the breathing rhythm of the infant (Hanley, 2008). Based on the natural multimodal stimulation in the womb, it is the most natural way not only to sing for a baby but also to hold, rock, or touch the baby. The music therapist assesses the "music" of the preterm infant – the breathing pattern, the most fundamental rhythm of a human being, together with the infant's facial expressions and gesticulations – and transforms it into infant-directed improvised humming that is constantly adjusted to the fragile rhythms and subtle expressions of the preterm infant. The singing is entrained to the breathing rhythm of the infant, e.g., by singing one long note on three breaths of the infant. The minimal movements of the infants are assessed in a musical understanding, e.g., by assessing if a movement is going up or down. Often this transformation of affects and rhythms into music takes place in a synchronous way; e.g., when the infant's eyebrows lift, the music therapist steers the melody upward (Haslbeck, 2013a). Conversely, when the infant is too aroused, the music therapist moves in the opposite way, e.g., bringing the melody downward and slowing its tempo so as to soothe the baby with sedative musical parameters (Loewy, Hallan, Friedmann, & Martinez, 2005). Moreover, the infant-directed humming or singing is kept as simple as possible, since preterm infants can easily be overwhelmed. Humming fluently using rich overtones in a lullaby and infant-directed style, keeping the music calm and soft (approx. 55 dB), simple, predictable, and repetitive, is warranted as also recommended in existing guidelines on music therapy in the NICU (Hanson-Abromeit et al., 2008). It is also the responsibility of the special trained music therapist to avoid reverberation when singing to an infant that is still placed in the incubator.

How to work with the family depends upon the circumstances (of the unit) and their wishes regarding how often music therapy sessions involving them will take place. Some parents are able to spend a lot of time in the NICU (or all the time) and enjoy the sessions that are conducted together, mostly and preferably during skin-to-skin contact.

When offering music therapy during skin-to-skin contact, the first author largely uses a monochord as accompanying instrument. A monochord is a single-stringed wooden instrument designed for the therapeutic purpose of generating relaxing sounds and vibro-acoustic stimulation. It is especially lacquered to meet the hygiene requirements of the NICU and tune in the key of the NICU environment (the key of monitors, alarms, air conditioners, etc.) to mask environmental noise (Hanson-Abromeit et al., 2008Loewy, 2000). To allow for the replication of live womb sounds (Loewy et al., 2013), the monochord is used to mimic the deep intrauterine vibratory fluid sounds. The monochord is placed next to the kangaroo care chair, so that the parents can touch the instrument with their elbow and feel the instrument's relaxing vibrations conducted through the parent's body; the vibration may then smoothly reach the infant. Since many parents are also very stressed during SSC, due to posttraumatic reactions, the relaxing sound of the monochord may be an opportunity for parents and infants to effectively calm down, relax, and perceive each other more intensely (Lee et al., 2012). Since the monochord is characterized by an open sound without chord or harmony limitations, it provides a perfect background against which to sing along calmly and vibrantly in all musical styles and keys, as preferred by the parents. For many parents, it is much easier to sing along with this accompanying instrument, because "this doesn't feel quite so naked" (a mother's quote). Also while working with the infant-parent-environment triad, CMT aims to incorporate as many of the child's and parents' rhythms, signs, and affects as possible. To honor the family's culture and choices, parents' favorite musical style and/or song(s) or the favorite song(s) of siblings, grandparents, or other family members are integrated to transform a meaningful classical or well-known melody into a "song of kin" (Loewy, 2015; Loewy et al., 2013).

Family-Centered Music Therapy in Switzerland

At University Hospital in Bern and Zurich, Switzerland, where CMT is offered, all levels of NICU are built as an open space. Visiting hours for parents are limited to the time during the day and evening. There is no general rooming-in for parents, but they are encouraged to be present, to be involved in the care of their baby, and to kangaroo in comfortable chairs next to the infant's incubator. They can close a curtain for some privacy. Music therapy takes place three times each week for the infants and the parent-infant triad until discharge, so that an intense therapeutic process can develop over time. In the sense of family-centered care (Gooding et al., 2011), once each month, a parent-to-parent support group is also being offered in collaboration with a dedicated premature mother, chaplains, and psychologists.

For the purpose of family-centered care, the University Hospital in Bern, Switzerland, was the first hospital in Europe to implement and adapt the COPE program – Creating Opportunities for Parent Empowerment – to the Swiss context. COPE is an educational-behavioral intervention program for parents. With this program, the neonatal team offers supervision and educational guidance for parents, while supporting close contact between the parents and infant and preparing them for the transition from hospital to home. Findings indicate that the COPE program reduces parental stress (Melnyk & Feinstein, 2009). At the University Hospital in Zurich, no Cope program is provided, but the neonatal unit integrates many components of the NIDCAP approach and family-centered care approach.

Case Vignette
Annett and Peter[1] were a young married academic couple with a good social network and good relationships with family. The only thing still missing was a child. Since Annett was born with meningomyelocele and tied to her wheelchair, giving birth was associated with risks from the very beginning. When Annett became pregnant, the couple was overjoyed but also worried. In the 26th week of pregnancy, Annett felt very ill and had to be admitted to the hospital. Two weeks later, a cesarean section had to be performed because of childlike indications. Michael[2] was born at 28 weeks of gestational age, weighing 740 g. He suffered from infant respiratory distress syndrome, apnea-bradycardia syndrome, hyperglycemia, anemia, hyperbilirubinemia, a poor Apgar score, and persistent ductus arteriosus. The couple was joyful and thankful that Michael was alive but also very anxious and uncertain about the health complications being experienced by Michael. They felt helpless, shaken, and stressed. This was reinforced by the fact that Peter had to go back to work soon, which meant to be away in London for 4 days of the week. Thus, Annett and Peter had to deal with a challenging mixture of emotions and circumstances at the same time.

The NICU team referred Michael for music therapy with the aims of relaxing and stabilizing Michael, especially to help him achieve more regular, deep breathing and to support the parents to relax and to find (self-)confidence. At the very beginning, I conducted the music therapy sessions during kangaroo care with the mother. Before the first session, Annett seemed stressed and skeptical. I hummed for mother and infant accompanied with the monochord. Michael reacted positively to the music, demonstrating enhanced relaxation, more regular breathing, and increased stabilization and awareness (e.g., eyebrow lifting, smiling). Annett was very touched by the music and the positive reactions of Michael. She smiled back at her son, caressed him tenderly, and seemed to be intimately connected. Also the next sessions, she preferred just listening to some improvised music. With the aim of providing a blanket of relaxing, nurturing sound for the mother and to offer meaningful interaction with her son, this was a perfect start. Since the mother especially remained tense and stressed even during kangaroo care, it was already a huge plus that she reported feeling less anxious and stressed combining kangaroo care with singing and relaxing smooth vibrations by the monochord.

Since she told me that she would be too shy to sing but that perhaps her husband would sing for Michael, we scheduled a session with the father as soon as possible. When I asked him for a special song (song of kin) he proposed "Hallelujah" from

---

[1] Names changed to protect their anonymity.
[2] Name changed to protect his anonymity.

Leonard Cohen as one of his favorite songs being nurtured by which he often plays along with his bass guitar. We sang the song together while the father was in kangaroo care, entrained to the breathing rhythm of Michael and accompanied with the monochord. Michael reacted with smiling, soft finger, and mouth movements, so the father smiled back, caressed him tenderly, and seemed fulfilled with joy. He wrote in his diary: "….we sang Hallelujah, and you seemed to try and join in the singing too. Love you so much, daddy" (see illustration). Especially for the father who had to struggle with the circumstances that he was not able to visit his son every day, this was a very important and valuable "moment of meeting" for parenting and bonding.

Illustration: Diary note of Peter

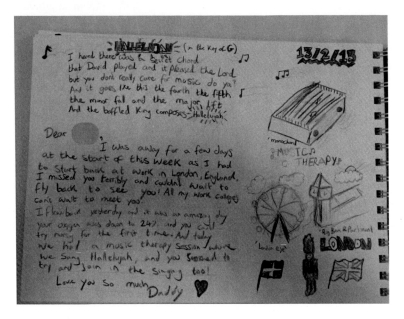

From now on, the father sang regularly "Hallelujah" for Michael during kangaroo care and reported that it helped him to calm down and feel connected and that Michael continued to react positively to his singing. I also encouraged the mother to sing for Michael during kangaroo care, and she started humming softly when she felt less observed. However, when there were some health complications with Michael, the mother still worried a lot and she seemed to be stressed. There also seemed to be some tensions inherent to the couple's relationship. To support their relationship and to further help them to relax while drawing strength, I asked them if they would like to write a song, together with me, in which all their mixed feelings, individual experiences, and concerns could be given room.

The songwriting went very well. Using the melody of "Hallelujah," we drafted lyrics to incorporate the parents' individual experiences and feelings about the premature birth and their anxiety, but mainly their joy, hope, pride, love, and care were given room. The first verse was created and sung by the father from his personal perspective and the second by the mother and her perspective. While composing the lyrics, they shared their individual experiences, feelings, and struggles to become a premature parent. After giving room for each other's feelings, they then created and sang the third verse together – much the same as a reunion of their relationship, their points of view, and their new hope and reconnection. Once the song was written, they grinned from ear to ear, filled with pride and a new sense of strength and purpose.

Hallelujah for Michael[3]
Dad: *I remember the day*
That you were born
The doctors came to inform
That you are here and
You would like to meet me
My heart was jumping out my chest
I held my hand to my breast
And every breath I drew was Hallelujah
Refrain (both):
Hallelujah, Hallelujah.
Hallelujah, Hallelujah.
Mum: *I remember the day*
That I held you
The very first time in kangaroo
Your tiny fingers touched my skin and heart
I was overwhelmed by the love I felt
It melted away the fears I held
And every breath we drew was Hallelujah
Refrain (both)
Mum and Dad:
Every day you grow strong
In our hearts you belong
We cannot wait
Until we'll take you home
Every step makes us proud
Every gaze lets our heart sings loud
Thus, it's a bold and joyful Hallelujah.
Refrain (both)

From then on, they sang that song together for Michael as much as possible. They became more and more sensitive to their son's signs and affects and the meaningful shared interactions of the music. Altogether, we had 15 music therapy sessions.

---

[3] Lyrics composed by his parents in the melody of the Leonard Cohen song. Listen to the original song here: https://www.youtube.com/watch?v=WIF4_Sm-rgQ

Two weeks later, they could leave the hospital with the words "We will definitely continue singing for Michael. It was as if the sun sends its golden rays. It is such a valuable resource. And we look forward to sing him to sleep in his own bed in our own home so much."

Family-Centered Music Therapy in Sweden

The neonatal intensive care units in Sweden provide family-centered care on different levels. In short, it means that the parents have the opportunity to attend their preterm-born baby 24 h/day. Parents also have the possibility to take part in the care of their baby as much as they can based on their unique situation, encouraged and supported by the staff (Craig et al., 2015; Gooding et al., 2011; Griffin, 2006; McGrath, 2001). The neonatal unit at the Karolinska University Hospital/Danderyds Hospital in Stockholm, Sweden, is one of three units in Stockholm which all three together comprise the biggest regional center for neonatal care in Scandinavia. The ward is a family-centered developmentally supportive care unit where all the medical staff are skilled in supporting and encouraging the parents as the primary caregivers with the infant's well-being, development, and possibility to attach in focus (Westrup, 2015). The neonatal unit at Danderyds Hospital was one of the first units in Sweden to implement the developmental supportive and family-centered care model NIDCAP (Westrup, Kleberg, von Eichwald, Stjernqvist, & Lagercrantz, 2000; Westrup, 2007; Örtenstrand, Westrup, Broström, et al., 2010).

At the unit, there is room for 24 infants and their parents. The ward carries two acute care rooms with four beds. In adherence to each bed is an armchair available for the parents, and the family can easily get some privacy by putting a shield in front of their corner of the room. There are also several family rooms where the parents and their baby move when the infant is stable enough. Here, the family stays until the baby is ready for discharge. In the family rooms, the parents have the whole responsibility for taking care of their baby 24 h around the clock supported and coached by the nurses. Music therapy takes place two times per week and can take place both in the acute care rooms and in the family rooms.

Case Vignette: Feelings of Closeness

I knock on the door and hear a tiny voice that says "" "Come in." When I enter the room, I see the mother sitting in the armchair with her baby girl on her naked chest. She looks at me with tired eyes and says "Oh, it's you." The room is shadowed and the air feels a bit stuffy. I ask her if I can come in for a moment, and she says yes. Beside the armchair is a stool and I settled down. When I gently ask her how it is and how her baby girl is feeling today, she answers that she is so tired that she hasn't any energy to talk about it. So we just sit together for a while, looking at the baby and following her breathing and small movements. After a while, the mother asks me if I can sing for her and her baby girl. "Can't you sing the one that we sang the last time we met?" she asks. I start to hum on the well-known lullaby with a smooth and gentle voice, very quiet and attentive to the signs from the baby. The mother closes her eyes, and I can see that her body relaxes and that her face loses its tension. The baby seems to adjust to her mother's more relaxed posture, and the saturation of the oxygen that has been quite irregular stabilizes for a while. After some minutes, the mother opens her eyes and smiles "I love when you sing to us, it gets me so relaxed!" she says. "Do you want us to sing it together?" I ask. "Yes, please!" So, we sing together on the same lullaby and now she is looking at her baby girl with a smile and some tears in her eyes and says: "My wonderful, pretty daughter you are so strong. You are struggling all the time but Mommy is here to help you, always!" After a pause, she starts to sing on a song that she has invented and that she invents just now in the moment. The melody consists of just a few tones and is very simple. It's about how her daughter is running in their garden trying to catch a small rabbit that she wants to keep as her own, but Mommy says no, no, no, and (child's name) says yes, yes, yes. The mother invents the text while singing about how wonderful it is to be with her daughter in the garden. Afterward, we can talk about how it is and she reveals how she sometimes feels such hopelessness and that she never can rest because everything can change from moment to moment. I put her attention to the song that she just sang, how it was about their future and of what will come and mediates the importance of having dreams of the future and how it can help her in the present moment and give strength to the relation between her and her daughter. She smiles and some tears are falling. I also mediate what I observe is happening when she is singing: a smile in her face, glitter in her eyes, more energy around her and her baby, and maybe the most important – a closeness between them that is difficult to put in words but that is very strongly felt in the room. "Yes, I can feel that she likes when I sing to her!" she says. When I after a while leave them, the room seems brighter and once again I think of how absolutely invaluable it is to have the possibility to share feelings and how clearly they express themselves through our bodies, facial expressions, and voices.

Summary and Discussion

Both case vignettes illustrate how family-centered music therapy can facilitate the attachment and bonding process between the preterm infant and their parents from the very beginning through music and through parental singing (compare Fig. 13.1). Even if the infants are placed in an open space, NICU (parental) singing has the potential to facilitate a personal and safe place of intimate contact and growing relationship. Or in the words of a mother: "Singing helped me to build a bubble around us during the kangaroo sessions, a bubble that was oblivious to the surrounding world and that could shut out the disturbing going-ons. There were only the two of us. Singing helped me to build intimacy."

Within the finely attuned infant-directed singing, parents and infants are able to share a "neonatal moment of meeting" that Bruschweiler-Stern (2009) describes as essential after birth to unfold the mother-infant attachment process.

As demonstrated in a micro-video analysis (Haslbeck, 2013b), even for parents who have problems to connect with their infant, singing can lure out hidden parental capabilities of attunement and sensitivity to infant cues. This experience may result in increased numbers of appropriate parent-infant interactions and secure attachments, as argued by several authors (Fig. 13.1) (Edwards, 2011; Stern et al., 1998; Whipple, 2000).

Supporting parents in singing during SSC while holding their infant in their arms is not only the most natural way of singing lullabies, but it is also the most natural way for the infant to learn about affects and stimuli in an already-interactive and multisensory manner. When parents sing for their infant in SSC, the babies can "bathe" in this vibro-acoustic-olfactory experience that may facilitate the most natural way of relaxation, sensory perception, and attachment. However, parental stress can block these relaxing effects since stress, for instance, changes breathing patterns into small, shallow breaths and inhibits a fluently soothing vibratory voice and inner balance (Brown, 1977). And also, the infants are often very stressed and have therefore struggles to breathe calmly and deeply (Pediatrics, A. A. of, 2007). Unfortunately, stress also acts easily in a transference-countertransference dynamic and blocks relationship building (Diamond, 2015). It is therefore even more important to facilitate relaxation in both, the infants and their parents, e.g., by offering a blanket of relaxing and nurturing sound for the traumatized and stressed parents and infants during SSC and guiding the parents to breathe deeply and relax (Fig. 13.1).

Affording parents the opportunity to actively interact with their baby by singing may be an effective way of reducing feelings of guilt, fear, and lost self-esteem. Supporting parents' singing offers the opportunity for music to be a continuously stabilizing factor – a bridge from the prenatal to neonatal period and even throughout childhood. However, not all parents are comfortable to sing; they can feel exposed and worried about someone hearing them singing. The role of the music therapist is therefore to support and motivate the parents to use their voice individually, and if singing seems (not yet) appropriate, also talking in a responsive way with "motherese" is effective and powerful for both, e.g., as demonstrated by Filippa, Devouche, Arioni, Imberty, and Gratier (2013). The aim should be neither to force nor to teach the parents in singing but rather to give parents the opportunity to playfully and creatively lure out endogenous capabilities of using their voice to reconnect with their baby.

The initial conversation about family songs and musical background may also act as key to inspire parents to start singing for their infants. When the therapeutic process proceeds and the parents have been getting more confidence in singing, they often share experiences of different situations where they have been using singing or where singing has been a way to be near and to connect with their baby emotionally. Through sensitive and perceptive coaching, the music therapist can help the parents to gain a deeper understanding of their baby's emotional needs and how the singing and talking to their baby support the baby's development in different stages (Hanson-Abromeit, 2003; Malloch et al., 2012; Shoemark & Dearn, 2008; Shoemark et al., 2015). It is a reciprocal dialogue, both musical and conversational, between the parents and the music therapist where they share their knowledge, observations, and experiences (Malloch et al., 2012; Shoemark & Dearn, 2008; Shoemark et al. 2015).

Exposure to repeated stress in preterm infants is associated with altered brain development, function, and neurodevelopmental outcomes (Radley & Morrison, 2005; Vinall & Grunau, 2014). On the other side, individualized interactive and multisensory experiences support brain development in preterm infants (Als, 2009). Also, music promotes neurobiological processes and neuronal learning and modulates synaptic plasticity in the human brain (McMahon et al., 2012; Xu et al., 2009). This begs the question if creative music therapy promotes preterm infants' brain development by facilitating relaxation, individualized interaction, and finely attuned auditory experiences at the same time. Therefore, two trials, one in Scandinavia and one in Switzerland (Haslbeck, 2015a; Haslbeck, 2014; Hugoson et al., 2015), currently examine if preterm infants who experience infant-directed singing by a music therapist and their parents during their neonatal intensive care period demonstrate improved short- and long-term neurological development. To our knowledge, these are the first randomized controlled clinical trials worldwide to systematically examine the effects of (parental) infant-directed singing on brain structure and function in preterm infants as well as their long-term neurological behavior, particularly socio-emotional and language outcomes. New insights into the potential of music on brain function and development may be gained, and a low-cost, low-risk family-centered intervention found to support brain development and well-being and secure attachment in this vulnerable group from the very beginning.

Key Messages
- Family-centered music therapy can facilitate parental singing.
- Parental singing during SSC is the most natural way for premature infants to learn about affects and stimuli in an interactive and multisensory manner that is essential for further neurobehavioral development.
- Family-centered music therapy can relax and empower both the infants and the parents.
- Family-centered creative music therapy supports bonding through experiencing communicative musicality from the very beginning.

References

Aarnoudse-Moens, C. S., Weisglas-Kuperus, N., van Goudoever, J. B., & Oosterlaan, J. (2009). Metaanalysis of neurobehavioral outcomes in very preterm and/or very low birth weight children. *Pediatrics, 124*, 717–728.

Adams-Chapman, I., Bann, C., Carter, S. L., Stoll, B. J., & for the NICHD neonatal research network. (2015). Language outcomes among ELBW infants in early childhood. *Early Human Development, 91*, 373–379.

Ådén, U. (2014). Maternal singing during kangaroo care comforts both the mother and the baby. *Acta Paediatrica, 103*(10), 995–996.

Aldridge, D. (1996). *Music therapy research and practice in medicine: From out of the silence.* London, England: Jessica Kingsley Publishers.

Aldridge, D., Gustorff, D., & Hannich, H. J. (1990). Where am I? Music therapy applied to coma patients. *Journal of the Royal Society of Medicine, 83*, 345–346.

Als, H. (1983). Toward a synactive theory of development: Promise for the assessment and support of infant individuality. *Infant Mental Health Journal, 3*(4), 229–243.

Als, H. (2009). NIDCAP: Testing the effectiveness of a relationship-based comprehensive intervention. *Pediatrics, 124*(4), 1208–1210.

American Academy of Pediatrics. (2003). Family-centered care and the pediatrician's role. *Pediatrics, 112*(3), 691–696.

Arnon, S., Diamant, C., Bauer, S., Regev, R., Sirota, G., & Litmanovitz, I. (2014). Maternal singing during kangaroo care led to autonomic stability in preterm infants and reduced maternal anxiety. *Acta Paediatrica, 103*(10), 1039–1044.

Bialoskurski, M., Cox, C. L., & Hayes, J. A. (1999). The nature of attachment in a neonatal intensive care unit. *The Journal of Perinatal and Neonatal Nursing, 13*(1), 66–77.

Boukydis, Z. (2012). *Collaborative consultation with parents and infants in the perinatal period.* Baltimore, MD: Brookes Publishing.

Boundy, E. O., Dastjerdi, R., Spiegelman, D., et al. (2016). Kangaroo mother care and neonatal outcomes; a meta-analysis. *Pediatrics, 137*(1), e20152238.

Brisch, K. H., Bechinger, D., Betzler, S., & Heinemann, H. (2003). Early preventive attachment-oriented psychotherapeutic intervention program with parents of a very low birthweight premature infant: Results of attachment and neurological development. *Attachment & Human Development, 5*(2), 120–135.

Brown, B. (1977). *Stress and the art of biofeedback.* Oxford, England: Harper & Row.

Bruns-Neumann, E. (2006). Das Erleben von Eltern nach der Frühgeburt ihres Kindes. *Pflege, 19*(3), 146–155.

Bruschweiler-Stern, N. (2009). The neonatal moment of meeting – Building the dialogue, strengthening the bond. *Child and Adolescent Psychiatric Clinics of North America, 18*(3), 533–544.

Buber, M. (1958). *I and thou* (2nd ed.). New York, NY: Charles Scribner's Sons.

Charpak, N., Ruiz-Palaez, J. G., & de Calume, Z. F. (1996). Current knowledge of kangaroo mother intervention. *Pediatrics, 8*, 108–112.

Cho, E.-S., Kim, S.-J., Kwon, M. S., Cho, H., Kim, E. H., Jun, E. M., & Lee, S. (2016, in press). The effects of kangaroo care in the neonatal intensive care unit on the physiological functions of preterm infants, maternal–infant attachment, and maternal stress. *Journal of Pediatric Nursing.*

Craig, J. W., Glick, C., Phillips, R., Hall, S. L., Smith, J., & Browne, J. (2015). Recommendations for involving the family in developmental care of the NICU baby. *Journal of Perinatology, 35*, 5–8.

de l'Étoile, S. (2006). Infant-directed singing: A theory for clinical intervention. *Music Therapy Perspectives, 24*(1), 22–29.

Diamond, L. (2015). Stress and attachment. In J. A. Simpson & W. Rholes (Eds.), *Attachment theory and research: New directions and emerging themes* (pp. 97–123). New York, NY: Guilford Publications.

Edwards, J. (2011). *Music therapy and parent-infant bonding.* Oxford: Oxford University Press.

EFCNI. (2011). Caring for tomorrow. In *EFCNI white paper on maternal and newborn health and aftercare services.* Karlsfeld, Gemany: European Foundation for the Care of Newborn Infants.

Eulau, L. (2007). Visor i livets början för barn och föräldrar i intensivvården. Rapport från Kultur i vården och vården som kultur, 2007:1. Stockholm, Sweden: Stockholms Universitet. Institutionen för musik och teatervetenskap. (In swedish).

Feldman, R., Rosenthal, Z., & Eidelman, A. I. (2014). Maternal-preterm skin-to-skin contact enhances child physiologic organization and cognitive control across the first 10 years of life. *Biological Psychiatry, 75*, 56–64.

Feldman, R., Weller, A., Sirota, L., & Eidelman, A. I. (2002). Skin-to-skin (kangaroo care) promotes self-regulation in premature infants: Sleep-wake cyclicity, aurosal modulation and sustained exploration. *Developmental Psychology, 38*(2), 194–207.

Filippa, M., Devouche, E., Arioni, C., Imberty, M., & Gratier, M. (2013). Live maternal speech and singing have beneficial effects on hospitalized preterm infants. *Acta Paediatrica, 102*(10), 1017–1020.

Fischer, G., & Riedesser, P. (2009). *Lehrbuch der Psychotraumatologie [Textbook of psychotraumatology]* (4th ed.). Munich, Germany: Ernst Reinhardt Verlag.

Gooding, J. S., Cooper, L. G., Blaine, A. I., Franck, L. S., Howse, J. L., & Berns, S. D. (2011). Family support and family-centered care in the neonatal intensive care unit: Origins, advances, impact. *Seminars in Perinatology, 35*(1), 20–28.

Graven, S. N. (2000). Sound and the developing infant in the NICU: Conclusions and recommendations for care. *Journal of Perinatology, 20*, 88–93.

Griffin, T. (2006). Family-centered care in the NICU. *The Journal of Perinatal & Neonatal Nursing, 20*(1), 98–102.

Ham, J., & Tronick, E. (2009). Relational psychophysiology: Lessons from mother-infant physiology research on dyadically expanded states of consciousness. *Psychotherapy Research, 19*(6), 619–632.

Hanley, M. A. (2008). Therapeutic touch with preterm infants: Composing a treatment. *Explore, 4*(4), 253–258.

Hanson-Abromeit, D. (2003). The newborn individualized developmental care and assessment program (NIDCAP) as a model of music therapy interventions with premature infants. *Music Therapy Perspectives, 21*, 60–68. doi:10.1093/mtp/21.2.60

Hanson-Abromeit, D., Shoemark, H., & Loewy, J. (2008). Music therapy with pediatric units: Newborn intensive care unit (NICU). In D. Hanson-Abromeit & C. Colwell (Eds.), *Medical music therapy for pediatrics in hospital settings. Using music to support medical interventions* (pp. 15–69). Silver Spring, MD: AMTA.

Hart, S. (2011). *The impact of attachment-Developmental neuroaffective psychology*. New York, NY: WW Norton & Company.

Hartling, L., Shaik, M. S., Tjosvold, L., Leicht, R., Liang, Y., & Kumar, M. (2009). Music for medical indications in the neonatal period: A systematic review of randomised controlled trials. *Archives of Disease in Childhood. Fetal and Neonatal Edition, 94*, F394–F354.

Haslbeck, F. (2004). Music therapy with preterm infants – Theoretical approach and first practical experience. *Music Therapy Today*.

Haslbeck, F. (2015a). ClinicalTrials.gov. *Creative music therapy for premature infants*. ClinicalTrials.gov identifier: NCT02434224.

Haslbeck, F. (2015b). Empowerment and empowering self: Using creative music therapy to reconnect premature infants and their mothers. In C. Dileo (Ed.), *Advanced practice in medical music therapy: Case reports* (pp. 20–32). Jeffrey Books.

Haslbeck, F. (2016, in press). Three little wonders. Music therapy with families in neonatal care. In S. Lindahl Jacobsen & G. A. Thompson (Eds.), *Models of music therapy with families*. London, England: Jessica Kingsley Publishers.

Haslbeck, F. B. (2012). Music therapy for premature infants and their parents: An integrative review. *Nordic Journal of Music Therapy, 21*(3), 203–226.

Haslbeck, F. B. (2013a). Creative music therapy with premature infants: An analysis of video footage. *Nordic Journal of Music Therapy, 23*(1), 5–35.

Haslbeck, F. B. (2013b). The interactive potential of creative music therapy with premature infants and their parents: A qualitative analysis. *Nordic Journal of Music Therapy, 23*(1), 36–70.

Haslbeck, F. B. (2014). Creative music therapy in premature infants: Testing its possible influence on brain development. *Music Therapy Today (online), 10*(1), 116–117.

Haslbeck, F. B. (2015a). Frühstart ins Leben: Musik al Therapie für frühgeborene Kinder und ihre Eltern. *Musik, Spiel Und Tanz, 2*, 40–42.

Hugoson, P., Westrup, B., Erkkilä, J., Haslbeck, F., Huotilainen, M., Fellman, V., Lagercrantz, H., Ådén, U. (2015). Singing kangaroo-a family centered music therapy intervention with infants born preterm. Poster presentation at the Berzelius symposium 90 *Neurobiology of Parenting*, Stockholm august 19-21 2015.

Jotzo, M., & Poets, C. F. (2005). Helping parents cope with the trauma of premature birth: An evaluation of a trauma-preventive psychological intervention. *Pediatrics, 115*(4), 915–919.

Lagercrantz, H. (2012). I barnets hjärna. Stockholm, Sweden: Riviera förlag. (In swedish).

Lai, H.-L., Chen, C.-J., Peng, T.-C., Chang, F.-M., Hsieh, M.-L., Huang, H.-Y., & Chang, S.-C. (2006). Randomized controlled trial of music during kangaroo care on maternal state anxiety and preterm infants' responses. *International Journal of Nursing Studies, 43*(2), 139–146.

Lee, E. J., et al. (2012). Monochord sounds and progressive muscle relaxation reduce anxiety and improve relaxation during chemotherapy: A pilot EEG study. *Complementary Therapies in Medicine, 20*(6), 409–416.

Lenz, G., & von Moreau, D. (2004). Coming together - Resonance and synchronization as a regulating factor in relationships. In M. Nöcker-Ribaupierre (Ed.), *Music therapy for premature and newborn infants* (pp. 67–81). Barcelona, Spain: Gilsum, NH.

Lickliter, R. (2000). Atypical perinatal sensory stimulation and early perceptual development: Insights from developmental psychobiology. *Journal of Perinatology, 20*, 45–54.

Lind, J. (1980). Music and the small human being. *Acta Paediatrica Scandinavia., 69*, 131–136.

Loewy, J. (2000). *Music therapy in neonatal care unit*. New York, NY: Satchnote Press.

Loewy, J. (2015). NICU music therapy: Song of kin as critical lullaby in research and practice. *Annals of the New York Academy of Sciences, 1337*(1), 178–185.

Loewy, J., Hallan, C., Friedmann, E., & Martinez, C. (2005). Sleep/sedation in children undergoing EEG-testing: A comparison of chloral hydrate and music therapy. *Journal of Perinatal Anesthesia Nursing, 20*(5), 323–332.

Loewy, J., Stewart, K., Dassler, A. M., Telsey, A., & Homel, P. (2013). The effects of music therapy on vital signs, feeding, and sleep in premature infants. *Pediatrics, 31*(5), 902–919.

Lopez-Teijon, M., Garcia-Faura, A., & Prats-Galino, A. (2015). Fetal facial expression in response to intravaginal music emission. *Ultrasound, 216*–223.

Malloch, S., Shoemark, H., Crncec, R., Newnham, C., Paul, C., Prior, M., … Butnham, D. (2012). Music therapy with hospitalized infants – Arts and science of communicative musicality. *Infant Mental Health Journal, 33*(4), 386–399.

Malloch, S., & Trevarthen, C. (2009a). Communicative musicality. Exploring the basis of human championship. In S. Malloch & C. Trevarthen (Eds.), *Communicative musicality. Exploring the basics of human championship*. Oxford: Oxford University Press.

Malloch, S., & Trevarthen, C. (2009b). Musicality: Communicating the vitality and interests of life. In S. Malloch & C. Trevarthen (Eds.), *Communicative musicality. Exploring the basis of human championship* (pp. 1–11). Oxford: Oxford University Press.

McGrath, J. M. (2001). Building relationships with families in the NICU: Exploring guarded alliance. *The Journal of Perinatal & Neonatal Nursing, 15*(3), 74–83.

McMahon, E., Wintermark, P., & Lahav, A. (2012). Auditory brain development in premature infants: The importance of early experience. *New York Academy of Sciences, 1252*, 17–24.

Melnyk, B. M., & Feinstein, N. F. (2009). Reducing hospital expenditures with the COPE (Creating Opportunities for Parent Empowerment) program for parents and premature infants: An analysis of direct healthcare neonatal intensive care unit costs and savings. *Nursing Administration Quarterly, 33*(1), 32–37.

Moon, C. (2011). The role of early auditory development in attachment and communication. *Clinics in Perinatology, 38*(4), 657–669.

Moon, C. M., & Fifer, W. P. (2000). Evidence of transnatal auditory learning. *Journal of Perinatology, 20*(8), 37–44.

Moore, E. R., Anderson, G. C., Bergman, N., & Dowswell, T. (2014). Early skin-to-skin contact for mothers and their healthy newborn infants. *The Cochrane Database of Systematic Reviews, 5*, CD003519. doi:10.1002/14651858.CD003519.pub3

Mörelius, E. (2006). *Stress in infants and parents. Studies of salivary cortisol behavior and psychometric measures*. (Dissertation). Linköping: Linköping University.

Nordoff, P., & Robbins, C. (1977). *Creative music therapy: Individualized treatment for the handicapped child*. New York, NY: John Day Company.

O'Gorman, S. (2005). The infant's mother: Facilitating an experience of infant-directed singing with the mother in mind. *British Journal of Music Therapy, 19*(2), 22–30.

O'Gorman, S. (2006). Theoretical interfaces in the acute paediatric context: A psychotherapeutic understanding of the application of infant-directed singing. *American Journal of Psychotherapy, 60*(3), 271–283.

Örtenstrand, A., Westrup, B., Broström, E., et al. (2010). The Stockholm neonatal family-centered care study: Effects on lengths of stay and infant morbidity. *Pediatrics, 125*, 278–285.

Papousek, M. (2012). Resilience, strengths, and regulatory capacities: Hidden resources in developmental disorders of infant mental health. *Infant Mental Health Journal, 32*(1), 29–46.

Papousek, M., & Papousek, H. (1991). The meanings of melodies in motherese in tone and stress languages. *Journal of Infant Behavior & Development, 14*, 415–440.

Pediatrics, A. A. of. (2007). *Prevention and management of pain in the neonate. An update.*

Philbin, K. M. (2000). The influence of auditory experience on the behavior of preterm newborns. *Journal of Perinatology, 20*, 76–86.

Radley, J. J., & Morrison, J. H. (2005). Repeated stress and structural plasticity in the brain. *Ageing Research Reviews, 4*(2), 271–287.

Rock, A. M., Trainor, L. J., & Addison, T. L. (1999). Distinctive messages in infant-directed lullabies and play songs. *Developmental Psychology, 35*, 527–534.

Schlez, A., Litmanovitz, I., Bauer, S., Dolfin, T., Regev, R., & Arnon, S. (2011). Combining kangaroo care and live harp music therapy in the neonatal intensive care unit setting. *The Israel Medical Association Journal, 13*, 354–358.

Schore, A. N. (2003). Minds in the making: Attachment, the self-organising brain, and developmentally oriented psychoanalytic psychotherapy. In J. Corrigall & H. Wilkinson (Eds.), *Revolutionary connections: Psychotherapy & neuroscience* (pp. 7–52). London, England: Karnac Books.

Serenius, F., Källèn, K., Blennow, M., Ewald, U., Fellman, V., Holmström, G., Lindberg, E., Lundqvist, P., Marsál, K., Norman, M., Olhager, E., Stigson, L., Stjernqvist, K., Vollmer, B., Strömberg, B. for the Express group (2013). Neurodevelopmental outcome in extremely preterm infants at 2,5 years after active perinatal care in Sweden. FREE

Shoemark, H. (2011). Translating "infant-directed singing" into a strategy for the hospitalized family. In J. Edwards (Ed.), *Music therapy and parent-infant bonding* (pp. 161–178). Oxford: Oxford University Press.

Shoemark, H. (2014). The fundamental interaction of singing. *Nordic Journal of Music Therapy, 23*(1), 2–4.

Shoemark, H., & Arnup, S. (2014). A survey of how mothers think about and use voice with their hospitalized newborn infant. *Journal of Neonatal Nursing, 20*(3), 115–121.

Shoemark, H., & Dearn, T. (2008). Keeping parents at the centre of family centered music therapy with hospitalised infants. *The Australian Journal of Music Therapy, 19*, 3–24.

Shoemark, H., Hanson-Abromeit, D., & Stewart, L. (2015). Constructing optimal experience for the hospitalized newborn through neuro-based music therapy. *Frontiers in Human Neuroscience, 9*, 487. doi:10.3389/fnhum.2015.00487

Shoemark, H., Music, N., & Roundtable, T. (2015). Culturally transformed music therapy in the perinatal and paediatric neonatal intensive care unit : an international report. *Music and Medicine, 7*(2), 2014–2016.

Shoemark, H., & the WCMT 2014 NICU Music Therapy Roundtable Group. (2014). Culturally transformed music therapy in the perinatal and paediatric neonatal intensive care unit: An international report. *Music and Medicine, 7*(2), 34–36.

Standley, J. (2012). Music therapy research in the NICU: An updated meta-analysis. *Neonatal Network, 31*(5), 311–316.

Stern, D. N. (1985). *The interpersonal world of the infant.* New York, NY: Basic Books.

Stern, D. N. (2010a). *Forms of vitality.* Oxford: Oxford University Press.

Stern, D. N. (2010b). The issue of vitality. *Nordic Journal of Music Therapy, 19*(2), 88–102.

Stern, D. N., Bruschweiler-Stern, N., Harrison, A., Lyons-Ruth, K., Morgan, A., ... Tronick, E. Z. (1998). The process of therapeutic change involving implicit knowledge: Some implications of developmental observations for adult psychotherapy. *Infant Mental Health Journal, 19*(3), 300–308.

Teckenberg-Jansson, P., Huotilainen, M., Pölkki, T., Lipsanen, J., & Järvenpää, A.-L. (2011). Rapid effects of neonatal music therapy combined with kangaroo care on prematurely-born infants. *Nordic Journal of Music Therapy, 20*(1), 22–42.

Thomas, K. A., & Martin, P. A. (2000). NICU sound environment and the potential problems for caregivers. *Journal of Perinatology, 20*, 93–98.

Trainor, L. J., Clark, E. D., Huntley, A., & Adams, B. A. (1997). The acoustic basis of preferences for infant-directed singing. *Infant Behavior & Development, 20*, 383–396.

Trehub, S. E., & Trainor, L. J. (1998). Singing to infants: Lullabies and playsongs. In C. Rovee-Collier, L. P. Lipsitt, & H. Hayne (Eds.), *Advances in infancy research* (Vol. 12, pp. 43–77). Norwood, NJ: Ablex.

Trondalen, G., & Skarderud, F. (2007). Playing with affects ….. and the importance of "affect attunement". *Nordic Journal of Music Therapy, 16*(2), 100–111.

Tuomi, K-M. (2014). *The effects of combining kangaroo care and parental singing on premature infant's and parent's wellbeing and development of parent-infant relationship* (Master thesis in music therapy). Department of Music, University of Jyväskylä, Finland.

Unyk, A. M., Trehub, S. E., Trainor, L. J., & Schellenberg, E. G. (1992). Lullabies and simplicity: A cross-cultural perspective. *Psychology of Music, 20*, 15–28.

Vinall, J., & Grunau, R. E. (2014). Impact of repeated procedural pain-related stress in infants born very preterm. *Pediatric Research, 75*(5), 584–587. doi:10.1038/pr.2014.16

Westrup, B. (2007). Newborn individualized developmental care and assessment program (NIDCAP) – Family-centered developmentally supportive care. *Early Human Development, 83*, 443–449.

Westrup, B. (2015). Family-centered developmentally supportive care: The Swedish example. *Archives de Pediatrie, 2015,* 22:1086-1091 0929-693X.

Westrup, B., Kleberg, A., von Eichwald, K., Stjernqvist, K., & Lagercrantz, H. (2000). A randomized controlled trial to evaluate effects of NIDCAP (newborn individualized developmental care and assessment program) in a Swedish setting. *Pediatrics, 105*, 66–72.

Whipple, J. (2000). The effect of parent training in music and multimodal stimulation on parent-neonate interactions in the neonatal intensive care unit. *Journal of Music Therapy, 37*(4), 250–268.

Xu, J., Yu, L., Cai, R., Zhang, J., & Sun, X. (2009). Early auditory enrichment with music enhances auditory discrimination learning and alters NR2B protein expression in rat auditory cortex. *Behavioural Brain Research, 196*(1), 49–54.

Part V
Early Family-Based Interventions in the NICU

Chapter 14
Stress-Sensitive Parental Brain Systems Regulate Emotion Response and Motivate Sensitive Child Care

James E. Swain

Abstract The mother-child relationship is central to early human development and provides the foundation that supports socioemotional functioning. Mothers with trauma exposure and mental illness histories are at risk for higher stress and impaired parental sensitivity. Sensitive parenting of children requires complex regulation of thoughts and behaviors such as vocalization. These form the first social bond that furnishes each individual with their capacity to flourish. After covering some basic neuroimaging design issues, this review concentrates on a selection of brain imaging studies, which examine the brain systems that govern human parenting – operationalized mostly as brain activity responses to infant cues – largely cries and pictures. Research highlights brain circuits that govern reflexive parenting behaviors, emotion response and regulation, executive function, empathy, and reflective function. Accordingly presented are recent studies that include fathers, mothers affected by psychopathology and treated with parenting intervention, circumstances of stress, poverty and issues of feeding and delivery, and also new methods including complex stimuli and hormone measures. Finally, future directions will be discussed, including the study interventions that influence parenting and support the importance of optimizing perinatal and neonatal care – future interventions may focus on optimizing maternal voice from a mechanistic brain perspective.

J.E. Swain (✉)
Department of Psychiatry and Psychology, Stony Brook University Medical Center,
HSC, T10-020, Stony Brook, NY 11794-8101, USA
e-mail: james.swain@stonybrookmedicine.edu

© Springer International Publishing AG 2017
M. Filippa et al. (eds.), *Early Vocal Contact and Preterm Infant Brain Development*, DOI 10.1007/978-3-319-65077-7_14

Abbreviations

ACC   Anterior cingulate cortex
DA   Dopamine
fMRI   Functional magnetic resonance imaging   .
HPA   Hypothalamic-pituitary axis
NAcc   Nucleus accumbens
OFC   Orbitofrontal cortex
OT   Oxytocin
PFC   Prefrontal cortex
PTSD   Post-traumatic stress disorder

Parental Sensitivity and Child Attachment

Mary Ainsworth first defined maternal sensitivity as a mother's ability to attend and respond to her child in ways that are contingent to the infant's needs (Ainsworth, Blehar, Waters, & Wall, 1978). In the naturalistic context, sensitive maternal care behaviors show a great deal of variation between individual mothers, despite being relatively stable in the same mothers across time and contexts (Behrens, Hart, & Parker, 2012; Jaffari-Bimmel, Juffer, van IJzendoorn, Bakermans-Kranenburg, & Mooijaart, 2006; Wan et al., 2013). Maternal sensitivity represents a pattern of behavior that provides the infant with its primary social experience. This suggests that it is important for organizing and regulating the infant's emotional, social, and cognitive systems. Indeed, this idea is consistent with an impressive accumulation of evidence that maternal sensitivity predicts many child socioemotional outcomes – including the quality of each child's future attachment relationships (Bakermans-Kranenburg, van IJzendoorn, and Juffer, 2003; De Wolff & van Ijzendoorn, 1997), emotional self-regulation (Eisenberg et al., 2001), social functioning (Kochanska, 2002; Van Zeijl et al., 2006), socioemotional development (De Wolff & van Ijzendoorn, 1997), and cognitive and language competence (Bernier, Carlson, & Whipple, 2010; Tamis-LeMonda, Bornstein, & Baumwell, 2001). In supportive contrast, the absence of skills needed to respond sensitively to child signals has been linked to risk for maltreatment (Milner, 1993, 2003). Poor maternal sensitivity in infancy predicts later harsh parenting (Joosen, Mesman, Bakermans-Kranenburg, and van IJzendoorn, 2012) and attitudes toward punishment (Engfer & Gavranidou, 1987). Frightening and anomalous maternal behavior confers profound risk to the parent-infant attachment relationship (Schuengel, Bakermans-Kranenburg, & Van, 1999) to subsequent child outcomes and future parenting of their own children.

The conceptual development of the central role of parent-infant attachment represents a landmark in contemporary developmental psychology (Bowlby, 1969, 1973). In fact, John Bowlby formulated his attachment theory after studying associations between maternal deprivation and juvenile delinquency, postulating a universal human need to form close, affect-laden bonds, primarily between mother and infant. He strongly argued, from an evolutionary perspective, that attachment represents an innate biological system promoting proximity seeking between an infant and a conspecific attachment figure. This proximity then logically increases the likelihood of survival to reproductive age.

Because of this powerful biological instinct for attachment, and in response to the patterns of attachment identified in the Ainsworth mother-infant studies (Ainsworth et al., 1978), Bowlby hypothesized that all human infants attach to their caregiver but that children manifest different patterns of attachment "security" depending on the quality of the care they receive (Bowlby, 1977). Indeed, a vast literature in the study of attachment over the last several decades has established that infants of caregivers who are available, responsive, and sensitive to their emotional and physical needs tend to manifest patterns of "secure attachment." Conversely, chaotic, unpredictable, rejecting, or neglectful care in which noncontingent responses to the child occur frequently results in insecure or disorganized patterns of attachment (Shaver, Schwartz, Kirson, & O'Connor, 1987).

Understanding the neurobiology of attachment formation through parental sensitivity may help to formulate and ameliorate pervasive and complex social problems such as child abuse and neglect. However, little is known about the cognitive or neurobiological mechanisms that underpin healthy sensitivity, let alone poor sensitivity in mothers with mental illness. This may explain why some promising interventions targeted at improving parenting through improved sensitivity have shown inconsistent findings and generally small effect sizes thus far (Bakermans-Kranenburg et al., 2003; Wan, Warren, Salmon, & Abel, 2008).

Introduction to the Brain Imaging of Parenting: Approaches and Design Issues

In this chapter, we present a selection of studies in support of a model to encompass human parental behavior and thoughts. The attempt to formulate a brain basis of human parenting that could connect with child outcome, despite the limitations of current neuroimaging methods, was perhaps audacious at first. Nevertheless, a consistent literature is emerging. Most of the key studies use infant stimuli to measure brain activity using the high-resolution and noninvasive brain imaging technique of blood-oxygen-dependent functional magnetic resonance imaging (fMRI) to localize signals to the millimeter. fMRI assays brain activity by indirectly measuring changes in regional blood oxygenation, which changes magnetic properties of protons. The differences between a region's oxygenated and deoxygenated hemoglobin, between states of action vs. inaction, for instance, provide characteristic magnetic signals that are detected by scanners positioned around each subject's head without using ionizing radiation. An important caveat throughout the interpretation of parenting fMRI studies, however, is that that brain activity measurements represent an integration of electrical brain activity that may be instantaneous – yet, the related blood flow change lags behind over seconds. Furthermore, experimental design captures brain activity over periods of a few seconds or 10's of seconds. On the one hand, short blocks or events may capture briefly held mental states but miss bigger changes such as sustained emotion, while on the other hand, longer blocks may capture more complex brain responses but also average them out making subtle responses more difficult to detect. Brain activity during these blocks may then be measured and compared between periods of attending to stimuli of interest and control stimuli to generate maps of the brain indicating differences in brain activity that may be important for one set of perceptions and thoughts versus another.

Dissecting Brain Mechanisms for Parental Sensitivity

For sensitive caregiver responses to infant cues, complex brain systems must manage an array of complex drives, emotions, thoughts, and behaviors contingent on feedback from the child. These include recognition and acknowledgment of child signals, attribution of salience to child cues, maintenance of visual contact, expression of positive affect, appropriate mirroring and vocal quality, resourcefulness in handling child distress or expanding the interaction, consistency of style, and display of an affective range that matches the child's readiness to interact. Such behaviors are the result of complex neural networks involved in organizing the sensorimotor input, in managing emotional responses (Kober et al., 2008), as well as in attention and executive function. Evolving models (Kim, Strathearn, & Swain, 2016; Swain, 2011b; Swain, Kim, et al., 2014; Swain, Leckman, et al., 2008; Swain, Lorberbaum, Kose, & Strathearn, 2007) all contain the major caveat of presenting brain systems as separate – quite different from the actual way in which the brain operates – on fire with activity across all of these circuits all the time. However, for the purpose of some heuristic reductionism, we will continue with such a model, though encourage the reader to keep in mind that all circuits are simultaneously active and influencing each other in ways that we are just beginning to understand.

"Reflexive" Salience, Motivation, and Reward Circuits

Some brain systems appear to be conserved across many species including ours. Indeed, both animal and human research (Numan, 2014; Numan & Woodside, 2010; Strathearn, Fonagy, Amico, & Montague, 2009) suggest that responses to infants utilize the brain's motivational systems, dopamine (DA) and oxytocin (OT). DA contributes to many reward-motivated behaviors, reinforcement learning, and drug addiction. Dopaminergic neurons, which originate in the brainstem's "primitive" deep brain structures including the ventral tegmental area and substantia nigra, project to the ventral and dorsal portions of the striatum, as well as to the medial prefrontal cortex (PFC), via mesocorticolimbic and nigrostriatal pathways. Natural reward-related stimuli, including food and social cues such as faces of one's sexual partner or child, activate the brain's "reward" system (Aharon et al., 2001; Delgado, Nystrom, Fissell, Noll, & Fiez, 2000; Melis & Argiolas, 1995; Panksepp, 1998; Stoeckel et al., 2008; Strathearn, Li, Fonagy, & Montague, 2008). In mothers, the initial experiences of pleasure and activity in these brain circuits when exposed to their own infants' cues may increase the salience of their infants' stimuli and promote greater attention and bond formation to ensure continuous engagement in sensitive caregiving (Strathearn et al., 2008; Strathearn, Mamun, et al., 2009). Such reward pathways may be relevant very early in the postpartum period, as a mother's positive feelings toward her unborn fetus, as well as her perception of her fetus, have been associated with greater maternal sensitivity to the infant's signals and more affectionate vocalizations and touch (Keller, Lohaus, Völker, Elben, & Ball, 2003; Keren, Feldman, Eidelman, Sirota, & Lester, 2003).

Structural Change in Maternal Motivation Circuits

In recent years, human parents have been shown to exhibit structural changes during adaptation to the new role as parents. Among mothers, from the first to fourth months postpartum, several brain regions involved in maternal motivation and reward processing, including the striatum, amygdala, hypothalamus, and the substantia nigra, exhibited structural growth (Kim, Leckman, Mayes, Feldman, et al., 2010). Structural growth was also observed in areas involved in processing sensory information and empathy, including the superior temporal gyrus, thalamus, insula, and pre- and postcentral gyri. Finally, regions associated with regulating emotions, such as the inferior and medial frontal gyri and the anterior cingulate cortex (ACC), also showed structural increases. Interestingly, no neural regions showed reduction in gray matter during this time period. The evidence suggests that neural plasticity, particularly growth, occurs in a wide range of brain regions, each serving important aspects of child caregiving in human mothers during the first few months postpartum. Furthermore, the greater the observed structural growth in the midbrain region (involved in reward and motivation), the stronger the positive emotions a mother reported having about her baby in the third and fourth months postpartum. This finding further supports the existence of a bidirectional association between maternal experience and neural plasticity during the first few months postpartum.

Father Brain

Despite much less research attention, the role of the father in child development may be thought to require brain activity in support of the following domains: (1) positive and direct engagement (e.g., play, soothing) with the child in ways that promote healthy development, (2) parental warmth and responsiveness directed toward the child, and (3) activities that serve to monitor and make decisions on behalf of the child in order to control his/her environment (Lamb, Pleck, Charnov, & Levine, 1985; Pleck, 2010). Auxiliary domains may include (4) indirect care such as arranging child care and medical care and contributing to home safety and environmental richness and (5) process responsibility that includes monitoring activities to ensure that the child's needs within the first four domains are being met.

One might expect similar brain regions to be active for fathers during the early postpartum. Over those same first several months postpartum as above, a recent study of fathers demonstrated growth in the hypothalamus, amygdala, and other regions that regulate emotion, motivation, and decision-making. Furthermore, dads with more growth in these brain areas were less likely to show depressive symptoms. Thus, some physiological brain changes seem to be similar for new moms and dads, while other changes seem different and could relate to the roles of respective parents (P. Kim et al., 2014; Kim et al., 2014).

Thus, a very recent literature on the father brain is evolving (Swain, Dayton, Kim, Tolman, & Volling, 2014). So far, healthy father brain activity in response to infant stimuli involves motivation and emotion response/regulation circuits much the same as those that we focus on for mothers below. Interesting differences are just now emerging in terms of the way brain function may be tuned. For example, vasopressin seems to tune amygdala response to complex child video stimuli for fathers instead of OT for mothers. It also appears that different brain circuits are at play for fathers as compared to mothers for different types of thoughts as they impact child development (Kim, Rigo, et al., 2015) discussed below (section "Does Parental Brain Function Relate to Child Outcome"). These are very early days in the study of sex differences among parents according to sex or other factors and will require replication and studies that include both fathers and mothers.

Emotion Response: Fear and Joy

Central to emotion response circuitry of the brain is the amygdala; given its established central roles in social cognition (Adolphs, 2010), social-cognitive-emotional value-based decision-making (Ho, Gonzalez, Abelson, & Liberzon, 2012), vicarious pain (Krishnan et al., 2016), face-based emotional processing (Sergerie, Chochol, & Armony, 2008), and task-dependent processing positive and negative salience signals (Morrison & Salzman, 2010; Santos, Mier, Kirsch, & Meyer-Lindenberg, 2011), it is not surprising that the amygdala also interacts with the reward circuit to motivate maternal behaviors. In response to infant stimuli, infant cry and smiles activate the amygdala (Barrett et al., 2012; Seifritz et al., 2003; Swain, Tasgin, et al., 2008), which has often been interpreted as a sign of emotional salience (Seifritz et al., 2003; Strathearn & Kim, 2013) or positive emotion associated with attachment (Leibenluft, Gobbini, Harrison, & Haxby, 2004). On the other hand, in virgin rats, activation in the medial nucleus of the amygdala was associated with reduced maternal behaviors (Morgan, Watchus, Milgram, & Fleming, 1999; Oxley & Fleming, 2000). Thus, while increased activation of the amygdala to infant stimuli is interpreted as a more negative response to infants among typical adults (Riem et al., 2011), in mothers, it can be associated with more positive responses to one's own infant (Barrett et al., 2012b).

Another perspective on parental thoughts that influence behaviors involves so-called postpartum preoccupations that may be part of healthy maternal responses to their infants that draw them close in order to meet the infant's physical and psychological needs (Bowlby, 1969; Winnicott, 1956) – perhaps even providing a reasonable explanation of why obsessional disorders have survived evolution (Feygin, Swain, & Leckman, 2006). Thus, the "checking and worrying" brain circuits may overlap with those hyperactive in obsessional anxiety in parents (Leckman et al., 2004). Indeed, parental anxiety peaks immediately after childbirth and then begins to diminish during the first 3–4 months postpartum (Feldman, Weller, Leckman, Kuint, & Eidelman, 1999; Kim, Mayes, Feldman, Leckman, & Swain, 2013; Leckman et al., 1999). This also fits with apparent increased responses to infant crying in postpartum anxiety circuits including the basal ganglia, orbitofrontal cortex, and insula that diminish over the first 4 months postpartum (Swain, Kim, et al., 2014). Perhaps persistently high or low activity in these circuits around parenting may predict psychopathology and inform treatments.

Parent Psychopathology

Brain activity is indeed proving to be abnormal in mothers with psychopathology. The brain basis of psychopathology for parents has been recently reviewed in detail (Moses-Kolko, Horner, Phillips, Hipwell, & Swain, 2014). Briefly, mothers with syndromal levels of depression have blunted amygdala and insula activity to negative emotional stimuli and infant distress stimuli, which is the opposite of that described in non-postpartum depressed samples. Heightened intrusive/anxious responses that accompany subsyndromal affective symptoms in very early (3 weeks) postpartum mothers, associated with medial PFC and lenticular nucleus activity to infant cry, may change over time and serve an adaptive role that may fail in the development of syndromal depression. Recently, depressed mother's amygdala has been shown to be hyporesponsive to certain standard cognitive neuroimaging challenges (Moses-Kolko et al., 2014) and that dampened amygdala response may be shown among mothers with unresolved attachment trauma after viewing their own (but not unknown) infant's crying faces (Kim, Fonagy, Allen, & Strathearn, 2014). Using a child face empathy task (Lenzi et al., 2016), depressed compared to healthy mothers displayed greater reactivity of the right amygdala – perhaps related to emotional dysregulation. Finally, amygdala reactivity was increased in a self-focused baby-cry task designed to provoke brain responses in participants with a history of adverse early life experiences sometimes described as a malevolent background "shark music" (Ho & Swain, 2017). Thus, amygdala responses related to parenting seem to be a function of the personal relevance of the stimuli.

Reward-related neural responses to non-baby stimuli, such as positive words and monetary gain that are known to be affected by depression in nonparents, are noted to be reduced in depressed mothers. Mothers, more than 1 year postpartum, who have postpartum post-traumatic stress disorder (PTSD), have a neurobiology which resembles that in non-postpartum populations, characterized by hyperactivity within the fear circuitry (amygdala and anterior insula) and alternatively decreased or increased (dissociative-type) voluntary ventromedial PFC/ventral ACC regulation of subcortical activity. Circuits that support social cognition, mentalization, and empathy (discussed below) in healthy mothers are hyporesponsive to infant stimuli in mothers with insecure attachment and substance use disorders. Specific interventions currently being given and still being refined may benefit from brain-based analyses.

Parent Intervention

For example, parent intervention programs including the Circle of Security (Hoffman, Marvin, Cooper, & Powell, 2006; Powell, Cooper, Hoffman, & Marvin, 2014), Triple P (Positive Parenting Program) (Sanders, Kirby, Tellegen, & Day, 2014), Video Interaction for Promoting Positive Parenting Programme (Van Zeijl et al., 2006), and Mom Power (Muzik et al., 2015) have been validated according to randomized clinical trial approaches but lack well-developed grounding in brain function. In the first study of its kind, mothers 2–7 years postpartum, who have suffered at least one trauma, were studied with fMRI and child empathy and baby-cry response tasks before and after Mom Power intervention. This intervention includes sessions devoted to improve reflective emotion response, emotion regulation, and empathic function related to parenting. Brain activity for empathy to own-child stimuli was increased in the amygdala and inversely related to parenting stress (Swain, Ho, Dayton, Rosenblum, & Muzik, 2014). Mom Power-treated mothers, as compared to control group, also showed decreased parenting stress and increased child-focused responses in social brain areas highlighted by the precuneus and its functional connectivity with subgenual anterior cingulate cortex – key components of social cognition in response to own baby cry (Swain et al., 2017). In this paper, time-dependent reduction in parenting stress was related to concomitant increasing child- vs. self-focused baby-cry responses in amygdala-temporal pole functional connectivity, which may facilitate maternal ability to take her child's perspective. In further work on Mom Power-treatment brain mechanisms, maternal amygdala's response when mothers were instructed to emotionally attune and empathize the emotions expressed by their own child (versus unknown child) was increased (Muzik et al., 2017). Furthermore, the greater the maternal amygdala activity in response to positive versus negative child emotions, the more reduction in their parenting stress was observed from pretreatment to posttreatment. Taken together, these results suggest that enhancing child-oriented altruism can protect mothers from adverse effects of distress and stress related to caregiving, consistent with the hypothesis that prosocial motivation improves caregivers' well-being (Brown & Brown, 2015).

The findings and ideas provide neural mechanisms to stimulate brain-based research on parenting interventions that may benefit from understanding when, how, and for whom therapies may work best. One possibility, consistent with the theme of this book, is that specific aspects of parental sensitivity, such as parental vocalizations, may be studied as a function of intervention – perhaps with specific language brain areas in mind. So far, however, work has focused on the mechanisms that act on parental brain circuits at the intersection of emotion response as well as regulation and empathy circuits covered below. Figure 14.1 illustrates the model.

Emotion Regulation and Integration

During healthy interactions, it is critical for mothers to perceive the cues of infants appropriately and manage their own potential distress in response to their infants' negative emotions. Indeed, mother's sensitivity to distress has been a better predictor of the child's outcome than her sensitivity to non-distress cues (Joosen et al., 2012; Leerkes, 2011; Leerkes, Nayena Blankson, & O'Brien, 2009; McElwain & Booth-Laforce, 2006).

The medial and lateral PFC and ACC are well known to operate in emotion regulation – often suppression of the amygdala responses to strong negative emotional information (Ochsner, Silvers, & Buhle, 2012) – and play this role for parents and parenting stimuli as well. Indeed, activation of the medial and lateral PFC and ACC has been consistently observed among new mothers in response to an infant's stimuli: including own vs. baby cry (Heidemarie K Laurent & Ablow, 2012; Lorberbaum et al., 2002), videos of a distressed infant (Noriuchi, Kikuchi, & Senoo, 2008), and to one's own child greater than to familiar/unknown faces (Leibenluft et al., 2004).

Exposure to Stress and Childhood Adversity

Early life adversity and current stress may decrease parental sensitivity and adversely affect child development through identifiable brain circuits. Concurrent levels of parenting-related stress in mothers were associated with individual differences in neural responses to infants (Barrett et al., 2012). In this experiment, mothers at 3 months postpartum viewed images of their own versus an unrelated infant. Lower levels of parental distress and more positive attachment-related feelings about their own infants were associated with increased responses in the amygdala to their own infants' versus unrelated infants' positive images (e.g., smiling).

Early life stress also shapes later brain function (McGowan et al., 2009). Exposure to stress activates the hypothalamic-pituitary-adrenal (HPA) axis and increases cortisol levels, which may reduce neural responses of mothers to an infant's cry, perhaps due to difficulties in regulation of emotions. Mothers with infants aged 18 months old had their cortisol levels measured following a strange

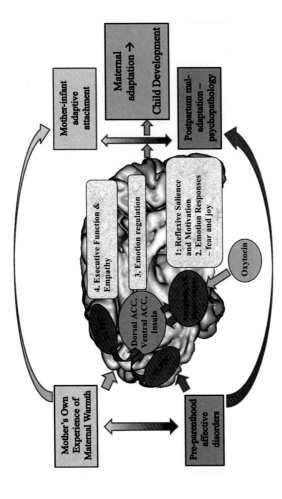

Fig. 14.1 Parental brain: In this heuristically oversimplified model, circuits are roughly dissected according to brain imaging literature indicating parental brain circuit activity in response to child stimuli is a function of individual differences and groupings of parents and fir with the broader human neuroimaging literature. Plastic or adaptable circuits, some of which are overlapping, include structures that serve in (1) "reflexive" salience and motivation processing and (2) emotion response (including the amygdala, NAcc, hippocampus, and other limbic structures), (3) emotion regulation and integration (insula and ACC), and (4) executive function (OFC, DLPFC) and related empathy and mentalization circuits (MPFC, precuneus, and temporal cortex). Parental brain function is influenced by hormones such as OT and cortisol in addition to early life factors, such as experience of parental warmth and previous mental health. Adaptive engagement of these circuits toward sensitive parenting by regulating parental thoughts, behaviors, affective regulation capacity, and caregiving outcomes (Adapted from Kim et al., 2016) contributes to child outcome

situation, a task that can elicit stress reactivity in the HPA axis to mother-child separation (Laurent, Stevens, & Ablow, 2011). Mothers then participated in a neuroimaging session while listening to their own infant's cry versus an unrelated infant's cry sounds. Reduced reactivity to stress in the HPA axis was associated with greater activation in the midbrain and striatum, areas involved in maternal motivation; the insula and orbitofrontal cortex (OFC), areas involved in negative emotional processing; and the dorsolateral PFC and ACC, areas involved in emotion regulation. Thus, poor physiological stress regulation can contribute to diminished neural responses to infants' cry sounds among mothers.

In addition to current stress levels, early adversity may have long-term effects on stress regulation and maternal motivation in humans based on clear demonstrations of exactly that effect in the animal literature (Champagne, Weaver, Diorio, Sharma, & Meaney, 2003; Fleming et al., 2002). In one human study, mothers with infants aged 1 month old were divided into two groups based on retrospective self-reported quality of maternal care received during childhood (P. Kim, Leckman, Mayes, Newman, et al., 2010). Mothers with high vs. low scores on maternal care were compared on neural structure and functional responses to infants' cries. High quality of maternal care in childhood was associated with increased gray matter volumes in regions involved in regulation of emotions and social and sensory information processing, including the superior frontal gyrus, the OFC, the superior and middle temporal gyri, and the fusiform gyrus. Furthermore, higher levels of neural responses to infants' cry sounds were found in these same regions. The only region that was more active in mothers who reported low quality of maternal care in childhood was the hippocampus. The hippocampus is particularly rich in the glucocorticoid receptors and critically involved in stress regulation (Bruce S McEwen, 2001). Increased hippocampal activation has been observed in response to both acute and chronic exposure to stress in human and animals (Tottenham & Sheridan, 2009; van Hasselt et al., 2012). Thus, the increased activation in the hippocampus in response to infants' cries among mothers with lower-quality childhood experiences may reflect greater stress responses to the cries or greater encoding of negative information. Therefore, the findings suggest that differences in maternal neural responses to infants are influenced by mothers' own childhood experiences, which contribute to baseline differences in terms of neural structure and functions.

Differences in adult classification are likely related to environment-biology interactions during childhood caregiving experience (Shah, Fonagy, & Strathearn, 2010). Previous studies have shown that mothers with an insecure/dismissing type of adult attachment show diminished OT response to mother-infant interaction, which is associated with reduced activation in the hypothalamus and the nucleus accumbens (NAcc). Mothers from this attachment group also show reduced activation of the mesocorticolimbic DA system, including the NAcc and ventromedial PFC, when viewing images of their own versus unknown infants' faces (Strathearn, Fonagy, et al., 2009; Strathearn, Mamun, et al., 2009). Furthermore, this pattern of attachment is associated with differences in maternal behavior, including less attuned mother-to-infant vocalization at 7 months postpartum (Kim et al., 2014).

Further effects of attachment of parents that may impact child development may be fruitful avenues to grapple with devastating and common but complex phenomena such as childhood poverty (Kim, Fonagy et al., 2014).

Chronic Childhood Poverty

Childhood poverty is a major detriment to childhood potential to flourish across many domains, including increased risk of psychopathology (N.E. Adler & Rehkopf, 2008; Bradley & Corwyn, 2002; Grant et al., 2003) and physical illness in adulthood (Chen, Matthews, & Boyce, 2002; Cohen, Janicki-Deverts, Chen, & Matthews, 2010). Furthermore, childhood poverty predicts adult morbidity irrespective of adult socioeconomic status (Blair & Raver, 2012; Cohen et al., 2010; Poulton et al., 2002) – suggesting that damage is done early in life and some aspects may be difficult to reverse. One possible mechanism to explain the far-reaching effects of childhood poverty on health is chronic stress (Evans, 2004) and associated harsh parenting and family conflict (Repetti, Taylor, & Seeman, 2002). Indeed, insensitive parenting appears to be trans-generationally transmitted to offspring when they become parents (Belsky et al., 2005; Capaldi, Pears, Patterson, & Owen, 2003; Kaufman & Zigler, 1989). There are many long-term adverse effects on physiological stress regulatory systems (Evans, Chen, Miller, & Seeman, 2012; Evans & Kim, 2010; Lupien, King, Meaney, & McEwen, 2000; McEwen, 1998), believed to ultimately lead to pathology (N. E. Adler, Marmot, McEwen, & Stewart, 1999; Kessler, Price, & Wortman, 1985). Growing evidence suggests exposure to chronic stress and socioeconomic adversity leaves damage as lasting neurobiological differences (Boyce, Sokolowski, & Robinson, 2012; McEwen, 2012). The mechanisms through which childhood poverty affects brain physiology over time are just beginning to be studied – with emerging effects on brain systems for emotion response and regulation (Evans et al., 2016; Javanbakht et al., 2015; Kim, Evans, et al., 2013; Liberzon et al., 2015), stress reactivity (Sripada, Swain, Evans, Welsh, & Liberzon, 2014), pleasure, (Silverman, Muennig, Liu, Rosen, & Goldstein, 2009), and, finally, caregiving responses to baby cry.

In the latter study, baby-cry stimuli were employed in a prospective study of individuals who grew up in poverty (Kim, Ho, Evans, Liberzon, & Swain, 2015b). Among nonparents, females showed increased neural activations in emotion regulation and motivation areas. For males, childhood poverty was associated with reduced levels of neural responses to infant cry in the same regions. In all regions irrespective of gender, neural activation was associated with higher levels of feeling annoyed by the cry sound and reduced desire to approach a crying infant. In a separate analysis of parents that all grew up in low SES, but varied in a measure of subjective SES, which has been recently linked with many psychiatric disorders (Scott et al., 2014), responses to own vs. other baby cry were directly proportional responses in the insula (emotion regulation) and inversely proportional in the habenula (learned helplessness and stress) (Swain, Ho, et al., 2012). Thus, as subjective SES goes down, baby cry activates a pattern of brain activity consistent with less regulation and more stress. These findings may ultimately help us understand how individuals who grow up in harsh environments including family conflict and insensitive parenting are at risk for a host of adverse developmental outcomes (Repetti et al., 2002) including the apparent intergenerational transmission of insensitive parenting from harsh parents to their children when they become parents (Barnett & The Family Life Project Key, 2008; Belsky et al., 2005; Capaldi et al., 2003; Hoff, Laursen, & Tardif, 2002; Kaufman & Zigler, 1989; Simons, Whitbeck, Conger, & Wu, 1991). It also suggests that interventions to decrease the subjective experience of poverty may decrease the adverse effects.

Executive Functions

Executive functions, including attention control, working memory, and flexible task switching, are also important to parental sensitivity. Accordingly, deficits in attention set shifting, spatial working memory, and a sustained attention measure have been linked with poor maternal sensitivity to non-distress infant cues (Gonzalez, Jenkins, Steiner, & Fleming, 2012). In closely related work, mothers with a classification of disorganized attachment responded more slowly to negative attachment words, and the speed of response to such stimuli was correlated with disorganization, suggesting negative associations with attachment stimuli that may contribute to ongoing cognitive difficulties during mother-infant interactions (Atkinson et al., 2009). Greater attention bias to infant distress cues in late pregnancy has also been associated with better scores on a parental bonding questionnaire (Pearson, Cooper, Penton-Voak, Lightman, & Evans, 2010), raising the question of how attention deficit disorder affects parenting – another common yet largely unstudied issue. Attention bias to infant distress has been compared between breastfeeding ($n = 27$) and formula feeding ($n = 24$) mothers of 3–6-month-old infants and observed to be greater in breastfeeding mothers (Pearson, Lightman, & Evans, 2011). It is plausible that reduced attention bias toward emotional stimuli (specifically infant distress) is associated with low maternal sensitivity in some mothers. However, other mothers with low sensitivity may show a selectively exaggerated attention bias to infant distress which results in the mother becoming overwhelmed by the stimuli; this may be particularly relevant for mothers and fathers with schizophrenia or in those with little social supports in deprived circumstances. In depressed patients, evidence suggests a tendency to pay *more* attention to negative emotional stimuli (Elliott, Zahn, Deakin, & Anderson, 2011), an effect mediated by *enhanced* response in the ventral anterior cingulate, which may contribute to the maintenance of low mood. Ultimately, depression may involve responses that are too much to some negative stimuli not enough to other negative stimuli.

Brain Connections with Birth and Feeding

To explain individual differences in the human maternal brain that affect child development, birth and feeding methods have been examined. Vaginal delivery provides sensory stimulation that increases release of OT, and so it is believed to help establish maternal behaviors (Morgan, Fleming, & Stern, 1992). Such sensory stimulation is absent in cesarean section delivery. In a small fMRI study, significant associations between birth method and neural responses to cry sounds from mothers' own babies (Swain, Tasgin, et al., 2008) emerged. During the first month postpartum, mothers from the vaginal delivery group exhibited greater neural responses to their own babies' cries (vs. control babies' cries) compared to mothers who delivered via cesarean section. Vaginal delivery was indeed associated with greater responses in brain circuits typically important for motivation (striatum, hypothalamus, amygdala), sensory information processing (the superior and middle temporal gyri, fusiform gyrus, and thalamus), and cognitive and emotional control regions (superior frontal gyrus), compared to the cesarean section. Interestingly, further plasticity among healthy mothers is exhibited by the disappearance of significant functional difference between vaginal and cesarean delivering – in response to baby cry – by 3 to 4 months postpartum (Swain, 2011a) suggesting that healthy humans (e.g., nondepressed) can compensate for different circumstances of delivery.

During the first month postpartum, feeding methods may also be significantly associated with maternal neural responses to cries of one's own baby. Breastfeeding, perhaps also operating at least in part through OT, is associated with higher maternal sensitivity and reduced levels of child neglect in some studies (Britton, Britton, & Gronwaldt, 2006; Strathearn, Mamun, Najman, & O'Callaghan, 2009). In an fMRI study, exclusive breastfeeding was associated with greater neural responses to cries of one's own baby (vs. unrelated baby's cry sounds), compared to exclusive formula feeding (Kim et al., 2011). Interestingly, brain regions associated with breastfeeding vs. formula feeding largely overlapped those associated with vaginal vs. cesarean delivery. The neural regions showing greater activation among breastfeeding mothers included those related to maternal motivation (striatum, amygdala), sensory information processing (superior and middle temporal gyri), and cognitive and emotional control (superior frontal gyrus). Furthermore, greater neural responses in the striatum/amygdala and superior frontal gyrus to one's own infant's cries at the first month postpartum were positively associated with maternal sensitivity, observed during mother-infant interactions at 3–4 months postpartum – a major key to child flourishing. Thus, both delivery and feeding methods, which are potentially associated with maternal hormones such as OT, may enhance neural sensitivity to cries of one's own baby in brain regions involved in maternal motivation, sensory information processing, and emotion regulation.

Empathy and Reflective Function

Parental empathy (the appropriate perception, experience, and response to another's emotion) may be especially relevant for the eventual flourishing of preverbal children. Experiencing pain of a loved one activates relatively focused anterior area of the dorsal ACC – perhaps a subset of a broader circuit for experiencing personal pain that also includes brainstem, cerebellum, and sensorimotor cortex. Such partial overlap of representations of empathy for others with self-related processing in cortical structures such as in the anterior insula is postulated as necessary for a theory of mind (Saxe, 2006), namely, our ability to understand the thoughts, beliefs, and intentions of others in relation to ourselves (Frith & Frith, 2003; Hein & Singer, 2008). Humans may utilize separate circuitry to "decouple" representations of external vs. internal information in order to understand many social exchanges. Indeed, considerable brain imaging research on empathy, largely related to the imitation of others' emotions using stimuli such as emotional faces, images of others in pain, or crying sounds (Fan, Duncan, de Greck, & Northoff, 2011), has highlighted the functional importance of medial PFC, precuneus/posterior cingulate cortex, temporoparietal junction, and posterior superior temporal sulcus (Frith & Frith, 2006; Mitchell, 2009). Additional regions including the anterior insula, orbitofrontal cortex, and amygdala may be important for emotion information processing but also for both sharing and explicitly considering affectively charged states (Decety, 2015; Zaki & Ochsner, 2012) .

Such ability to share and understand others' emotional state is of importance for parental caring responses to own baby cry (Swain, Mayes, & Leckman, 2004) and other stimuli. For example, a complex set of brain responses was reported in a recent study of mothers responding to child visual feedback after a caring decision (Ho, Konrath, Brown, & Swain, 2014). Responses that correlated with dimensions of empathy included the aforementioned amygdala and ventrolateral PFC. Experiments using a parenting-empathy task will shed light on maternal brain function when actually asked to empathize with their infant. In another approach, brain responses to own vs. other baby cry were correlated with maternal mental state talk coded from transcriptions of mother-infant interactions (Hipwell, Guo, Phillips, Swain, & Moses-Kolko, 2015). Results showed higher functional activity in the right fronto-insular cortex (RFIC) correlated with subcortical brain activity for personal mental state talk rather than global aspect of observed caregiving. In sum, preliminary brain-based experiments suggest that parenting may be one instance of altruistic functions that apply to particular social situations (Preston, 2013; Swain, Konrath, et al., 2012) and further research will tell if neural markers are predictive of parent-child functioning.

Does Parental Brain Function Relate to Child Outcome

The first study to look for parental brain markers in the early postpartum to predict child outcomes within the first 2 years of infancy was recently published (P. Kim, Rigo, et al., 2015). In this study, relationships between parental thoughts/actions and brain responses to baby stimuli for mothers and fathers in the neonatal period were studied in relation to the child's social and emotional development at the toddler age. Investigators looking at own vs. other baby-cry responses at 2–4 weeks postpartum found that for mothers, anxious thoughts were associated with differences in motor cortex and substantia nigra responses and decreased child socioemotional functioning at 18 months. In contrast for fathers, lower positive perception of parenthood was associated with lower socioemotional functioning and higher function in the auditory cortex and caudate. If replicated, these results may inform therapies according to parent sex or other factors to target aspects of mood or parental thought that have long-term impact of child development.

Complex Baby Stimuli, Brain Response, and Hormones

Since fMRI techniques were first used to examine maternal neural activation for parenting, researchers have looked for associations between neural and behavioral sensitivity to infants using very specific stimuli. A new direction involves the use of less well-controlled and multimodal stimuli, such as video clips, that are closer to "real life" – but contain more noise. In one of these studies, mothers at 4 to 6 months postpartum were divided into two groups: mothers with high synchronous scores and low intrusiveness scores (synchronous mothers) and mothers with low synchronous scores and high intrusiveness scores (intrusive mothers) based on observed interactions (Atzil, Hendler, & Feldman, 2011). Synchronous maternal behaviors, including coordination of gaze, touch, and vocalizations with infants, are interpreted as more sensitive parenting behaviors and are associated with positive infant outcomes. Contrariwise, intrusive maternal behaviors include lack of coordination and more directedness with the infant, and they tend to be associated with maternal anxiety and the HPA and stress responses (Ruth Feldman, 2007). During a neuroimaging session, mothers were presented with video clips of their own infants and an unfamiliar infant. The main contrast between responses to their own versus the unfamiliar infant was greater activation in the NAcc, a key reward/motivation region, and the amygdala, a key stress and negative emotion processing area. When intrusive and synchronous mothers were compared, intrusive mothers showed greater responses in the amygdala to their own babies, whereas synchronous mothers showed greater activation in the NAcc. Furthermore, functional connectivity in the whole brain using the NAcc and the amygdala as seed regions was examined, and the intrusive and synchronous mothers were compared. In synchronous mothers, activity in the NAcc was correlated with activity in attention and social information processing regions, including the inferior frontal gyrus, the medial frontal gyrus, visual and motor areas, and the parietal cortex. Contrariwise, intrusive mothers showed greater connectivity between the amygdala and the OFC, which is characteristic of elevated anxiety. Thus, reward-related neural responses to one's own infant were associated with enhanced neural connectivity for attention and social information processing, which may further support synchronous mother-infant interactions. Anxiety-related neural responses to one's own infant were associated with more disrupted and intrusive mother-infant interactions.

In another study, the same group of researchers demonstrated that among mothers, plasma OT levels correlated positively with activations in the ventral ACC, the left NAcc, the inferior parietal lobule, and the temporal and frontal gyri in response to videos of their own infants (Atzil, Hendler, Zagoory-Sharon, Winetraub, & Feldman, 2012). When mothers watched videos of various mother-infant interactions, they exhibited greater neural responses to synchronous interactions compared to abnormal interactions (such as between depressed or anxious mothers and their infants), particularly in the dorsal ACC (Atzil, Hendler, & Feldman, 2013). Additionally, greater activation in the dorsal ACC in response to synchronous interactions was positively associated with mothers' own synchronous scores. The dorsal ACC is involved in integrating affective and social processes as well as regulating social pain such as social rejection. Thus, greater activation in the dorsal ACC may contribute to more sensitive processing of social cues, which may be further associated with highly synchronous behaviors among mothers interacting with their own infants (Musser et al., 2012).

Although not using complex video stimuli, other researchers have found associations between parenting behaviors and greater responses to infant stimuli in neural regions important for regulating emotions and processing social information as first shown using a standard measure of maternal sensitivity from free play at 3–4 months described above (Kim et al., 2011). With a similar design, though at 18 months postpartum, maternal sensitivity and intrusiveness were assessed and combined with a similar baby-cry task (Musser, Kaiser-Laurent, & Ablow, 2012). When neural responses to their own versus a control infant's cry were examined, the observed maternal sensitivity was associated with prefrontal activations (superior and inferior frontal gyri), regions involved in regulation of emotions. This suggests that the field will have to contend with an apparent "moving target" of brain circuit activity being different at different postpartum time points.

In another study of mothers with infants aged 4–10 months, the observation of positive mother-infant interactions was associated with increased response to videos of their own infants (vs. control infants) in the putamen and the inferior and middle frontal gyri, areas involved in maternal motivation and regulation of emotions (Wan et al., 2014). Self-reported maternal warmth was associated with greater neural responses to videos of their own infants in the precuneus, visual areas, the insula, and the medial frontal gyrus. The findings suggest that positive parenting behaviors are associated with greater responses to mothers' own infants compared to unfamiliar infants in brain areas involved in social and sensory information processing.

Future Directions

There has been significant improvement in our understanding of the human maternal brain based on a growing number of fMRI studies with human parents. However, important questions remain unanswered:

First, although most of the studies with human mothers have focused on understanding neural functions, little work has been done regarding structural changes. Although human evidence suggests structural growth occurs in the maternal brain (Kim, Leckman, Mayes, Feldman, et al., 2010), animal evidence suggests mixed findings on reduced neurogenesis in the hippocampus but increased synaptic density in the prefrontal cortex during the postpartum period (Leuner, Glasper, & Gould, 2010). Furthermore, current literature suggests mixed evidence in the direction of the anatomical and functional correlations. While training-induced increased gray matter volumes have been associated with increased activation in the hippocampus (Hamzei, Glauche, Schwarzwald, & May, 2012), decreased gray matter volumes were associated with increased activation in the amygdala among trauma-exposed individuals (Ganzel, Kim, Glover, & Temple, 2008). Therefore, it would be important to clarify hormone-related and experienced-based anatomical changes and how they interact with neural functions among human mothers during the early postpartum period, which will provide deeper understanding of the neural plasticity of the maternal brain.

Second, prospective and longitudinal studies across important transition periods for parenting are important to map the temporal processes of neural changes in the human maternal brain. Existing findings of the human maternal brain are based primarily on studies with women during the postpartum period or the first few years of a child's life. However, measures in these studies, such as maternal mood, hormones, neural activation, and parenting behaviors, are measured cross-sectionally, providing only correlative associations that must be interpreted with caution. Thus, causal or temporal conclusions cannot be drawn on how these factors are related to each other. Therefore, prospective studies, particularly studying women during pregnancy and/or even before conception with follow-up until the postpartum periods, may help determine if hormonal changes during the pregnancy prime and enhance neural activation in response to infants during the early postpartum period, which will be further associated with more sensitive maternal behavioral responses to infants during later postpartum periods. In addition, a full understanding of these biological substrates will ultimately also be informed by genetic and epigenetic factors.

Third, negative environments such as living in poverty, being a single or teenage mother, high marital conflict and impaired attachment are significant risk factors for psychopathology and maternal insensitivity toward their children (Magnuson & Duncan, 2002; Sturge-Apple, Davies, & Cummings, 2006). However, little is known about whether such negative environments can increase risk for negative maternal outcomes through changes in the neurobiological processes of parenting and mood regulation. This would be highly expected, given that early life environments are so well established to affect gene expression in animals. Understanding these genetic and neurological factors that are influenced by environment will be critical to determining the most effective interventions to optimize child development. Future parental brain research must include mothers in at-risk environments – especially given recent reports that women with male-perpetrated interpersonal violence-related PTSD (IPV-PTSD) differed in their brain activation from healthy controls (HC) when exposed to scenes of male-female interaction of differing emotional content (Moser, Aue, et al., 2015). Using video stimuli of male-female interactions, IPV-PTSD participants compared with HC showed correlations between brain function, maternal behavior, and stress-related methylation of the glucocorticoid receptor promoter gene NR3C1 – likely associated with higher circulating cortisol and parenting stress (Schechter et al., 2015), BDNF (Moser, Paoloni-Giacobino, et al., 2015) – and serotonin 3A receptor gene (HTR3A), which has been linked to child maltreatment and adult psychopathology (Schechter et al., 2016).

Fourth, we have discussed findings in mothers with defined psychopathology in the previous section, including postpartum depression and substance abuse. Larger and more targeted samples may help to identify specific neural mechanisms that are most affected in specific psychopathologies. For instance, dysfunctions in the regulation of the emotion network may be associated with postpartum depression, whereas the reward/motivation network may be more associated with substance abuse. Alternately, as proposed in the National Institute of Mental Health's Research Domain Criteria (RDoC) (Cuthbert, 2014), continuous symptom spectra, which may overlap across defined psychopathologies, may better align with neurobiological systems. Such specificity can be critical for developing targeted interventions and treatments that are more effective in preventing psychopathology and improving symptoms of psychopathology that may be different for new mothers vs. fathers as suggested by recent research (Kim, Rigo, et al., 2015). Perhaps training parent vocalization can be incorporated into interventions as part of increasing parental sensitivity.

Fifth, the field will benefit from continuing to move toward combining well-established paradigms known to probe certain aspects of brain function, such as executive functions and emotion response/regulation with naturalistic and personally salient infant information. This is especially important as it seems that brain physiology is changing according to child stage – itself adapting to child development. Consensus on brain imaging methodology and expectations as we examine specific links between neural regions/networks and behaviors throughout pregnancy and the postpartum period will be important to generate a consistent picture. Next steps may include examining whether activation in specific neural regions/circuits such as the hippocampus and precuneus/posterior cingulate cortex, which are parts of the neural memory circuits, changes over time across pregnancy and the postpartum period, for example, verbal recall memory declines during pregnancy and the postpartum period (Glynn, 2010). This research does raise interesting possibilities of investigating cultural differences – at the intersection of evolutionary biology and developmental cultural psychology – where candidate behavioral universals may be embedded in the nervous systems of human caregivers. This could also shed light on other domains of caregiving that could be encouraged or optimized.

Sixth, many research reports point to the need to move to more natural and personally relevant stimuli. In addition to the use of movies and decision-making tasks, for example, future experiments might include the child, using forms of neuroimaging that allow for some natural movement, such as with functional near-infrared spectroscopy (fNIRS) and electroencephalography (EEG). This may yield brain-based models that reflect real-life parental planning, responding, and decision-making and perhaps avoid neuroimaging problems in other fields that have typically been difficult to replicate or interpret, perhaps because of not using personally tailored or particularly compelling stimuli close to reality. Along these lines, alternate neuroimaging methods will also be needed to incorporate brain structure, resting state and functional neural activation, and parenting behaviors. Such multimodal approaches that use machine learning methods promise diagnostic and prognostic models for healthy maternal adaptation vs. psychopathology (Orru, Pettersson-Yeo, Marquand, Sartori, & Mechelli, 2012) that may not be possible with any one method. Perhaps in the future, a routine brain scan – with advanced post-processing – will provide biomarkers for earlier assessment and correction of parenting problems toward breaking trans-generational mental health problems and healthier children, whose developing brains are themselves another frontier of research.

Acknowledgments The author is currently supported by the University of Michigan, Department of Psychiatry, and grants from the National Center for Advancing Translational Sciences via the University of Michigan Institute for Clinical Health Research UL1 TR000433, Centers for Disease Control & Prevention Award Number via the University of Michigan Injury Center U49/CE002099, and Brain & Behavior Research Foundation.

References

Adler, N. E., Marmot, M., McEwen, B. S., & Stewart, J. (Eds.). (1999). *Socioeconomic status and health in industrial nations*. New York, NY: New York Academy of Sciences.

Adler, N. E., & Rehkopf, D. H. (2008). U.S. disparities in health: Descriptions, causes, and mechanisms. *Annual Review of Public Health, 29*, 235–252.

Adolphs, R. (2010). What does the amygdala contribute to social cognition? *Annals of the New York Academy of Sciences, 1191*(1), 42–61. doi:10.1111/j.1749-6632.2010.05445.x

Aharon, I., Etcoff, N., Ariely, D., Chabris, C. F., O'Connor, E., & Breiter, H. C. (2001). Beautiful faces have variable reward value: fMRI and behavioral evidence. *Neuron, 32*(3), 537–551.

Ainsworth, M. S., Blehar, M. C., Waters, E., & Wall, S. (1978). *Patterns of attachment: A psychological study of the strange situation*. Oxford, England: Erlbaum.

Atkinson, L., Leung, E., Goldberg, S., Benoit, D., Poulton, L., Myhal, N., … Kerr, S. (2009). Attachment and selective attention: Disorganization and emotional Stroop reaction time. *Development and Psychopathology, 21*(1), 99–126. doi:10.1017/S0954579409000078

Atzil, S., Hendler, T., & Feldman, R. (2011). Specifying the neurobiological basis of human attachment: Brain, hormones, and behavior in synchronous and intrusive mothers. *Neuropsychopharmacology, 36*(13), 2603–2615. doi:10.1038/npp.2011.172

Atzil, S., Hendler, T., & Feldman, R. (2013). The brain basis of social synchrony. *Social Cognitive and Affective Neuroscience*. doi:10.1093/scan/nst105

Atzil, S., Hendler, T., Zagoory-Sharon, O., Winetraub, Y., & Feldman, R. (2012). Synchrony and specificity in the maternal and the paternal brain: Relations to oxytocin and vasopressin. *Journal of the American Academy of Child and Adolescent Psychiatry, 51*(8), 798–811. doi:10.1016/j.jaac.2012.06.008

Bakermans-Kranenburg, M. J., van IJzendoorn, M. H., & Juffer, F. (2003). Less is more: Meta-analyses of sensitivity and attachment interventions in early childhood. *Psychological Bulletin, 129*(2), 195–215.

Barnett, M. A., & The Family Life Project Key, I. (2008). Mother and grandmother parenting in low-income three-generation rural households. *Journal of Marriage and Family, 70*(5), 1241–1257. doi:10.1111/j.1741-3737.2008.00563.x

Barrett, J., Wonch, K. E., Gonzalez, A., Ali, N., Steiner, M., Hall, G. B., & Fleming, A. S. (2012). Maternal affect and quality of parenting experiences are related to amygdala response to infant faces. *Social Neuroscience, 7*(3), 252–268. doi:10.1080/17470919.2011.609907

Behrens, K. Y., Hart, S. L., & Parker, A. C. (2012). Maternal sensitivity: Evidence of stability across time, contexts, and measurement instruments. *Infant and Child Development, 21*(4), 348–355. doi:10.1002/Icd.1747

Belsky, J., Jaffee, S. R., Sligo, J., Woodward, L., & Silva, P. A. (2005). Intergenerational transmission of warm-sensitive-stimulating parenting: A prospective study of mothers and fathers of 3-year-olds. *Child Development, 76*, 384–396.

Bernier, A., Carlson, S. M., & Whipple, N. (2010). From external regulation to self-regulation: Early parenting precursors of young children's executive functioning. *Child Development, 81*(1), 326–339. doi:10.1111/j.1467-8624.2009.01397.x

Blair, C., & Raver, C. C. (2012). Child development in the context of adversity: Experiential canalization of brain and behavior. *American Psychologist, 67*(4), 309–318. doi:10.1037/a0027493

Bowlby, J. (1969). *Attachment* (2nd ed., Vol. 1). New York, NY: Basic Books.

Bowlby, J. (1973). *Attachment and loss* (Vol. 2, Separation: Anxiety and anger). London, England: Basic Books.

Bowlby, J. (1977). The making and breaking of affectional bonds. I. Aetiology and psychopathology in the light of attachment theory. An expanded version of the Fiftieth Maudsley Lecture, delivered before the Royal College of Psychiatrists, 19 November 1976. *The British Journal of Psychiatry, 130*, 201–210.

Boyce, W. T., Sokolowski, M. B., & Robinson, G. E. (2012). Toward a new biology of social adversity. *Proceedings of the National Academy of Sciences of the United States of America, 109*(Suppl 2), 17143–17148. doi:10.1073/pnas.1121264109

Bradley, R. H., & Corwyn, R. F. (2002). Socioeconomic status and child development. *Annaul Review of Psychology, 53*(1), 371–399.

Britton, J. R., Britton, H. L., & Gronwaldt, V. (2006). Breastfeeding, sensitivity, and attachment. *Pediatrics, 118*, e1436–e1443.

Brown, S. L., & Brown, R. M. (2015). Connecting prosocial behavior to improved physical health: Contributions from the neurobiology of parenting. *Neuroscience and Biobehavioral Reviews, 55*, 1–17. doi:10.1016/j.neubiorev.2015.04.004

Capaldi, D. M., Pears, K. C. P., Patterson, G. R., & Owen, L. D. (2003). Continuity of parenting practices across generations in an at-risk sample: A prospective comparison of direct and mediated associations. *Journal of Abnormal Child Psychology, 31*, 127–142.

Champagne, F. A., Weaver, I. C., Diorio, J., Sharma, S., & Meaney, M. J. (2003). Natural variations in maternal care are associated with estrogen receptor alpha expression and estrogen sensitivity in the medial preoptic area. *Endocrinology, 144*(11), 4720–4724.

Chen, E., Matthews, K. A., & Boyce, W. T. (2002). Socioeconomic differences in children's health: How and why do these relationships change with age? *Psychological Bulletin, 128*, 295–329.

Cohen, S., Janicki-Deverts, D., Chen, E., & Matthews, K. A. (2010). Childhood socioeconomic status and adult health. *Annals of the New York Academy of Sciences, 1186*, 37–55. doi:10.1111/j.1749-6632.2009.05334.x

Cuthbert, B. N. (2014). The RDoC framework: Facilitating transition from ICD/DSM to dimensional approaches that integrate neuroscience and psychopathology. *World Psychiatry, 13*(1), 28–35. doi:10.1002/wps.20087

De Wolff, M., & van Ijzendoorn, M. H. (1997). Sensitivity and attachment: A meta-analysis on parental antecedents of infant attachment. *Child Development, 68*(4), 571–591. doi:10.2307/1132107

Decety, J. (2015). The neural pathways, development and functions of empathy. *Current Opinion in Behavioral Sciences, 3*, 1–6.

Delgado, M. R., Nystrom, L. E., Fissell, C., Noll, D. C., & Fiez, J. A. (2000). Tracking the hemodynamic responses to reward and punishment in the striatum. *Journal of Neurophysiology, 84*(6), 3072–3077.

Eisenberg, N., Cumberland, A., Spinrad, T. L., Fabes, R. A., Shepard, S. A., Reiser, M., … Guthrie, I. K. (2001). The relations of regulation and emotionality to children's externalizing and internalizing problem behavior. *Child Development, 72*(4), 1112–1134.

Elliott, R., Zahn, R., Deakin, J. F., & Anderson, I. M. (2011). Affective cognition and its disruption in mood disorders. *Neuropsychopharmacology, 36*(1), 153–182. doi:10.1038/npp.2010.77

Engfer, A., & Gavranidou, M. (1987). Antecedents and consequences of maternal sensitivity: A longitudinal study. In H. Rauh, H.-C. Steinhausen (Eds.), *Psychobiology and early development* (Vol. 46, pp. 71–99). North Holland, The Netherlands. Elsevier Science Publishers B.V.

Evans, G. W. (2004). The environment of childhood poverty. *American Psychologist, 59*, 77–92.

Evans, G. W., Chen, E., Miller, G. E., & Seeman, T. E. (2012). How poverty gets under the skin: A life course perspective. In V. Maholmes & R. King (Eds.), *The Oxford handbook of poverty and child development* (pp. 13–36). New York, NY: Oxford University Press.

Evans, G. W., & Kim, P. (2010). Multiple risk exposure as a potential explanatory mechanism for the socioeconomic status-health gradient. *Annals of the New York Academy of Sciences, 1186*, 174–189. doi:10.1111/j.1749-6632.2009.05336.x

Evans, G. W., Swain, J. E., King, A. P., Wang, X., Javanbakht, A., Ho, S. S., … Liberzon, I. (2016). Childhood cumulative risk exposure and adult amygdala volume and function. *Journal of Neuroscience Research, 94*(6), 535–543. doi:10.1002/jnr.23681

Fan, Y., Duncan, N. W., de Greck, M., & Northoff, G. (2011). Is there a core neural network in empathy? An fMRI based quantitative meta-analysis. *Neuroscience and Biobehavioral Reviews, 35*(3), 903–911.

Feldman, R. (2007). Parent-infant synchrony and the construction of shared timing; physiological precursors, developmental outcomes, and risk conditions. *Journal of Child Psychology and Psychiatry, 48*(3–4), 329–354. doi:10.1111/j.1469-7610.2006.01701.x

Feldman, R., Weller, A., Leckman, J. F., Kuint, J., & Eidelman, A. I. (1999). The nature of the mother's tie to her infant: Maternal bonding under conditions of proximity, separation, and potential loss. *Journal of Child Psychology and Psychiatry, 40*(6), 929–939.

Feygin, D. L., Swain, J. E., & Leckman, J. F. (2006). The normalcy of neurosis: Evolutionary origins of obsessive-compulsive disorder and related behaviors. *Progress in Neuro-Psychopharmacology & Biological Psychiatry, 30*(5), 854–864.

Fleming, A. S., Kraemer, G. W., Gonzalez, A., Lovic, V., Rees, S., & Melo, A. (2002). Mothering begets mothering: The transmission of behavior and its neurobiology across generations. *Pharmacology, Biochemistry and Behavior, 73*(1), 61–75.

Frith, C. D., & Frith, U. (2006). The neural basis of mentalizing. *Neuron, 50*(4), 531–534. doi:10.1016/j.neuron.2006.05.001

Frith, U., & Frith, C. D. (2003). Development and neurophysiology of mentalizing. *Philosophical Transactions of the Royal Society of London. Series B, Biological Sciences, 358*(1431), 459–473.

Ganzel, B. L., Kim, P., Glover, G. H., & Temple, E. (2008). Resilience after 9/11: Multimodal neuroimaging evidence for stress-related change in the healthy adult brain. *NeuroImage, 40*(2), 788–795.

Glynn, L. M. (2010). Giving birth to a new brain: Hormone exposures of pregnancy influence human memory. *Psychoneuroendocrinology, 35*(8), 1148–1155. doi:10.1016/j.psyneuen.2010.01.015

Gonzalez, A., Jenkins, J. M., Steiner, M., & Fleming, A. S. (2012). Maternal early life experiences and parenting: The mediating role of cortisol and executive function. *Journal of the American Academy of Child and Adolescent Psychiatry, 51*(7), 673–682. doi:10.1016/j.jaac.2012.04.003

Grant, K. E., Compas, B. E., Stuhlmacher, A. F., Thurm, A. E., McMahon, S. D., & Halpert, J. A. (2003). Stressors and child and adolescent psychopathology: Moving from markers to mechanisms of risk. *Psychological Bulletin, 129*, 447–466.

Hamzei, F., Glauche, V., Schwarzwald, R., & May, A. (2012). Dynamic gray matter changes within cortex and striatum after short motor skill training are associated with their increased functional interaction. *NeuroImage, 59*(4), 3364–3372.

Hein, G., & Singer, T. (2008). I feel how you feel but not always: The empathic brain and its modulation. *Current Opinion in Neurobiology, 18*(2), 153–158.

Hipwell, A. E., Guo, C., Phillips, M. L., Swain, J. E., & Moses-Kolko, E. L. (2015). Right fronto-insular cortex and subcortical activity to infant cry is associated with maternal mental state talk. *The Journal of Neuroscience, 35*(37), 12725–12732. doi:10.1523/JNEUROSCI.1286-15.2015

Ho, S. S., Gonzalez, R. D., Abelson, J. L., & Liberzon, I. (2012). Neurocircuits underlying cognition-emotion interaction in a social decision making context. *NeuroImage, 63*(2), 843–857. doi:10.1016/j.neuroimage.2012.07.017

Ho, S. S., Konrath, S., Brown, S., & Swain, J. E. (2014). Empathy and stress related neural responses in maternal decision making. *Frontiers in Neuroscience, 8*, 152. doi:10.3389/fnins.2014.00152

Ho, S. S., & Swain, J. E. (2017, in press). Depression altered limbic response and functional connectivity related to self-oriented distress signals. *Behavioral Brain Research.*

Hoff, E., Laursen, B., & Tardif, T. (2002). Socioeconomic status and parenting. In M. H. Bornstein (Ed.), *Handbook of parenting* (2nd ed., pp. 231–252). Mahwah, NJ: Erlbaum.

Hoffman, K. T., Marvin, R. S., Cooper, G., & Powell, B. (2006). Changing toddlers' and preschoolers' attachment classifications: The Circle of Security intervention. *Journal of Consulting and Clinical Psychology, 74*(6), 1017–1026.

Jaffari-Bimmel, N., Juffer, F., van IJzendoorn, M. H., Bakermans-Kranenburg, M. J., & Mooijaart, A. (2006). Social development from infancy to adolescence: Longitudinal and concurrent factors in an adoption sample. *Developmental Psychology, 42*(6), 1143–1153. doi:10.1037/0012-1649.42.6.1143

Javanbakht, A., King, A. P., Evans, G. W., Swain, J. E., Angstadt, M., Phan, K. L., & Liberzon, I. (2015). Childhood poverty predicts adult amygdala and frontal activity and connectivity in response to emotional faces. *Frontiers in Behavioral Neuroscience, 9*, 154. doi:10.3389/fnbeh.2015.00154

Joosen, K. J., Mesman, J., Bakermans-Kranenburg, M. J., & van IJzendoorn, M. H. (2012). Maternal sensitivity to infants in various settings predicts harsh discipline in toddlerhood. *Attachment & Human Development, 14*(2), 101–117. doi:10.1080/14616734.2012.661217

Kaufman, J., & Zigler, E. (1989). The intergenerational transmission of child abuse. In *Child maltreatment: Theory and research on the causes and consequences of child abuse and neglect* (pp. 129–150). Cambridge, UK/New York, NY: Cambridge University Press.

Keller, H., Lohaus, A., Völker, S., Elben, C., & Ball, J. (2003). Warmth and contingency and their relationship to maternal attitudes toward parenting. *Journal of Genetic Psychology, 164*, 275–292.

Keren, M., Feldman, R., Eidelman, A. I., Sirota, L., & Lester, B. (2003). Clinical interview of high-risk parents of premature infants (CLIP): Relations to mother-infant interaction. *Infant Mental Health Journal, 24*, 93–110.

Kessler, R. C., Price, R. H., & Wortman, C. B. (1985). Social factors in psychopathology: Stress, social support, and coping processes. *Annual Review of Psychology, 36*, 531–572. doi:10.1146/annurev.ps.36.020185.002531

Kim, P., Evans, G. W., Angstadt, M., Ho, S. S., Sripada, C. S., Swain, J. E., ... Phan, K. L. (2013). Effects of childhood poverty and chronic stress on emotion regulatory brain function in adulthood. *Proceedings of the National Academy of Sciences of the United States of America, 110*(46), 18442–18447. doi:10.1073/pnas.1308240110

Kim, P., Feldman, R., Mayes, L. C., Eicher, V., Thompson, N., Leckman, J. F., & Swain, J. E. (2011). Breastfeeding, brain activation to own infant cry, and maternal sensitivity. *Journal of Child Psychology and Psychiatry, 52*(8), 907–915.

Kim, P., Ho, S. S., Evans, G. W., Liberzon, I., & Swain, J. E. (2015). Childhood social inequalities influences neural processes in young adult caregiving. *Developmental Psychobiology, 57*(8), 948–960. doi:10.1002/dev.21325

Kim, P., Leckman, J. F., Mayes, L. C., Feldman, R., Wang, X., & Swain, J. E. (2010). The plasticity of human maternal brain: Longitudinal changes in brain anatomy during the early postpartum period. *Behavioral Neuroscience, 124*(5), 695–700. doi:10.1037/a0020884

Kim, P., Leckman, J. F., Mayes, L. C., Newman, M.-A., Feldman, R., & Swain, J. E. (2010). Perceived quality of maternal care in childhood and structure and function of mothers' brain. *Developmental Science, 13*(4), 662–673. doi:10.1111/j.1467-7687.2009.00923.x

Kim, P., Mayes, L., Feldman, R., Leckman, J. F., & Swain, J. E. (2013). Early postpartum parental preoccupation and positive parenting thoughts: Relationship with parent-infant interaction. *Infant Mental Health Journal, 34*(2), 104–116. doi:10.1002/Imhj.21359

Kim, P., Rigo, P., Leckman, J. F., Mayes, L. C., Cole, P. M., Feldman, R., & Swain, J. E. (2015). A prospective longitudinal study of perceived infant outcomes at 18-24 months: Neural and psychological correlates of parental thoughts and actions assessed during the first month postpartum. *Frontiers in Psychology, 6*, 1772. doi:10.3389/fpsyg.2015.01772

Kim, P., Rigo, P., Mayes, L. C., Feldman, R., Leckman, J. F., & Swain, J. E. (2014). Neural plasticity in fathers of human infants. *Social Neuroscience, 9*(5), 522–535. doi:10.1080/17470919.2014.933713

Kim, P., Strathearn, L., & Swain, J. E. (2016). The maternal brain and its plasticity in humans. *Hormones and Behavior, 77*, 113–123. doi:10.1016/j.yhbeh.2015.08.001

Kim, S., Fonagy, P., Allen, J., Martinez, S. R., Iyengar, U., & Strathearn, L. (2014). Mothers who are securely attached during pregnancy show more attuned infant mirroring at 7 months postpartum. *Infant Behavior & Development*.

Kim, S., Fonagy, P., Allen, J., & Strathearn, L. (2014). Mothers' unresolved trauma blunts amygdala response to infant distress. *Social Neuroscience, 9*(4), 352–363. doi:10.1080/17470919.2014.896287

Kober, H., Barrett, L. F., Joseph, J., Bliss-Moreau, E., Lindquist, K., & Wager, T. D. (2008). Functional grouping and cortical-subcortical interactions in emotion: A meta-analysis of neuroimaging studies. *NeuroImage, 42*(2), 998–1031. doi:10.1016/j.neuroimage.2008.03.059

Kochanska, G. (2002). Mutually responsive orientation between mothers and their young children: A context for the early development of conscience. *Current Directions in Psychological Science, 11*(6), 191–195. doi:10.1111/1467-8721.00198

Krishnan, A., Woo, C.-W., Chang, L. J., Ruzic, L., Gu, X., López-Solà, M., ... Wager, T. D. (2016). Somatic and vicarious pain are represented by dissociable multivariate brain patterns. *eLife, 5*, e15166. doi:10.7554/eLife.15166

Lamb, M. E., Pleck, J. H., Charnov, E. L., & Levine, J. A. (1985). Paternal behavior in humans. *American Zoologist, 25*, 883–894. doi:10.1093/icb/25.3.883

Laurent, H. K., & Ablow, J. C. (2012). A cry in the dark: Depressed mothers show reduced neural activation to their own infant's cry. *Social Cognitive and Affective Neuroscience, 7*(2), 125–134.

Laurent, H. K., Stevens, A., & Ablow, J. C. (2011). Neural correlates of hypothalamic-pituitary-adrenal regulation of mothers with their infants. Biological Psychiatry, 70(9), 826–832. doi:10.1016/j.biopsych.2011.06.011. S0006-3223(11)00610-X [pii]

Leckman, J. F., Feldman, R., Swain, J. E., Eicher, V., Thompson, N., & Mayes, L. C. (2004). Primary parental preoccupation: Circuits, genes, and the crucial role of the environment. *Journal of Neural Transmission, 111*(7), 753–771.

Leckman, J. F., Mayes, L. C., Feldman, R., Evans, D., King, R. A., & Cohen, D. J. (1999). Early parental preoccupations and behaviors and their possible relationship to the symptoms of obsessive-compulsive disorder. *Acta Psychiatrica Scandinavica, 100*, 1–26.

Leerkes, E. M. (2011). Maternal sensitivity during distressing tasks: A unique predictor of attachment security. *Infant Behavior & Development, 34*(3), 443–446. doi:10.1016/j.infbeh.2011.04.006

Leerkes, E. M., Nayena Blankson, A., & O'Brien, M. (2009). Differential effects of maternal sensitivity to infant distress and nondistress on social-emotional functioning. *Child Development, 80*(3), 762–775. doi:10.1111/j.1467-8624.2009.01296.x

Leibenluft, E., Gobbini, M. I., Harrison, T., & Haxby, J. V. (2004). Mothers' neural activation in response to pictures of their children and other children. *Biological Psychiatry, 56*, 225–232.

Lenzi, D., Trentini, C., Macaluso, E., Graziano, S., Speranza, A. M., Pantano, P., & Ammaniti, M. (2016). Mothers with depressive symptoms display differential brain activations when empathizing with infant faces. *Psychiatry Research, 249*, 1–11. doi:10.1016/j.pscychresns.2016.01.019

Leuner, B., Glasper, E. R., & Gould, E. (2010). Parenting and plasticity. *Trends in Neurosciences, 33*(10), 465–473.

Liberzon, I., Ma, S. T., Okada, G., Ho, S. S., Swain, J. E., & Evans, G. W. (2015). Childhood poverty and recruitment of adult emotion regulatory neurocircuitry. *Social Cognitive and Affective Neuroscience, 10*(11), 1596–1606. doi:10.1093/scan/nsv045

Lorberbaum, J. P., Newman, J. D., Horwitz, A. R., Dubno, J. R., Lydiard, R. B., Hammer, M. B., … George, M. S. (2002). A potential role for thalamocingulate circuitry in human maternal behavior. *Biological Psychiatry, 51*, 431–445.

Lupien, S. J., King, S., Meaney, M. J., & McEwen, B. S. (2000). Child's stress hormone levels correlate with mother's socioeconomic status and depressive state. *Biological Psychiatry, 48*, 976–980.

Magnuson, K. A., & Duncan, G. J. (2002). Parents in poverty. In M. H. Bronstein (Ed.), *Handbook of parenting* (2nd ed., Vol. 4, pp. 95–121). Mahwah, NJ: Erlbaum.

McElwain, N. L., & Booth-Laforce, C. (2006). Maternal sensitivity to infant distress and nondistress as predictors of infant-mother attachment security. *Journal of Family Psychology, 20*(2), 247–255. doi:10.1037/0893-3200.20.2.247

McEwen, B. S. (1998). Protective and damaging effects of stress mediators. *New England Journal of Medicine, 338*, 171–179.

McEwen, B. S. (2001). Plasticity of the hippocampus: Adaptation to chronic stress and allostatic load. *Annals of the New York Academy of Sciences, 933*(1), 265–277.

McEwen, B. S. (2012). Brain on stress: How the social environment gets under the skin. *Proceedings of the National Academy of Sciences of the United States of America, 109*(Suppl 2), 17180–17185. doi:10.1073/pnas.1121254109

McGowan, P. O., Sasaki, A., D'Alessio, A. C., Dymov, S., Labonte, B., Szyf, M., … Meaney, M. J. (2009). Epigenetic regulation of the glucocorticoid receptor in human brain associates with childhood abuse. Nature Neuroscience, 12(3), 342–348. https://doi.org/10.1038/nn.2270.

Melis, M. R., & Argiolas, A. (1995). Dopamine and sexual behavior. *Neuroscience and Biobehavioral Reviews, 19*(1), 19–38.

Milner, J. S. (1993). Social information-processing and physical child-abuse. *Clinical Psychology Review, 13*(3), 275–294. doi:10.1016/0272-7358(93)90024-G

Milner, J. S. (2003). Social information processing in high-risk and physically abusive parents. *Child Abuse & Neglect, 27*(1), 7–20.

Mitchell, J. P. (2009). Inferences about mental states. *Philosophical Transactions of the Royal Society of London. Series B, Biological Sciences, 364*(1521), 1309–1316. doi:10.1098/rstb.2008.0318

Morgan, H. D., Fleming, A. S., & Stern, J. M. (1992). Somatosensory control of the onset and retention of maternal responsiveness in primiparous Sprague-Dawley rats. *Physiology and Behavior, 51*(3), 549–555.

Morgan, H. D., Watchus, J. A., Milgram, N. W., & Fleming, A. S. (1999). The long lasting effects of electrical simulation of the medial preoptic area and medial amygdala on maternal behavior in female rats. *Behavioural Brain Research, 99*(1), 61–73. Doi: http://dx.doi.org/10.1016/S0166-4328(98)00070-9

Morrison, S. E., & Salzman, C. D. (2010). Re-valuing the amygdala. Current Opinion in Neurobiology, 20(2), 221–230. doi:10.1016/j.conb.2010.02.007. S0959-4388(10)00029-2 [pii]

Moser, D. A., Aue, T., Suardi, F., Kutlikova, H., Cordero, M. I., Rossignol, A. S., … Schechter, D. S. (2015). Violence-related PTSD and neural activation when seeing emotionally charged male-female interactions. *Social Cognitive and Affective Neuroscience, 10*(5), 645–653. doi:10.1093/scan/nsu099

Moser, D. A., Paoloni-Giacobino, A., Stenz, L., Adouan, W., Manini, A., Suardi, F., … Schechter, D. S. (2015). BDNF methylation and maternal brain activity in a violence-related sample. *PLoS One, 10*(12), e0143427. doi:10.1371/journal.pone.0143427

Moses-Kolko, E. L., Horner, M. S., Phillips, M. L., Hipwell, A. E., & Swain, J. E. (2014). In search of neural endophenotypes of postpartum psychopathology and disrupted maternal caregiving. *Journal of Neuroendocrinology, 26*(10), 665–684. doi:10.1111/jne.12183

Musser, E. D., Kaiser-Laurent, H., & Ablow, J. C. (2012). The neural correlates of maternal sensitivity: An fMRI study. *Developmental Cognitive Neuroscience, 2*(4), 428–436. doi:10.1016/j.dcn.2012.04.003

Muzik, M., Ho, S. S., Morelen, D., Rosenblum, K. L., King, A. C., Zubieta, J. K., & Swain, J. E. (2017, under review). Amygdala's role in maternal child-oriented empathy and parenting stress was revealed in a pre- and post-intervention fMRI study. *Neuropsychopharmacology, .*

Muzik, M., Rosenblum, K. L., Alfafara, E. A., Schuster, M. M., Miller, N. M., Waddell, R. M., & Kohler, E. S. (2015). Mom power: Preliminary outcomes of a group intervention to improve mental health and parenting among high-risk mothers. *Archives of Women's Mental Health.* doi:10.1007/s00737-014-0490-z

Noriuchi, M., Kikuchi, Y., & Senoo, A. (2008). The functional neuroanatomy of maternal love: mother's response to infant's attachment behaviors. *Biological Psychiatry, 63*(4), 415–423.

Numan, M. (2014). *Neurobiology of social behavior: Toward an understanding of the prosocial and antisocial brain* (1st ed.). Academic. London.

Numan, M., & Woodside, B. (2010). Maternity: Neural mechanisms, motivational processes, and physiological adaptations. *Behavioral Neuroscience, 124*(6), 715–741. doi:10.1037/a0021548

Ochsner, K. N., Silvers, J. A., & Buhle, J. T. (2012). Functional imaging studies of emotion regulation: A synthetic review and evolving model of the cognitive control of emotion. *Annals of the New York Academy of Sciences, 1251*(1), E1–E24. doi:10.1111/j.1749-6632.2012.06751.x

Orru, G., Pettersson-Yeo, W., Marquand, A. F., Sartori, G., & Mechelli, A. (2012). Using support vector machine to identify imaging biomarkers of neurological and psychiatric disease: A critical review. *Neuroscience and Biobehavioral Reviews, 36*(4), 1140–1152. doi:10.1016/j.neubiorev.2012.01.004

Oxley, G., & Fleming, A. S. (2000). The effects of medial preoptic area and amygdala lesions on maternal behavior in the juvenile rat. *Developmental Psychobiology, 37*(4), 253–265. doi:10.1002/1098-2302(2000)37:4<253::AID-DEV6>3.0.CO;2-Q

Panksepp, J. (1998). *Affective neuroscience: The foundation of human and animal emotions.* Oxford: Oxford University Press.

Pearson, R. M., Cooper, R. M., Penton-Voak, I. S., Lightman, S. L., & Evans, J. (2010). Depressive symptoms in early pregnancy disrupt attentional processing of infant emotion. *Psychological Medicine, 40*(4), 621–631. doi:10.1017/S0033291709990961

Pearson, R. M., Lightman, S. L., & Evans, J. (2011). The impact of breastfeeding on mothers' attentional sensitivity towards infant distress. *Infant Behavior & Development, 34*(1), 200–205. doi:10.1016/j.infbeh.2010.12.009

Pleck, J. H. (2010). Paternal involvement: Revised conceptualization and theoretical linkages with child outcome. In M. E. Lamb (Ed.), *The role of the father in child development* (pp. 58–93). Hoboken, NJ: Wiley.

Poulton, R., Caspi, A., Milne, B. J., Thomson, W. M., Taylor, A., Sears, M. R., & Moffitt, T. E. (2002). Association between children's experience of socioeconomic disadvantage and adult health: A life-course study. *Lancet, 360*, 1640–1645.

Powell, B., Cooper, G., Hoffman, K., & Marvin, B. (2014). *The circle of security intervention: Enhancing attachment in early parent-child relationships.* Guilford Press. New York

Preston, S. D. (2013). The origins of altruism in offspring care. *Psychological Bulletin, 139*(6), 1305–1341. doi:10.1037/a0031755

Repetti, R. L., Taylor, S. E., & Seeman, T. E. (2002). Risky families: Family social environments and the mental and physical health of offspring. *Psychological Bulletin, 128*(2), 330–366.

Riem, M. M., Bakermans-Kranenburg, M. J., Pieper, S., Tops, M., Boksem, M. A., Vermeiren, R. R., … Rombouts, S. A. (2011). Oxytocin modulates amygdala, insula, and inferior frontal gyrus responses to infant crying: A randomized controlled trial. *Biological Psychiatry, 70*(3), 291–297. doi:10.1016/j.biopsych.2011.02.006

Sanders, M. R., Kirby, J. N., Tellegen, C. L., & Day, J. J. (2014). The triple P-Positive Parenting Program: A systematic review and meta-analysis of a multi-level system of parenting support. *Clinical Psychology Review, 34*(4), 337–357. doi:10.1016/j.cpr.2014.04.003

Santos, A., Mier, D., Kirsch, P., & Meyer-Lindenberg, A. (2011). Evidence for a general face salience signal in human amygdala. *NeuroImage, 54*(4), 3111–3116. doi:http://dx.doi.org/10.1016/j.neuroimage.2010.11.024

Saxe, R. (2006). Why and how to study theory of mind with fMRI. *Brain Research, 1079*(1), 57–65.

Schechter, D. S., Moser, D. A., Paoloni-Giacobino, A., Stenz, L., Gex-Fabry, M., Aue, T., ... Rusconi Serpa, S. (2015). Methylation of NR3C1 is related to maternal PTSD, parenting stress and maternal medial prefrontal cortical activity in response to child separation among mothers with histories of violence exposure. *Frontiers in Psychology, 6*, 690. doi:10.3389/fpsyg.2015.00690

Schechter, D. S., Moser, D. A., Pointet, V. C., Aue, T., Stenz, L., Paoloni-Giacobino, A., ... Dayer, A. G. (2016). The association of serotonin receptor 3A methylation with maternal violence exposure, neural activity, and child aggression. *Behavioural Brain Research.* doi:10.1016/j.bbr.2016.10.009

Schuengel, C., Bakermans-Kranenburg, M. J., & Van, I. M. H. (1999). Frightening maternal behavior linking unresolved loss and disorganized infant attachment. *Journal of Consulting and Clinical Psychology, 67*(1), 54–63.

Scott, K. M., Al-Hamzawi, A. O., Andrade, L. H., Borges, G., Caldas-de-Almeida, J. M., Fiestas, F., ... Kessler, R. C. (2014). Associations between subjective social status and DSM-IV mental disorders: Results from the World Mental Health surveys. *JAMA Psychiatry, 71*(12), 1400–1408. doi:10.1001/jamapsychiatry.2014.1337

Seifritz, E., Esposito, F., Neuhoff, J. G., Luthi, A., Mustovic, H., Dammann, G., ... Di Salle, F. (2003). Differential sex-independent amygdala response to infant crying and laughing in parents versus nonparents. *Biological Psychiatry, 54*(12), 1367–1375.

Sergerie, K., Chochol, C., & Armony, J. L. (2008). The role of the amygdala in emotional processing: A quantitative meta-analysis of functional neuroimaging studies. *Neuroscience & Biobehavioral Reviews, 32*(4), 811–830. doi:10.1016/j.neubiorev.2007.12.002

Shah, P. E., Fonagy, P., & Strathearn, L. (2010). Is attachment transmitted across generations? The plot thickens. *Clinical Child Psychology and Psychiatry, 15*(3), 329–346.

Shaver, P., Schwartz, J., Kirson, D., & O'Connor, C. (1987). Emotion knowledge: Further exploration of a prototype approach. *Journal of Personality and Social Psychology, 52*(6), 1061–1086.

Silverman, M. E., Muennig, P., Liu, X., Rosen, Z., & Goldstein, M. A. (2009). The impact of socioeconomic status on the neural substrates associated with pleasure. *Open Neuroimaging Journal, 3*, 58–63. doi:10.2174/1874440000903010058

Simons, R. L., Whitbeck, L. B., Conger, R. D., & Wu, C.-I. (1991). Intergenerational transmission of harsh parenting. *Developmental Psychology, 27*(1), 159.

Sripada, R. K., Swain, J. E., Evans, G. W., Welsh, R. C., & Liberzon, I. (2014). Childhood poverty and stress reactivity are associated with aberrant functional connectivity in default mode network. *Neuropsychopharmacology, 39*(9), 2244–2251. doi:10.1038/npp.2014.75

Stoeckel, L. E., Weller, R. E., Cook, E. W., 3rd, Twieg, D. B., Knowlton, R. C., & Cox, J. E. (2008). Widespread reward-system activation in obese women in response to pictures of high-calorie foods. *NeuroImage, 41*(2), 636–647. doi:10.1016/j.neuroimage.2008.02.031

Stratpearn, L., Fonagy, P., Amico, J., & Montague, P. R. (2009). Adult attachment predicts maternal brain and oxytocin response to infant cues. *Neuropsychopharmacology, 34*(13), 2655–2666.

Stratpearn, L., & Kim, S. (2013). Mothers' amygdala response to positive or negative infant affect is modulated by personal relevance. *Frontiers in Neuroscience, 7*(176), 1–10. doi:10.3389/fnins.2013.00176

Strathearn, L., Li, J., Fonagy, P., & Montague, P. R. (2008). What's in a smile? Maternal brain responses to infant facial cues. *Pediatrics, 122*(1), 40–51.

Strathearn, L., Mamun, A. A., Najman, J. M., & O'Callaghan, M. J. (2009). Does breastfeeding protect against substantiated child abuse and neglect? A 15-year cohort study. *Pediatrics, 123*, 483–493.

Sturge-Apple, M. L., Davies, P. T., & Cummings, E. M. (2006). Impact of hostility and withdrawal in interparental conflict on parental emotional unavailability and children's adjustment difficulties. *Child Development, 77*(6), 1623–1641.

Swain, J. E. (2011a). Brain imaging of human parent-infant relationships. *Archives of Women's Mental Health, 14*(Suppl 2), s93–s94.

Swain, J. E. (2011b). The human parental brain: In vivo neuroimaging. *Progress in Neuro-Psychopharmacology & Biological Psychiatry, 35*(5), 1242–1254.

Swain, J. E., Dayton, C. J., Kim, P., Tolman, R. M., & Volling, B. L. (2014). Progress on the paternal brain: Theory, animal models, human brain research, and mental health implications. *Infant Mental Health Journal, 35*(5), 394–408. doi:10.1002/imhj.21471

Swain, J. E., Ho, S. S., Dayton, C. J., Rosenblum, K. L., & Muzik, M. (2014). Brain activity in empathy and approach-motivation domains for high-risk parents is increased by intervention and inversely related to parenting stress. *Neuropsychopharmacology, 39*, S523–S524.

Swain, J. E., Ho, S. S., Evans, G. W., Wang, X., Varney, R., & Liberzon, I. (2012). Parents of low socioeconomic status: Brain function and structure is affected by perceived social status and early life experience. *Neuropsychopharmacology, 37*(Suppl 1S), S365–S366.

Swain, J. E., Ho, S. S., Rosenblum, K. L., Morelen, D., Dayton, C. J., & Muzik, M. (2017). Parent-child intervention decreases stress and increases maternal brain responses and connectivity in response to own baby-cry. *Development and Psychopathology, 29*, 535–553.

Swain, J. E., Kim, P., Spicer, J., Ho, S. S., Dayton, C. J., Elmadih, A., & Abel, K. M. (2014). Approaching the biology of human parental attachment: Brain imaging, oxytocin and coordinated assessments of mothers and fathers. *Brain Research, 1580*, 78–101. doi:10.1016/j.brainres.2014.03.007

Swain, J. E., Konrath, S., Brown, S. L., Finegood, E. D., Akce, L. B., Dayton, C. J., & Ho, S. S. (2012). Parenting and beyond: Common neurocircuits underlying parental and altruistic caregiving. *Parenting, Science and Practice, 12*(2–3), 115–123. doi:10.1080/15295192.2012.680409

Swain, J. E., Leckman, J. F., Mayes, L. C., Feldman, R., Constable, R. T., & Schultz, R. T. (2008, in submission). First-time mothers and fathers show differential activation of the right orbital frontal and insular cortices in response to listening to their own infant's cries. *Biological Psychiatry*.

Swain, J. E., Lorberbaum, J. P., Kose, S., & Strathearn, L. (2007). Brain basis of early parent-infant interactions: Psychology, physiology, and in vivo functional neuroimaging studies. *Journal of Child Psychology and Psychiatry, 48*(3–4), 262–287.

Swain, J. E., Mayes, L. C., & Leckman, J. F. (2004). The development of parent-infant attachment through dynamic and interactive signaling loops of care and cry. *Behavioral and Brain Sciences, 27*(4), 472–473.

Swain, J. E., Tasgin, E., Mayes, L. C., Feldman, R., Constable, R. T., & Leckman, J. F. (2008). Maternal brain response to own baby-cry is affected by cesarean section delivery. *Journal of Child Psychology and Psychiatry, 49*(10), 1042–1052.

Tamis-LeMonda, C. S., Bornstein, M. H., & Baumwell, L. (2001). Maternal responsiveness and children's achievement of language milestones. *Child Development, 72*(3), 748–767.

Tottenham, N., & Sheridan, M. A. (2009). A review of adversity, the amygdala and the hippocampus: A consideration of developmental timing. *Frontiers in Human Neuroscience, 3*, 68. doi:10.3389/neuro.09.068.2009

van Hasselt, F. N., Cornelisse, S., Yuan Zhang, T., Meaney, M. J., Velzing, E. H., Krugers, H. J., & Joëls, M. (2012). Adult hippocampal glucocorticoid receptor expression and dentate synaptic plasticity correlate with maternal care received by individuals early in life. *Hippocampus, 22*(2), 255–266.

Van Zeijl, J., Mesman, J., Van IJzendoorn, M. H., Bakermans-Kranenburg, M. J., Juffer, F., Stolk, M. N., ... Alink, L. R. A. (2006). Attachment-based intervention for enhancing sensitive discipline in mothers of 1-to 3-year-old children at risk for externalizing behavior problems: A randomized controlled trial. *Journal of Consulting and Clinical Psychology, 74*(6), 994–1005. doi:10.1037/0022-006x.74.6.994

Wan, M. W., Downey, D., Strachan, H., Elliott, R., Williams, S. R., & Abel, K. M. (2014). The neural basis of maternal bonding. *PLoS One, 9*(3), e88436. doi:10.1371/journal.pone.0088436

Wan, M. W., Green, J., Elsabbagh, M., Johnson, M., Charman, T., Plummer, F., & Team, B. (2013). Quality of interaction between at-risk infants and caregiver at 12-15months is associated with 3-year autism outcome. *Journal of Child Psychology and Psychiatry, 54*(7), 763–771. doi:10.1111/Jcpp.12032

Wan, M. W., Warren, K., Salmon, M. P., & Abel, K. M. (2008). Patterns of maternal responding in postpartum mothers with schizophrenia. *Infant Behavior & Development, 31*(3), 532–538. doi:10.1016/j.infbeh.2008.04.003

Winnicott, D. W. (1956). Primary maternal preoccupation. In D. W. Winnicott (Ed.), *Through paediatrics to psycho-analysis.* London, England: Hogarth.

Zaki, J., & Ochsner, K. N. (2012). The neuroscience of empathy: Progress, pitfalls and promise. *Nature Neuroscience, 15*(5), 675–680.

Chapter 15
Mother/Infant Emotional Communication Through the Lens of Visceral/Autonomic Learning

Martha G. Welch and Robert J. Ludwig

Abstract *Introduction*: The benefits of early mother/infant vocal communication are widely acknowledged, but the mechanisms underlying the phenomenon remain unclear.

Aims: In this chapter, the authors aim to describe the methods, strategy, and theory behind *Family Nurture Intervention (FNI),* a nurture-based therapy that breaks from conventional brain-based strategies, methods, and theories. FNI emphasizes vocal exchange of deep emotion in order to create and maintain emotional connection. During FNI dyadic holding sessions, family members are encouraged to maintain close physical contact and persist through the full range of verbal expression of emotions until the pair achieves deep mutual physiological and psychological calm. Following a randomized controlled trial comparing Standard Care vs. Standard Care plus FNI in the NICU, FNI mothers showed better maternal care giving behavior in the hospital and significantly fewer symptoms of anxiety and depression at 4 months. FNI infants showed greatly improved brain activation at term age and neurobehavioral outcomes at 18 months, including a significant decrease in scores on a standard measure of risk for autism. In an attempt to explain the efficacy of FNI's vocal approach, the authors discuss mother/infant vocal behavior through the lens of Calming Cycle Theory. The theory posits that emotional connection between mother and infant is the key to adaptive visceral/autonomic learning via Pavlovian conditioning mechanisms. The discussion is organized around Tinbergen's four levels of analysis: causation, ontogeny, function, and evolution. Pavlovian conditioning is a highly conserved subconscious learning mechanism that lies at the root of survival, adaptation, and drive.

M.G. Welch (✉) • R.J. Ludwig
Department of Pediatrics, Columbia University Medical Center, New York, NY, USA
e-mail: mgw13@columbia.edu; robertjludwig@gmail.com

© Springer International Publishing AG 2017   271
M. Filippa et al. (eds.), *Early Vocal Contact and Preterm Infant Brain Development*, DOI 10.1007/978-3-319-65077-7_15

Conclusion: The authors propose that the emotional relationship between mother and infant is shaped by visceral/autonomic state, which determines the effect each one has on the physiology and behavior of the other, including their vocal communication. When negative vocal communication between mother and infant occurs, a counterconditioning intervention such as FNI can be exploited to change negative vocal communication to positive when it occurs.

Introduction

Ethologists have shown that mother/infant communication, especially immediately after birth, is the key to survival in many species (Tinbergen, 1951). Although there is an extremely wide range of successful parenting communication behaviors and strategies that have evolved in many species, including humans (i.e., bi-parenting, same-sex parenting, and alloparenting), for purposes of this book, we will focus our discussion on the vocal communication between mother and infant.

Other chapters in this book review what is currently known about mother/infant speech in the perinatal period. Taken together, research indicates that language development begins before birth, involves learning, and is closely tied to mother/infant communication during gestation and after birth. Indeed, mother/infant vocal interactions have been studied by physiologists, psychologists, and ethologists for the past 6 or 7 decades (Numan, Fleming, & Levy, 2006). It is clear that such vocal interactions in the perinatal period can have profound influence on the development of the infant and on the behavior of both the infant and mother. When reciprocal communication between mother and infant is robust and positive, normal development and adaptive behavior follows. When communication between mother and infant is absent or negative, the adverse effects on development and behavior can be profound and long-lasting (Arpi & Ferrari, 2013).

Nowhere has this fact become more evident than with prematurely born infants and their mothers (Vohr, 2014), a population that has been on the rise since the 1950s. Approximately one in ten infants in the USA are less than 37 weeks gestation at the time of delivery (Hamilton, Hoyert, Martin, Strobino, & Guyer, 2013). Despite continued success in overcoming the medical challenges of keeping ever younger preterm infants alive, the long-term negative neurodevelopmental and socio-emotional outcomes for infant, mother, and family remain stubbornly high and resistant to intervention.

As reported elsewhere in this book, interventions within the neonatal intensive care unit (NICU), such as skin-to-skin contact, live and recorded mother reading programs, and others have been designed to increase maternal vocal exposure to the infant. However, despite evidence showing that such interventions promote "bonding and attachment" and benefit both infant and mother, there remains much confusion about the actual mechanisms involved. Consequently, many questions remain unanswered about the origins and nature of mother/infant communication. Arguably, the field of infant development is no closer to understanding the underlying biological mechanisms of mother/infant communication than it was in the 1950s.

In this chapter, we will describe a new intervention, *Family Nurture Intervention* that targets emotional communication between mother and infant in the NICU (FNI-NICU), and summarize published results thus far from a randomized controlled trial of the intervention. We will then discuss the intervention's theoretical basis, *Calming Cycle Theory*, including the Pavlovian conditioning mechanism hypothesized to underlie autonomic co-conditioning of mother and infant through FNI. Finally, in an attempt to arrive at an integrated understanding of mother/infant speech, we will discuss visceral/autonomic learning and Calming Cycle Theory within the context of Tinbergen's four questions (causation, ontogeny, function, and phylogeny).

Family Nurture Intervention

Family Nurture Intervention in the NICU (FNI-NICU) is aimed at reestablishing emotional connection and co-regulation between the mother and infant while the infant is still in the hospital, following traumatic separation from the mother caused by premature birth (Welch et al., 2012). The intervention is facilitated by trained nurture specialists and the central activity of FNI is the "calming session." Within the calming session, FNI employs mutual scent cloth exchange, skin-to-skin contact and holding, comfort touch, eye contact, vocal soothing, listening, and deep emotional expression on the part of the mother. The main goal of the intervention is to facilitate emotional connection between mother and infant and a mutual physiological state of appropriately varied levels of arousal including calm arousal. Mothers are helped to express their deepest emotions to the infant, including sense of loss, dashed hopes, fears, future hopes, and dreams. Mothers can be reluctant to openly express their emotions, fearing strong emotional affect might have a negative impact on the infant. However, a positive response is typically observed when the prosody of strong emotion is conveyed by the mother in her primary language (i.e., the language spoken to her by her mother as a baby). Families have been very moved to observe this responsivity, and many mothers describe their very first feelings of deep connection with her infant when the infant responds to her emotions.

Accurate facial emotion recognition in children has been shown to be associated with positive autonomic state (i.e., higher vagal tone and lower heart rate) (Bal et al., 2010). Additionally, the amount of affectionate "motherese" vocalizations and the expression of positive affect between mother and infant during the first 6 months can impact hormonal changes (i.e., higher oxytocin levels in the mother) (Gordon, Zagoory-Sharon, Leckman, & Feldman, 2010). Intonation is a critical aspect of affectionate maternal vocalizations, and studies have shown that intonation is negatively impacted by maternal depression (Bettes, 1988). The importance of intonation in vocalizations is demonstrated in some languages, such as Chinese, where single words can express very different meaning depending on tone. A recent study found that musical expertise leads to facilitated recognition of angry prosody in sentences carrying no intelligible semantic information, providing support for the hypothesis that music and language share neural resources (Strait, Kraus, Skoe, & Ashley, 2009).

Interestingly, if the mother expresses feelings in her second or third language, there is little observed infant behavioral response. It is not surprising to us, then, that cross-cultural and intra-cultural research reports a positive relationship between the use of infant-directed native speech and rates of language development (Farran, Lee, Yoo, & Oller, 2016). When mothers are not certain of their primary language, we ask them to identify the language their mothers and grandmothers used when they were infants.

Case Vignette

One of our NICU study mothers was able to increase her baby's oxygen saturation by singing during skin-to-skin holding. Another fascinating case in point was a preterm infant whose mother, father, and grandmother reported having three different primary languages. One day the Italian-speaking grandmother, accompanied by her English-speaking daughter and Polish speaking son-in-law, was holding their infant while expressing severe anxiety about the infant's upcoming surgery. The infant was unresponsive to the grandmother's speech until upon prompting she began speaking Italian. I asked her to express her upset about the surgery. Nothing. Then she began speaking her native regional Sicilian dialect and immediately the baby opened her eyes and gazed directly at the grandmother. They tried this three times and each time the infant became alert to the emotional speech. Then the mother and father each spoke in respective native languages. The three were amazed by the new feeling of connection they experienced with their baby. The father was most surprised that the baby responded to his Polish that he assumed the baby had never heard. The baby is now a well-developed 5-year-old.

FNI employs some mother/infant activities that are the same as or similar to those employed by other NICU interventions. However, FNI differs substantially in its goal, strategy, and theoretical basis (Welch, 2016). Skin-to-skin contact and clothed holding, for instance, are component activities of FNI, but they are not the end goal. Rather, they are a means to establishing *emotional connection* and *visceral/autonomic co-regulation* between mother and infant. For instance, analyses controlling for the amount of skin-to-skin contact show that the positive effects of FNI are independent of the amount of skin-to-skin care and clothed holding (Welch et al., 2013).

The strategy of focusing on mother/infant emotional connection in the NICU was seen to have many benefits for both mother and infant. Results from a randomized controlled trial comparing FNI with Standard Care showed that FNI mothers had significantly improved caregiving behaviors at 36 weeks (Hane et al., 2015) and fewer depressive symptoms and less anxiety at 4 months (Welch et al., 2016).

FNI infants had greatly increased brain activation as measured by increases in power (Welch et al., 2014) and decrease in coherence at term age (Myers et al., 2015), the former indicative of increased brain activity and the latter of greater independence of activity in different areas of the brain. Together, increased EEG power and reduced EEG coherence are consistent with more advanced brain development with FNI. FNI infants also showed lower heart rate before, during, and after stress at 4 months (in prep). At 18-month follow-up, FNI infants had better language and cognition scores, fewer attention problems, as well as a significant decrease in scores on a standard measure of risk for autism (Welch et al., 2015).

An additional benefit of FNI strategy is that it provides the family with a parenting tool that can be continued when they return home with their baby. Families can learn to use the "calming cycle" routine to keep the family emotionally connected and physiologically co-regulated throughout development.

Summary
1. Family Nurture Intervention (FNI) aims at facilitating emotional connection and physiological co-regulation between mother and infant/child.
2. During FNI, family members are encouraged to express and tolerate the full range of emotions in their native language and to persist through the upset until each achieves deep calm.
3. A randomized controlled trial comparing Standard Care vs. Standard Care plus FNI in the NICU showed that FNI infants had significantly greater brain activation at term age and significantly improved behavior and neurodevelopment, including a significant decrease in scores on a standard measure of risk for autism at 18 months. FNI mothers showed better maternal caregiving behaviors in the NICU and less anxiety and depression at 4 months when the baby was safely home.

Calming Cycle Theory

Family Nurture Intervention is based on Calming Cycle Theory (Welch, 2016). The theory evolved from clinical observations treating families with children suffering from emotional, behavioral, and developmental disorders (Welch, 1988) and from findings in ethology (Tinbergen, 1951), physiology (Gantt, Newton, Royer, & Stephens, 1991), and psychology (James, 1884; Lang, 1994). The theory describes two new constructs as the basis for optimal development: *emotional connection* and *visceral/autonomic co-regulation*.

Calming Cycle Theory proposes that the quality and nature of the mother and infant/child emotional relationship is shaped by subconscious autonomic co-conditioning mechanisms. The theory parts with theories about mother/infant emotions that have dominated psychiatry and psychology for nearly a century (Wolff & Ferber, 1979). Specifically, it parts with the belief that control of emotional behavior resides within the cortex of the individual (Atzil, Hendler, & Feldman, 2011;

Hofer, 2016; Schore, 2005). The theory builds upon a phenomenon observed in dogs called *effect of person* (i.e., that autonomic physiological reflex that is triggered by physical contact with another animal) (Gantt et al., 1991). The effect was first reported by Pavlov in 1928 (Pavlov, 1928) and later studied extensively by one of his students, W. Horsley Gantt (Gantt, 1964). Gantt came to believe that the effect of person is a universal phenomenon and the basis for all emotional relationships. Calming Cycle Theory extends Gantt's ideas about autonomic conditioning and describes the mother and infant/child relationship in terms of autonomic co-conditioning. The theory provides the foundation for intervening in the emotional relationship between family members (viz., Family Nurture Intervention). In humans, specifically within the Calming Cycle construct of early development, we refer to the effect of person as the *co-effect of mother and infant* (e.g., the visceral/autonomic effect that each has on the other). The central hypothesis of the theory is that over time a disrupted mother and infant/child relationship can be changed from aversion and avoidance to one of approach and attraction by way of facilitated repeated calming sessions.

In order to understand co-conditioning as it is used in Calming Cycle Theory, one must rethink various terms that are used in much of conventional conditioning research. Calming Cycle Theory uses Pavlov's original terms "unconditional" and "conditional," as opposed to the current conventional terms "unconditioned" and "conditioned," which have come to be used in the conditioning literature since the 1970s. Gantt points out that the use of the past participle *conditioned* has led to a fundamental misunderstanding of Pavlovian conditioning (Gantt, 1968). Pavlov never considered the behavior fixed. The distinction is critical to a proper understanding of Pavlovian conditioning, since the point is that the stimulus and reflex are not fixed but always subject to conditions. This is a very important point, as it predicts the possibility of positive change through establishing emotional connection and co-regulation in a system that is not fixed or predetermined.

We have applied the principles of functional Pavlovian conditioning (Domjan, 2005) to the mother/infant perinatal experience. In our theoretical framework, the pairing of sensory and emotional experience with autonomic state during gestation produces an unconditional stimulus between mother and infant upon physical contact. This is often referred to as instinctive or innate behavior (Blumberg, 2017). Within our framework, however, the mother and infant behaviors, including speech, are seen as unconditional, and the behaviors are seen as unconscious conditional autonomic reflexes, with two biphasic conditions determining the type of behavior: emotional connection and emotional disconnection. Calming Cycle Theory predicts that upon sensory contact between mother and infant, there will occur one or more unconscious behavioral reflexes. In normal healthy birth, when the mother and infant are emotionally connected, the autonomic behavioral reflex is one of approach behaviors (i.e., motherese, infant sounds, smiling, eye contact, cuddling into each other, etc.). This behavioral reflex is not "fixed." The reflex can be changed. The behavioral reflex, which Pavlov called the social reflex, can be changed from avoidance to approach or approach to avoidance. As stated above, whether the behavioral reflex is one of avoidance or approach at any given point in time is determined by whether the two are emotionally connected or disconnected and physiologically co-regulated or dysregulated.

The pairing of the shared sensory stimuli and autonomic states of the growing fetus and the mother produces a preexisting "unconditional stimulus." The mother's voice becomes such an unconditional stimulus (i.e., the mother's voice produces a reflexive physiological and behavioral unconditional response in the infant). We term this reciprocal conditional physiological effect *visceral/autonomic co-regulation*. The mother/infant communication begins in utero and impacts the dyad via Pavlovian conditioning. The pairing of the sound and emotional content of the mother's voice with the infant's autonomic state during gestation produces the preexisting "unconditional stimulus." Following birth, the sound of the mother's voice produces a "conditional" autonomic reflex (i.e., the nature of the reflex is subject to the condition of the mother's voice) and the autonomic states (i.e., co-regulated or dysregulated) of the dyad (see Fig. 15.1).

The clinical relevance of Calming Cycle Theory is twofold. First, it provides the foundation for a straightforward physiological and behavioral measure of the mother/infant relationship that can be used to determine whether the relationship is adaptive or maladaptive. Second, it identifies a heretofore overlooked learning mechanism that can be utilized in therapies to prevent and overcome emotional, behavioral, and developmental disorders.

Summary

1. Calming Cycle Theory proposes that the primary mother and infant emotional relationship is shaped by subconscious co-conditioning mechanisms during gestation.

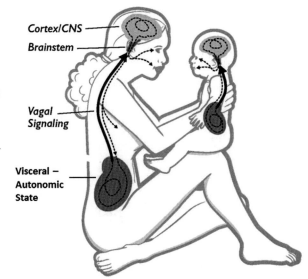

During normal gestation, the rhythmic and cyclical hormonal and sensory stimuli of mother and fetus result in Pavlovian co-conditioned physiology and behavior at the visceral-autonomic level.

Following normal birth, the autonomic states of mother and infant are reflexively (unconsciously) calmed upon sensory contact.

Vagal signaling of autonomic state produces attraction behavior, including positive vocal affect.

Cortex/CNS

Brainstem

Vagal Signaling

Visceral – Autonomic State

Fig. 15.1 Autonomic co-conditioning

2. A positive mother/infant emotional relationship is the foundation upon which are built all other emotional connections, one that leads to a "social reflex" that extends to others.
3. Breaks in emotional connection between mother and infant can be repaired, and behaviors can be changed from avoidance to attraction by employing interventions that take advantage of the autonomic co-conditioning learning mechanism (i.e., FNI).

Tinbergen's Four Questions

In his 1963 seminal paper on the study of animal behavior, "On aims and methods of ethology," Niko Tinbergen insisted that more attention be paid to studies of behaviors having "survival value." The paper is still relevant today and continues to have a profound effect on research (Barrett, Blumstein, Clutton-Brock, & Kappeler, 2013; Bateson & Laland, 2013; Honing, ten Cate, Peretz, & Trehub, 2015; Emergent et al., 2014).

Tinbergen framed four questions that need to be answered in order to form an integrated understanding of any particular behavior (Tinbergen, 1963). *First*, what is the *causation or mechanism* of the behavior, i.e., what stimuli elicit the response, and how is it modified by learning? *Second*, what is the *development or ontogeny* of the behavior, i.e., how does it change based on genetic code and the environment? *Third*, what is the *function or adaptation* of the behavior, i.e., how does it impact the animal's chances of survival and reproduction? *Fourth*, what is the *evolution or phylogeny* of the behavior, and how might it have arisen?

We now explain mother/infant speech by considering Tinbergen's four questions through the lens of Calming Cycle Theory (Welch, 2016).

What Is the Cause or Mechanism of Mother/Infant Speech?

What are the stimuli that elicit a response, and how can they be modified by learning?

The subject of causation in behavioral sciences with respect to early mother/infant interactions is a confusing one. One general problem with many of the proposed mechanisms is that they do not always qualify as a mechanism under a strict definition of the term. What constitutes a mechanism is not always clear, and there has been considerable revision and debate about the correct definition of mechanism over the last decade (Illari & Williamson, 2012). A mechanism, as it is used in biology, is a system of causally interacting processes that produce one or more predictable effects.

There have been numerous attempts to describe the mechanisms of nurture-based interventions (Atzil et al., 2011; Hofer, 2016; Mercer, 2011; Schore, 2000).

Many authors cite neuroscience findings when discussing mechanisms (Atzil, Hendler, & Feldman, 2014; Feldman, Weller, Sirota, & Eidelman, 2003). A review of Touch Therapy cites electrical, biochemical, and neurohormonal mechanisms, especially oxytocin (Field, 2014). A reductionist approach to mechanism has become common, as analyses of biological systems at the molecular and cellular level have become more feasible. While important, these approaches often fail to explain the multitude of antecedent influences and interacting consequences of human behavior.

It seems clear from recent research that "nurture" as a construct has moved well beyond the early criticisms of "idealism" that were leveled in the 1980s and 1990s (Lamb, 1982). Still, it is also clear that no consensus has emerged on a scientific causation for the powerful effects of nurture. Recognizing that nurture seems to involve many systems, some have taken a macro approach, proposing brain-mediated constructs such as "regulation" (Hofer, 1996) and "synchrony" (Feldman et al., 2003) between mother and infant. More recently, there has been growing interest in elucidating epigenetic mechanisms of infant development (Montirosso & Provenzi, 2015).

For the past 7 or 8 decades, with rare exception, it has been a scientific assumption that emotional behaviors, encompassing mother/infant behaviors (including speech), are controlled via operant conditioning mechanisms in the brain (Lang, 1994). This tendency to look only in the brain for biological mechanisms has seriously limited the scientific investigation of emotional behavior. Tinbergen wrote, "Because we human beings like to believe that our own behavior is entirely guided by in-sight or knowledge - a widespread fallacy due to overestimation of reason - the spectacle of behavior going wrong impresses and puzzles us" (Tinbergen, 1952). This has been especially true in the case of mother and infant behaviors stemming from premature birth. The answers to how and why early mother/infant behavior "goes wrong" – and when it does, why it leads to maladaptive behaviors in both the mother and infant – remain unresolved.

Clearly, there is some form of learning involved with mother/infant vocal communication during gestation: But what kind of learning? The fields of physiology and psychology have identified two distinct ways an organism learns from experience. Both involve the concept of conditioning, namely, learning to associate outcome with action through repetition.

On the one hand, since the 1920s, psychologists have explored how organisms learn cognitively through repeated experience with reinforcement and punishment, referred to as operant or instrumental conditioning (Skinner, 1988). This type of learning has come to dominate theories about behavior, behavioral interventions, and behavioral assessment. Current examples include revised attachment theory (Schore, 2005), cognitive behavioral therapy (Benjamin et al., 2011), and emotional availability theory (Saunders, Kraus, Barone, & Biringen, 2015).

On the other hand, physiologists, particularly from the Russian school, have revealed the way organisms learn subconsciously. Pavlov discovered a fundamental mechanism by which organisms learn behaviorally through repeated experience, without the need for higher cognitive function (Rescorla, 1988). Through this process, known as Pavlovian or classical conditioning, these behavioral responses are encoded as reflexes in the body. That is, the body reacts without input from the cortex. Just how the subconscious Pavlovian conditioning mechanism relates to the conscious operant conditioning mechanisms in the brain, especially with respect to emotional behavior, has been one of the most hotly contested topics in science since Pavlov's day (Gantt, 1953; Lang, 1994; Pavlov, 1941; Rescorla, 1988).

Pavlovian conditioning is often illustrated by Pavlov's famous experiment that elicits reflexive salivation in response to a bell tone after conditioning. This example illustrates how various conditions determine how the autonomic nervous system responds to paired stimuli, but it has led to a very limited view of such learning, especially the important and complicated ways that the visceral and enteric nervous system can learn via Pavlovian conditioning (Gantt, 1964). Within the autonomic nervous system, the enteric nervous system is quite independent, since it has its own reflexive activity. It learns and encodes memory on its own. This was first described in 1907 by a physician, Byron Robinson, in his book *The Abdominal and Pelvic Brain (Robinson, 1907)*, and more recently updated and expounded by Michael D. Gershon, M.D., in his book, *The Second Brain: The Gut Has a Mind of Its Own (Gershon, 1998)*. The reflexive activity of the ENS and its potential uses in medicine were extensively studied by the Russian schools of psychology and physiology (Gantt, 1960), though much of that literature is yet to be translated from Russian into other languages.

It is our position that *the cause* of early mother/infant speech behavior can be found by examining Pavlovian conditioning of the visceral/autonomic nervous system. It is well established that the fetus and newborn have a conditioned autonomic response (viz., decelerated heart rate) to the mother vocal communication (Fifer & Moon, 1994). What has not been studied is how autonomic conditioning affects the emotional relationship. By Pavlovian conditioning, we refer to what Pavlov termed a "social reflex," as opposed to the common definition of Pavlovian conditioning that is restricted to the release of saliva upon presentation of food. While Pavlovian conditioning has been demonstrated to produce numerous physiological effects in the individual, it is our position that the more important aspect of Pavlovian conditioning has to do with the interpersonal effects on behavior.

We contend that Pavlovian conditioning of the autonomic nervous system (learning, if you will) continues throughout life. Like all conditioning, either Pavlovian or operant, learning can be positive or negative and adaptive or maladaptive. A healthy mother and a healthy baby following full-term birth will experience the full range of hormonal and sensory stimuli that result in positive motherese-type vocalizations, emotional connection, and physical attraction to one another. If not interrupted, the emotional connection will likely lead to adaptive behaviors and adaptive socialization. On the other hand, if a mother and infant experience a break in their emotional connection, as can happen with premature birth, maladaptive behaviors, including negative or a paucity of vocal communications and poor socialization, can follow. In this case, negative emotional vocalizations can lead to emotional avoidance and maladaptive behavior in both the mother and infant. Premature birth can break or interrupt both emotional connection and visceral/autonomic co-regulation between the mother and infant, which results in maladaptive Pavlovian conditioning. In turn, this can lead to a cascade of adverse developmental and behavioral sequelae. This occurs if the normal types of sensory communication between infant and mother following birth are interrupted, delayed, or absent.

One expects the infant and mother to be attracted to one another following birth, but when attraction does not occur, as it sometimes does not following preterm birth, this can be "puzzling," as Tinbergen says. It is not puzzling, however, if one views symptomatic behavior as the result of breaks in emotional connection and visceral/autonomic co-regulation that normally results from negative autonomic co-conditioning mechanisms. More importantly, one can begin to design interventions that might be effective in helping the mother and infant overcome their traumatic separation.

Summary
1. Physiological and behavioral co-regulation at the visceral/autonomic level develops between mother and fetus/infant during the perinatal period via *co-conditioning* mechanisms.
2. Together, this autonomic "learning" forms the basis of the positive or negative nature of the *social reflex* (i.e., the physiological and behavioral response by mother and infant upon close physical contact).
3. Perinatal mother/infant speech is shaped by co-conditioning of the autonomic nervous systems of mother and infant(s).
4. The pairing of the shared sensory stimuli and autonomic states of the infant and the mother (co-conditioning) determines the vocal reflex (attraction or avoidance) and physiological reflex (co-regulated or dysregulated).

What Is the Development or Ontogeny of Mother/Infant Speech?

(How does the behavior change with age, and what early experiences influence the behavior?)

A crucial thesis of Calming Cycle Theory is that pairing of mother/infant contact with maternal vocal expression of deep emotions about her pregnancy, the birthing process, and the subsequent history will repair the relationship and set them on a path of optimal development. The development or ontogeny of mother/infant vocal communications is embedded in the development of emotions. It is through our emotions, positive and negative, that we convey the central aspects of our being, our sense of safety or threat and our joy at connection or fear of loss. These emotions are expressed in relation to other beings. And we contend, since all of us begin life inside the womb, that the first emotional learning experience for all humans, positive or negative, is with the mother during gestation.

The idea that the mother and fetus learn from one another and share an emotional relationship has until recently been largely conjecture, because relatively few experiments have directly tested the hypothesis. William James claimed that emotional feelings were the effects of physiological interoception but admitted that at the time he wrote his claim could not be subjected to direct test. Even now, emotions and feeling states are thought of as something that cannot be measured and therefore lie outside the realm of serious scientific study. Lang claims that whereas physiological events can be measured with objective precision, the target of those events – in this case the subjective feeling state – "does not yield to the scientist's clock, scale, or ruler" (Lang, 1994). We disagree with this statement. The fact that feeling states are imprecise and rough by nature does not preclude their measurement per se. We argue that, in fact, it is relatively easy to measure the subjective feeling state, if one equates feeling state to autonomic state and if one looks at the behavior associated with autonomic state. Such signs can be readily found in mother/infant affective speech, gaze, touch, and approach vs. avoidance behaviors.

The measurement of emotions actually has a long tradition. Observations starting with Darwin led to the idea within psychology (Craig, 1917; Lang, 1994) and ethology (Tinbergen, 1951) that emotional behavior is biphasic in nature, that is, it falls into two broad categories of "approach and avoidance" (Schur & Ritvo, 1970). Used in the perinatal context, we argue that the behaviors of the mother and infant fall between these two extremes. Avoidance behaviors for the infant might include arching the back, avoiding eye contact, closing the eyes, fussing, or crying. For the mother, avoidant vocal behavior ranges from vociferous anger to silence. Infant approach behaviors include nestling into the mother's body, looking into her eyes, cooing, making engaging facial expressions, or imitating mother's expressions, and for the mother, nestling into the infant's body, looking into the infant's eyes, cooing or engaging in motherese, making engaging facial expressions, or imitating her infant's vocal and facial expressions.

In the course of normal mother/infant interaction, vocalization is of paramount importance, often accompanying or even substituting for the other modes of contact. For example, a well-regulated hungry infant can be soothed vocally while mother prepares to feed the baby.

Case Vignette
One of our subject families in the NICU reacted with amusement and joy upon discovering how they sounded to one another when they spoke to the baby in Spanish. We began with the 7-year-old brother who was, we were told, being raised in an "English-only" home. However, the grandma living in the home did not speak English. The boy was asked to tell his baby sister how much he loved her, first in English and then in Spanish. The difference in affect was so pronounced that everyone broke out in laughter. Then the boy asked each parent to do the same exercise and with the same result. We all found it to be hilarious, because the difference was so obvious. Even staff who did not speak or understand Spanish could hear the difference in feeling.

Recent findings have begun to connect what we have long known about the mechanism controlling reflex-type reactions and the early emotional behavior of the infant. For instance, it is now proposed that the fetus encodes memory via subcortical networks (Dirix, Nijhuis, Jongsma, & Hornstra, 2009) and that such memory may have adaptive value (Hepper, 1996). Data suggest that fetal learning does not necessitate adult-like brain organization or even cortex (Robinson, 2015). Chemosensory stimuli occurring during gestation can promote the acquisition of long-term memories, which can affect behavior in the adult animal. These findings suggest that some likes and dislikes (e.g., a preference for licorice) expressed in adulthood can result from exposure (conditioning) in utero *(Gruest, Richer, & Hars, 2004)*. Finally, recent evidence suggests that innate anxiety and learned fear are both subject to modulation through abdominal vagal afferents (Klarer et al., 2014), adding further weight to theories emphasizing an important role of afferent visceral signals in the regulation of emotional behavior.

Collectively, this new research supports the idea that so-called instinctive or innate behavior between newborn infant and mother may be explained by Pavlovian conditioning that occurs during gestation. We theorize that many so-called instinctive behaviors of the infant after birth can be explained as conditional reflex behaviors and responses to preexisting associations formed in utero. For example, we hypothesize that the "breast crawl" phenomenon, first brought to the public's attention by Klaus and Kennell (Klaus, 1998), is an example of a conditional reflexive action by the baby. The breast crawl occurs when a healthy baby who is left quietly on the mother's abdomen in the first hours after birth will crawl to her breast, find the nipple, and begin to suckle. Notably, the baby will not crawl to the breasts if both breasts are washed. However, if only one breast is washed, the baby will crawl to the one that is not washed. If amniotic fluid is placed on a washed breast, the baby will crawl to it (Zanardo & Straface, 2015). We theorize that the breast crawl is a reflex behavior that is the result of Pavlovian conditioning to taste/scent molecules in the amniotic fluid during gestation.

The most important question is what environmental changes will change mother/infant communication when it is negative? Can avoidant negative behaviors, including speech, between mother and infant, be changed, and if so, how? Many attempts have been made to identify or isolate causal mechanisms that account for the effects of behaviors involved with mother/infant nurturing behaviors. Research in this area has been largely focused on demonstrating the beneficial effects of "nurture-related" interventions, such as skin-to-skin contact between parent and infant.

Recent studies have used cortisol levels of parent and infant as a way to determine "co-regulation." A randomized controlled trial was conducted to determine whether absolute cortisol levels of mother and prematurely born infant would decrease during three holding conditions in the NICU: facilitated skin-to-skin contact, facilitated clothed holding, or non-facilitated holding (Neu, Hazel, Robinson, Schmiege, & Laudenslager, 2014). Results supported the primary hypothesis. Interestingly, the author's second hypothesis, that over time the intervention would lead to improved "co-regulation" of cortisol levels, was not supported by the results. Co-regulation in this study was defined as progressive reduction in the absolute difference between mother and infant cortisol levels across holding sessions. The definition of co-regulation was based on a theory that each member of a dyad learns (presumably through operant conditioning) to expect behaviors of the other member through repeated reciprocal interactions (Fogel & Garvey, 2007).

In another study of cortisol in preterm infants, Morelius et al. demonstrated significant positive effects following near continuous skin-to-skin contact between mother and infant following birth (Morelius, Ortenstrand, Theodorsson, & Frostell, 2015). However, an integrative review of salivary cortisol reactivity studies of preterm infants in the NICU showed wide-ranging disparities in study design and methods (Morelius, He, & Shorey, 2016).

We see two problems with study design of current NICU interventions in general. The first is that current NICU interventions often do not clearly identify a learning mechanism. Therefore, hypotheses tend to be generated based on the unstated assumptions. For example, studies have for decades catalogued the negative outcomes associated with preterm birth and maternal separation. At the same time, studies of skin-to-skin contact have consistently catalogued the benefits to parent and preterm infant, especially if it is maintained continuously following birth. On the face of it, the answer to better outcomes is continuous skin-to-skin contact between parent and infant. In most cases it is true that continuous skin-to-skin contact will help facilitate emotional connection. However, without a clear underlying skin-to-skin contact mechanism, it is not clear what can be done when emotional connection does not occur following prolonged or continuous skin-to-skin contact. From our experience, which is limited so far to an urban American population, mothers or fathers often can't or won't maintain continuous skin-to-skin contact. In our study of FNI reported above, where control mothers engaged regularly in skin-to-skin contact, we did not see improved infant outcomes relative to outcomes of FNI infants.

The second problem has to do with outcome measures. Again, without a clear understanding of the biological processes underlying the prescribed intervention, it is difficult to be clear about what the outcome measure should be. The cortisol results reported in the first study above do not surprise us, because the assumption in this theory is that the act of placing the mother and infant together skin-to-skin will be sufficient to have a physiological effect over time. This is a common misunderstanding of both the learning mechanism involved and the factor mediating co-regulation.

We have proposed that Pavlovian, or in the case of FNI, co-conditioning determines the autonomic states of mother and infant (i.e., co-regulation or dysregulation). We have also proposed that *emotional connection* is the condition that will lead to co-regulated autonomic states and that *emotional disconnection* is the condition that will lead to dysregulated autonomic states. From our theoretical point of view, the autonomic co-conditioning mechanism is at work during skin-to-skin contact. The emotional relationship is being shaped, but that relationship could be positive or negative. The mechanism is agnostic. Our position is that skin-to-skin contact is not the crucial factor. Emotional connection is the critical factor. Without emotional connection, skin-to-skin contact or any other interaction between mother and infant could actually produce adverse co-conditioning.

In the case of mother/infant speech, mother/infant speech can be modified or changed through Pavlovian counterconditioning (i.e., FNI), but only to the extent that the mother and infant are emotionally connected. Indeed, Pavlovian counterconditioning is known to be effective in overcoming emotional disturbances (Bouton, Mineka, & Barlow, 2001; Pavlov, 1941). Since it has been shown that the fetus can be conditioned by the mother's voice and that the newborn recognizes and prefers the speech that he or she was exposed to in utero (Mariette & Buchanan, 2016), it seems logical to consider the ways in which the mother and infant learn via Pavlovian conditioning and to ask whether such conditioning might influence the ways in which a mother and infant communicate emotionally with one another following birth.

Intermediate Message

- Avoidant vocal behavior and dysregulated physiology can be changed to attraction vocal behavior via counterconditioning process (FNI).

We hypothesize that the mediating factor in the mother/infant relationship that determines approach or avoidant behavior, the fulcrum if you will, is *emotional connection* (see Fig. 15.2). The above-referenced Neu et al. cortisol study did not assess

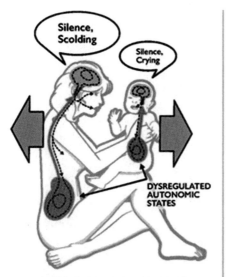
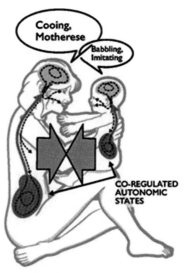

EMOTIONALLY DISCONNECTED

Dysregulated autonomic states of mother and infant are signaled to the brain via the vagus nerves, resulting in conflict behaviors, including negative vocal affect.

EMOTIONALLY CONNECTED

Co-regulated autonomic states of mother and infant are signaled to the brain via the vagus nerve, resulting in approach behaviors, including positive vocal affect.

Fig. 15.2 Emotional connection and disconnection

emotional connection. Nonetheless, the results suggest to us that the holding in that study may not have elicited an emotional connection and therefore did not produce the expected co-regulatory effect. This finding is consonant with our observation in the NICU that some mothers appeared to perform holding and skin-to-skin care without any sign of emotional connection or positive communication with their infants.

Case Vignette

Physical separation, such as occurs in preterm birth, can disrupt the emotional connection between mother and infant. Such a case occurred in our RCT when the mother's uterine rupture caused preterm birth and threatened the lives of both mother and child. The first skin-to-skin experience dramatically illustrated two points: the importance of infant-directed maternal speech for autonomic regulation of the infant and the importance of the primary language for communicating maternal emotion. When the infant was placed on the mother's chest skin to skin, the infant desaturated immediately. We asked the mother to speak in French, thinking that French was her primary language. The oxygen saturation rose from 60% to 85%. Then the mother told us that French was not her primary language and she began speaking in her true native dialect, whereupon the infant's oxygen level immediately reached 95%. Whenever the mother stopped speaking emotionally in her native tongue, the oxygen saturation dropped. When she resumed speaking emotionally in her native tongue, oxygen saturation rose again. She was able to maintain her infant's oxygen saturation at 95% for 2 h despite the infant's fragile condition.

Summary

1. Mother/preterm infant speech develops out of *Pavlovian co-conditioning* of the dyad's visceral and autonomic nervous systems during gestation.
2. The normal co-conditioning process produces *emotional connection*, *physiological co-regulation*, and attraction speech patterns between mother and infant following birth.
3. Mother/infant speech is not fixed. Breaks in emotional connection and physiological co-regulation produce avoidant or negative speech patterns and maladaptive behaviors.
4. FNI targets the Pavlovian co-conditioning mechanism to change avoidant speech to approach speech between mother and infant.

What Is the Function or Adaptation Value of Mother/Infant Speech?

(How does the mother/pre-infant speech impact chances of survival and reproduction?)

The common feature among successful mother/infant communications after birth is that it must elicit *attraction* behaviors between the two. Without attraction between mother and young, various types of avoidance, including aversive or absent affective speech, occur and can separate the pair. In the extreme, this situation can lead to maladaptive development in the young or abusiveness and neglect by the mother. If it is, as some have theorized, to promote survival and optimal development, why does it sometimes go wrong?

The functional strategy is employed in Family Nurture Intervention (Welch et al., 2013), in which the goal is to change the visceral/autonomic emotional response from avoidance to attraction using close physical contact combined with emotional vocalizations in repeated calming sessions. The idea behind this strategy is that the preexisting emotional connection that is established in utero forms the basis for reestablishing the emotional connection when it is disrupted after birth. This is true throughout life. Emotional connection is waiting to happen.

As discussed in the section on development and ontogeny above, emotional connection is the source of motivational drive that enables the infant to thrive and develop optimally. The quality of the emotional connection between the infant and mother shapes the developmental trajectory of the infant and of the mother with regard to her mothering of this child. An emotional connection can be broken and reformed between mother and infant or formed with others via visceral/autonomic conditioning. Such conditioning determines the nature of the social reflex, whether the infant is stressed or calmed by interaction with other humans.

Early vocal communication between mother and infant is ecologically critical (Mariette & Buchanan, 2016). To illustrate this point, consider the depressed mother with her infant and the nature of their emotional relationship. Depression among mothers of prematurely born infants is commonly reported as having negative effects on the relationship between the mother and infant (Tiffany Field).

Another recent study showed that infant learning was significantly related to maternal depression, even after demographic correlates of depression, antidepressant medication use, and extent of pitch modulation in maternal infant-directed speech had been taken into account (Kaplan, Danko, Cejka, & Everhart, 2015). The authors claim that the results support their hypothesis and that "associative learning-promoting effects of infant-directed speech depend on the infant's social experience." We do not agree that the results support the hypothesis as stated. We would restate the hypothesis: *The infant's social experience with the mother* (i.e., *whether there is an emotional connection*) *determines the effects of* infant-directed speech *on learning.*

Summary

1. The function of mother and infant emotional communication has evolved to ensure the survival of the infant. It provides the motivational drive to stay in physical proximity, which enables the infant not only to survive but also to thrive and develop optimally.
2. The quality of the emotional communication between mother and infant shapes the *social reflex* (viz., how the infant reacts subconsciously to physical/social interaction with others) and determines the growing child's ability to successfully socialize, mate, and parent.
3. Chronic negative emotional communication between mother and infant can lead to a maladaptive social reflex (a stress response of the visceral/autonomic nervous system upon contact with each other and with others).

4. Negative, including chronic negative emotional communication between mother and infant, can be changed to positive communication via visceral/autonomic co-conditioning (viz., FNI).

What Is the Evolution and Phylogeny of Mother/Infant Speech?

(How does the behavior compare with similar behavior in related species and how might it have arisen through the process of phylogeny?)

Human vocal expression evolved from the gill arches of fish, a fact that has been shown to be recapitulated in very early embryonic development (Gilbert, 2006) (see Fig. 15.3). Development of vocalization is closely tied to the development of the human nervous system. Humans share many primitive vocal characteristics with reptiles, especially concerning emotional response.

Porges, in his foundational book, the *Polyvagal Theory* (Porges, 2011), provides a comprehensive overview of the phylogenetic shift that occurred between reptiles and mammals in the neural regulation of the autonomic nervous system. The theory has several rules and assumptions:

1. Evolution has modified the structures of the autonomic nervous system.
2. Emotional experience and expression are functional derivatives of structural changes in the autonomic nervous system due to evolutionary processes.

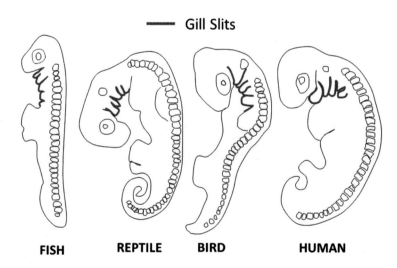

Fig. 15.3 The evolutionary origins of the larynx

3. The phylogenetic "level" of the autonomic nervous system determines affective states and range of social behavior.
4. In mammals, the autonomic nervous system response strategy to challenge follows a phylogenetic hierarch, starting with the newest structures and, when all else fails, reverting to the most primitive structural systems.

According to the theory, this evolutionary shift in neural regulation converged with greater regulation of the middle ear muscles to facilitate mammalian vocal communication, as well as the regulation of facial muscles (Porges, 67). Such vocal and facial communication, the Polyvagal theory contends, serve as the basis by which humans maintain self-control of autonomic function in response to social engagement. The theory clarifies the important distinction between two "tiers" of neural processes that function simultaneously within humans. Within Tier 1, the older unmyelinated vegetative vagal neural process gives rise to gross behaviors we would associate with reptiles (e.g., aggression and shutdown). The newer "smart" or "mammalian" myelinated vagal neural mechanisms control emotional behavior and give rise to socially adaptive behaviors (e.g., nurturance, empathy, etc.).

The Polyvagal theory builds upon Norbert Weiner's concept of a "closed system of feedback loops" (Wiener, 1961). This model provides a helpful explanation of how physiological homeostasis is maintained within the body's closed system. According to the theory, the newer Tier 1 "central regulators" serve to control Tier 1 emotional impulses (see Fig. 15.4, from Porges, ref. 67, figure 7.4).

There are several limitations to Weiner's and Porges' theories, in our opinion, which we address. We contend that mammalian emotional behavior is not controlled within an individual's closed physiological system, as the Weiner model contends. Calming Cycle Theory provides an alternative explanation for the control of human emotional behavior. Polyvagal theory does not account for the powerful and sometimes overriding effect that one being can have upon the physiology of another (i.e., Pavlov's effect of person), or the subcortical autonomic reflex that occurs upon

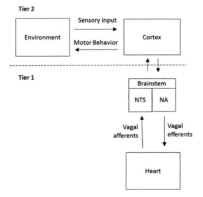

Fig. 15.4 Diagram of the Polyvagal Theory proposed closed homeostatic feedback loop

physical contact with a trusted other. Arguably, it is visceral/autonomic *co-regulation* that has allowed the human species to succeed: the ability to get along with one another, to mate, to care for, and to cooperate with one another. Such behavior is tied closely to survival, and while it may to some extent be subject to cortical inhibition, we argue that adaptively it is driven by visceral/autonomic conditional reflexes, such as "gut feelings."

This ability to have an effect on one another is the basis of mammalian sociality. It derives, we propose, from the highly conserved Pavlovian conditioning learning mechanism, which lies at the very root of survival, adaptation, and drive.

All animals are highly adaptable and rely on the modulation of gene expression, physiology, and behavior to continuously modify their phenotypes in response to environmental changes (Dukas, 2013). In many vertebrates, the young learn parental characteristics during gestation and later prefer or seek such features, a process termed imprinting (Lorenz, 1937). Polyvagal theory proposes a two-tiered closed neural system, where central regulators control emotional behavior via a vagal feedback loop. Calming Cycle Theory instead proposes that emotional behaviors of mother and infant are co-regulated at the visceral/autonomic level via the Pavlovian conditioning mechanism within an *open system of feedback loops*. Within this model, emotional behavior is determined by the conditional co-regulatory effect of mother-infant/child (see Fig. 15.5).

The evolution of mother/infant vocal communication from reptiles to mammals gave humans an ecological advantage. The development of the myelinated vagus nerve provided a mechanism by which visceral/autonomic states of two individuals could be co-regulated. This allowed cooperation, reciprocity, empathy, and reliance on one another to increase survivability. Co-regulation governs social interactions, including vocal communication. In this sense, we might say that the vocal communication, as well as touch and play, is the "gift" of the myelinated vagus. All are "governed" by autonomic state and "shaped" by emotional connection. Together, these highly conserved ecological mechanisms enable humans to get along with one another socially.

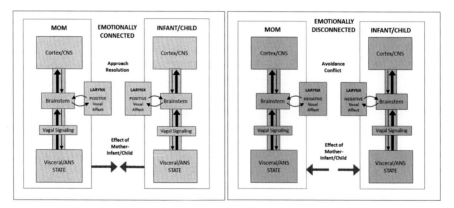

Fig. 15.5 Diagram of the Calming Cycle Theory open system of feedback loops

Summary
1. Mammalian socio-emotional behavior is the result of highly conserved co-conditioning mechanisms at work on the visceral/autonomic nervous systems within social groups.
2. The human species owes its survival and success to the *social reflex*, the ability to emotionally connect and physiologically co-regulate one another (viz., to modulate each other's state of arousal upon contact through physical and verbal communication and ensuing physiological response).
3. The visceral/autonomic co-conditioning that occurs between infant, mother, and other family members during the perinatal period can profoundly influence the social reflex throughout life.

References

Arpi, E., & Ferrari, F. (2013). Preterm birth and behaviour problems in infants and preschool-age children: A review of the recent literature. *Developmental Medicine and Child Neurology, 55*(9), 788–796. doi:10.1111/dmcn.12142

Atzil, S., Hendler, T., & Feldman, R. (2011). Specifying the neurobiological basis of human attachment: Brain, hormones, and behavior in synchronous and intrusive mothers. *Neuropsychopharmacology, 36*(13), 2603–2615. doi:10.1038/npp.2011.172

Atzil, S., Hendler, T., & Feldman, R. (2014). The brain basis of social synchrony. *Social Cognitive and Affective Neuroscience, 9*(8), 1193–1202. doi:10.1093/scan/nst105

Bal, E., Harden, E., Lamb, D., Van Hecke, A. V., Denver, J. W., & Porges, S. W. (2010). Emotion recognition in children with autism spectrum disorders: Relations to eye gaze and autonomic state. *Journal of Autism and Developmental Disorders, 40*(3), 358–370. doi:10.1007/s10803-009-0884-3

Barrett, L., Blumstein, D. T., Clutton-Brock, T. H., & Kappeler, P. M. (2013). Taking note of Tinbergen, or: The promise of a biology of behaviour. *Philosophical Transactions of the Royal Society of London. Series B, Biological Sciences, 368*(1618), 20120352. doi:10.1098/rstb.2012.0352

Bateson, P., & Laland, K. N. (2013). Tinbergen's four questions: An appreciation and an update. *Trends in Ecology & Evolution, 28*(12), 712–718. doi:10.1016/j.tree.2013.09.013

Benjamin, C. L., Puleo, C. M., Settipani, C. A., Brodman, D. M., Edmunds, J. M., Cummings, C. M., & Kendall, P. C. (2011). History of cognitive-behavioral therapy in youth. *Child and Adolescent Psychiatric Clinics of North America, 20*(2), 179–189. doi:10.1016/j.chc.2011.01.011

Bettes, B. A. (1988). Maternal depression and motherese: Temporal and intonational features. *Child Development, 59*(4), 1089–1096.

Blumberg, M. S. (2017). Development evolving: The origins and meanings of instinct. *Wiley Interdisciplinary Reviews: Cognitive Science, 8*(1–2), e1371.

Bouton, M. E., Mineka, S., & Barlow, D. H. (2001). A modern learning theory perspective on the etiology of panic disorder. *Psychological Review, 108*(1), 4–32.

Craig, W. (1917). Appetites and aversions as constituents of instincts. *Proceedings of the National Academy of Sciences of the United States of America, 3*(12), 685–688.

Dirix, C. E., Nijhuis, J. G., Jongsma, H. W., & Hornstra, G. (2009). Aspects of fetal learning and memory. *Child Development, 80*(4), 1251–1258. doi:10.1111/j.1467-8624.2009.01329.x

Domjan, M. (2005). Pavlovian conditioning: A functional perspective. *Annual Review of Psychology, 56*, 179–206. doi:10.1146/annurev.psych.55.090902.141409

Dukas, R. (2013). Effects of learning on evolution: Robustness, innovation and speciation. *Animal Behaviour, 85*, 1023–1030.

Emergent, P., Hofmann, H. A., Beery, A. K., Blumstein, D. T., Couzin, I. D., & Rubenstein, D. R. (2014). Nescent Working Group on Integrative Models of Vertebrate Sociality: Evolution, M. An evolutionary framework for studying mechanisms of social behavior. *Trends in Ecology & Evolution, 29*(10), 581–589. doi:10.1016/j.tree.2014.07.008

Farran, L. K., Lee, C. C., Yoo, H., & Oller, D. K. (2016). Cross-cultural register differences in infant-directed speech: An initial study. *PloS One, 11*(3), e0151518. doi:10.1371/journal.pone.0151518

Feldman, R., Weller, A., Sirota, L., & Eidelman, A. I. (2003). Testing a family intervention hypothesis: The contribution of mother-infant skin-to-skin contact (kangaroo care) to family interaction, proximity, and touch. *Journal of Family Psychology, 17*(1), 94–107.

Field, T. (2014). Massage therapy research review. *Complementary Therapies in Clinical Practice, 20*(4), 224–229. doi:10.1016/j.ctcp.2014.07.002

Fifer, W. P., & Moon, C. M. (1994). The role of mother's voice in the organization of brain function in the newborn. *Acta Paediatrica. Supplement, 397*, 86–93.

Fogel, A., & Garvey, A. (2007). Alive communication. *Infant Behavior & Development, 30*(2), 251–257. doi:10.1016/j.infbeh.2007.02.007

Gantt, W. H. (1953). Principles of nervous breakdown-schizokinesis and autokinesis. *Annals of the New York Academy of Sciences, 56*(2), 143–163.

Gantt, W. H. (1960). Pavlov and darwin, in evolution after Darwin. In S. Tax (Ed.), *The evolution of man: Mind, culture, and society* (pp. 219–238). Chicago, Il: University of Chicago press.

Gantt, W. H. (1964). Autonomic conditioning. *Annals of the New York Academy of Sciences, 117*, 132–141.

Gantt, W. H. (1968). The distinction between the conditional and the unconditional reflex. *Conditional Reflex, 3*(1), 1–3.

Gantt, W. H., Newton, J. E. O., Royer, F. L., & Stephens, J. H. (1991, Apr-Jun). Effect of person. 1966. *Integr Behav Physiol Sci, 26*, 145–160.

Gershon, M. D. (1998). *The second brain*. New York, NY: HarperCollins Publishers.

Gilbert, S. F. (2006). *Developmental Biology* (8th ed.). Sinauer associates.

Gordon, I., Zagoory-Sharon, O., Leckman, J. F., & Feldman, R. (2010). Oxytocin and the development of parenting in humans. *Biological Psychiatry, 68*(4), 377–382. doi:10.1016/j.biopsych.2010.02.005

Gruest, N., Richer, P., & Hars, B. (2004). Emergence of long-term memory for conditioned aversion in the rat fetus. *Developmental Psychobiology, 44*(3), 189–198. doi:10.1002/dev.20004

Hamilton, B. E., Hoyert, D. L., Martin, J. A., Strobino, D. M., & Guyer, B. (2013). Annual summary of vital statistics: 2010-2011. *Pediatrics, 131*(3), 548–558. doi:10.1542/peds.2012-3769

Hane, A. A., Myers, M. M., Hofer, M. A., Ludwig, R. J., Halperin, M. S., Austin, J., ... Welch, M. G. (2015). Family nurture intervention improves the quality of maternal caregiving in the neonatal intensive care. *Unit: Evidence from a Randomized Controlled Trial. J Dev Behav Pediatr*. doi:10.1097/DBP.0000000000000148

Hepper, P. G. (1996). Fetal memory: Does it exist? What does it do? *Acta Paediatrica. Supplement, 416*, 16–20.

Hofer, M. A. (1996). On the nature and consequences of early loss. *Psychosomatic Medicine, 58*(6), 570–581.

Hofer, M. A. (2016). Psychobiological roots of early attachment. *Current Directions in Psychological Science, 15*(2), 84–88.

Honing, H., ten Cate, C., Peretz, I., & Trehub, S. E. (2015). Without it no music: Cognition, biology and evolution of musicality. *Philosophical Transactions of the Royal Society of London. Series B, Biological Sciences, 370*(1664), 20140088. doi:10.1098/rstb.2014.0088

Illari, P. M., & Williamson, J. (2012). What is a mechanism? Thinking about mechanisms across the sciences. *Euro J Phil Sci, 2*, 119–135.

James, W. (1884). II. What is emotion? *Mind, os-IX*(34), 188–205.

Kaplan, P. S., Danko, C. M., Cejka, A. M., & Everhart, K. D. (2015). Maternal depression and the learning-promoting effects of infant-directed speech: Roles of maternal sensitivity, depression diagnosis, and speech acoustic cues. *Infant Behavior & Development, 41*, 52–63. doi:10.1016/j.infbeh.2015.06.011

Klarer, M., Arnold, M., Gunther, L., Winter, C., Langhans, W., & Meyer, U. (2014). Gut vagal afferents differentially modulate innate anxiety and learned fear. *The Journal of Neuroscience, 34*(21), 7067–7076. doi:10.1523/JNEUROSCI.0252-14.2014

Klaus, M. (1998). Mother and infant: Early emotional ties. *Pediatrics, 102*(5 Suppl E), 1244–1246.

Lamb, M. E. (1982). The bonding phenomenon: Misinterpretations and their implications. *The Journal of Pediatrics, 101*(4), 555–557.

Lang, P. J. (1994). The varieties of emotional experience: A meditation on James-Lange theory. *Psychological Review, 101*(2), 211–221.

Lorenz, K. Z. (1937). The companion in the bird's world. *The Auk, 3*, 245–273.

Mariette, M. M., & Buchanan, K. L. (2016). Prenatal acoustic communication programs offspring for high posthatching temperatures in a songbird. *Science, 353*(6301), 812–814. doi:10.1126/science.aaf7049

Mercer, J. (2011). Attachment theory and its vicissitudes: Toward an updated theory. *Theory Psychology, 21*, 25–45.

Montirosso, R., & Provenzi, L. (2015). Implications of epigenetics and stress regulation on research and developmental care of preterm infants. *Journal of Obstetric, Gynecologic, and Neonatal Nursing, 44*(2), 174–182. doi:10.1111/1552-6909.12559

Morelius, E., He, H. G., & Shorey, S. (2016). Salivary cortisol reactivity in preterm infants in neo-natal intensive care: An integrative review. *International Journal of Environmental Research and Public Health, 13*(3). doi:10.3390/ijerph13030337

Morelius, E., Ortenstrand, A., Theodorsson, E., & Frostell, A. (2015). A randomised trial of continuous skin-to-skin contact after preterm birth and the effects on salivary cortisol, parental stress, depression, and breastfeeding. *Early Human Development, 91*(1), 63–70. doi:10.1016/j.earlhumdev.2014.12.005

Myers, M. M., Grieve, P. G., Stark, R. I., Isler, J. R., Hofer, M. A., Yang, J., … Welch, M. G. (2015). Family nurture intervention in preterm infants alters frontal cortical functional connectivity assessed by EEG coherence. *Acta Paediatrica.* doi:10.1111/apa.13007

Neu, M., Hazel, N. A., Robinson, J., Schmiege, S. J., & Laudenslager, M. (2014). Effect of holding on co-regulation in preterm infants: A randomized controlled trial. *Early Human Development, 90*(3), 141–147. doi:10.1016/j.earlhumdev.2014.01.008

Numan, M., Fleming, A. S., & Levy, F. (2006). *Maternal behavior* (3rd ed.). New York, N.Y: Elsevier.

Pavlov, I. P. (1928). *Lectures on conditioned reflexes.* New York: International Publishers.

Pavlov, I. P. (1941). *Conditioned reflexes and psychiatry.* New York, N.Y: International.

Porges, S. W. (2011). *The polyvagal theory: Neurophysiological foundations of emotions, attachment, communication, and self-regulation.* New York, N.Y: W.W. Norton & Company.

Rescorla, R. A. (1988). Pavlovian conditioning. It's not what you think it is. *The American Psychologist, 43*(3), 151–160.

Robinson, B. (1907). The abdominal brain. In F. S. Betz (Ed.). Indiana: Hammond.

Robinson, S. R. (2015). Spinal mediation of motor learning and memory in the rat fetus. *Developmental Psychobiology, 57*(4), 421–434. doi:10.1002/dev.21277

Saunders, H., Kraus, A., Barone, L., & Biringen, Z. (2015). Emotional availability: Theory, research, and intervention. *Frontiers in Psychology, 6*, 1069. doi:10.3389/fpsyg.2015.01069

Schore, A. N. (2000). Attachment and the regulation of the right brain. *Attachment & Human Development, 2*(1), 23–47. doi:10.1080/146167300361309

Schore, A. N. (2005). Back to basics: Attachment, affect regulation, and the developing right brain: Linking developmental neuroscience to pediatrics. *Pediatrics in Review, 26*(6), 204–217.

Schur, M., & Ritvo, L. B. (1970). A principle of evolutionary biology for psychoanalysis. Schneirla's evolutionary and developmental theory of biphasic processes underlying approach and withdrawal and Freud's unpleasure and pleasure principles. *Journal of the American Psychoanalytic Association, 18*(2), 422–439.

Skinner, B. F. (1988). The operant side of behavior therapy. *Journal of Behavior Therapy and Experimental Psychiatry, 19*(3), 171–179.

Strait, D. L., Kraus, N., Skoe, E., & Ashley, R. (2009). Musical experience promotes subcortical efficiency in processing emotional vocal sounds. *Annals of the New York Academy of Sciences, 1169*, 209–213. doi:10.1111/j.1749-6632.2009.04864.x

Tinbergen, N. (1951). *The study on instincts*. New York, NY: Oxford Press.

Tinbergen, N. (1952). Derived activities; their causation, biological significance, origin, and emancipation during evolution. *The Quarterly Review of Biology, 27*(1), 1–32.

Tinbergen, N. (1963). On aims and methods of ethology. *Zeitshrift fur Tierpsychologie, 20*, 410–433.

Vohr, B. (2014). Speech and language outcomes of very preterm infants. *Seminars in Fetal & Neonatal Medicine, 19*(2), 78–83. doi:10.1016/j.siny.2013.10.007

Welch, M. G. (1988). *Holding time: How to eliminate conflict, temper tantrums, and sibling rivalry and raise happy, loving, successful children*. New York, NY: Simon and Schuster.

Welch, M. G. (2016). Calming cycle Theory: The Role of Visceral/Autonomic Learning in Early Mother and Infant/Child Behavior and Development. *Acta Paediatr*. doi:10.1111/apa.13547

Welch, M. G., Firestein, M. R., Austin, J., Hane, A. A., Stark, R. I., Hofer, M. A., … Myers, M. M. (2015). Family nurture intervention in the neonatal intensive care unit improves social-relatedness, attention, and neurodevelopment of preterm infants at 18 months in a randomized controlled trial. *Journal of Child Psychology and Psychiatry, 56*(11), 1202–1211. doi:10.1111/jcpp.12405

Welch, M. G., Halperin, M. S., Austin, J., Stark, R. I., Hofer, M. A., Hane, A. A., & Myers, M. M. (2016). Depression and anxiety symptoms of mothers of preterm infants are decreased at 4 months corrected age with family nurture intervention in the NICU. *Archives of Women's Mental Health, 19*(1), 51–61. doi:10.1007/s00737-015-0502-7

Welch, M. G., Hofer, M. A., Brunelli, S. A., Stark, R. I., Andrews, H. F., Austin, J., … Family Nurture Intervention Trial, G. (2012). Family nurture intervention (FNI): Methods and treatment protocol of a randomized controlled trial in the NICU. *BMC Pediatrics, 12*, 14. doi:10.1186/1471-2431-12-14

Welch, M. G., Hofer, M. A., Stark, R. I., Andrews, H. F., Austin, J., Glickstein, S. B., … Group, F. N. I. T, Group, F. N. I. T. (2013). Randomized controlled trial of family nurture intervention in the NICU: Assessments of length of stay, feasibility and safety. *BMC Pediatrics, 13*, 148. doi:10.1186/1471-2431-13-148

Welch, M. G., Myers, M. M., Grieve, P. G., Isler, J. R., Fifer, W. P., Sahni, R., … Group, F. N. I. T, Group, F. N. I. T. (2014). Electroencephalographic activity of preterm infants is increased by family nurture intervention: A randomized controlled trial in the NICU. *Clinical Neurophysiology, 125*(4), 675–684. doi:10.1016/j.clinph.2013.08.021

Wiener, N. (1961). *Cybernetics: Or Control and Communication in the Animal and the Machine* Hermann & Cie.

Wolff, P. H., & Ferber, R. (1979). The development of behavior in human infants, premature and newborn. *Annual Review of Neuroscience, 2*, 291–307. doi:10.1146/annurev.ne.02.030179.001451

Zanardo, V., & Straface, G. (2015). The higher temperature in the areola supports the natural progression of the birth to breastfeeding continuum. *PloS One, 10*(3), e0118774. doi:10.1371/journal.pone.0118774

Chapter 16
Implications of Epigenetics in Developmental Care of Preterm Infants in the NICU: Preterm Behavioral Epigenetics

Rosario Montirosso and Livio Provenzi

Abstract *Introduction*: Epigenetics is an emerging field of research at the interface between biological and environmental sciences, and it is suggesting that early adversities might be embedded into infants' developing biology through DNA functional processes (e.g., DNA methylation). Recent studies revealed an association between pain-related stress and epigenetic variations which can affect stress reactivity during early infancy. On the other hand, behavioral epigenetic studies on human subjects are suggesting that DNA methylation might be modified "for good" through caring interventions and protective environments.

Main aim of the chapter: This chapter will review the theoretical rationale and emerging findings related to the application of epigenetics to the field of prematurity (Preterm Behavioral Epigenetics, PBE).

Conclusions: The PBE research field holds promises to highlight the biological underpinnings of both NICU-related stressful and protective care in preterm infants.

Introduction

Preterm infants in neonatal intensive care unit (NICU) are exposed to numerous sources of stress, including high levels of physical (i.e., lights and sounds exposure) and painful stimulation (i.e., invasive skin-breaking procedures) which are thought to affect the neurodevelopment and the neuroendocrine systems (Aita, Johnston, Goulet, Oberlander, & Snider, 2013; Brummelte et al., 2012). For example, greater neonatal pain-related stress has been associated with decreased brain size of the frontal and parietal brain regions both at term equivalent post-menstrual age (Smith et al., 2011) and at school age (Ranger et al., 2013). Pain exposure during the hospitalization has been linked with downregulation of the hypothalamic-pituitary-adrenal (HPA) axis and with heightened cortisol levels at 18 months of age (Grunau,

R. Montirosso (✉) • L. Provenzi
0-3 Centre for the at-Risk Infant, Scientific Institute, IRCCS Eugenio Medea,
Bosisio Parini, LC, Italy
e-mail: rosario.montirosso@bp.lnf.it

© Springer International Publishing AG 2017
M. Filippa et al. (eds.), *Early Vocal Contact and Preterm Infant Brain Development*, DOI 10.1007/978-3-319-65077-7_16

2013). Furthermore, given the critical role of caregivers in early stress regulation, the prolonged separation from their mother deprives preterm infants of the protective role of maternal care, thus representing an additional source of stress during NICU stay (Gray, Watt, & Blass, 2000). Recently, it has been suggested that epigenetic mechanisms might play a role in the processes through which early stress exposure is embedded in the developmental phenotype of human infants. In the present chapter, we will provide a rationale and first evidence for the application of epigenetic research to the field of preterm birth and NICU stay. Preterm behavioral epigenetics (PBE; Montirosso & Provenzi, 2015) will be discussed as a novel approach to NICU-related stress exposure and protective developmental care (DC) practices. First, we will introduce the core concepts of epigenetics, highlighting biochemical mechanisms and their implications for stress regulation across human development. A specific focus will be devoted to DNA methylation, which is one of the most studied epigenetic mechanisms triggered by environmental cues and challenges, including stressful adverse experiences and variations in maternal care (Champagne & Curley, 2009). In the second section of the chapter, a clinically grounded model for PBE scientific research will be proposed. The model has been developed according to recent findings in human epigenetics and to NICU-related relevant issues for stress exposure and protective care (Provenzi, Borgatti, & Montirosso, 2016). In the third section, we will provide a brief review of the emergent evidence from PBE, which are primarily related to the association among NICU-related stress exposure, DNA methylation alterations, and behavioral outcomes in preterm infants. Finally, we will offer a potential perspective for future PBE research applied to the effects of DC practices.

What Is Epigenetics?

Introducing DNA Methylation

The genome is not a fixed structure. Rather, it dynamically interacts with the environment resulting in modifications of the chromatin structure in which the DNA is embedded (Hyman, 2009). Different chromatin shapes associate with different DNA accessibility to transcriptional factors, which are responsible for gene expression and protein synthesis. Epigenetics refers to processes that are capable of altering chromatin accessibility to transcriptional factors, thus leading to permanent alterations of gene expression and to phenotypic differences. Epigenetic mechanisms include DNA methylation, histone modification, and small noncoding RNA molecules (microRNAs). Nonetheless, DNA methylation is by far the main investigated epigenetic mechanism, at least in humans. DNA methylation consists in the binding of a methyl group to cytosine-rich dinucleotides (i.e., cytosine-phosphate-guanine (CpG) sites). When it occurs at clustered CpG sites (i.e., CpG islands) within the regulatory region of stress-related genes, DNA methylation results in an inhibition of the transcriptional activity, also known as gene silencing (Fig. 16.1). As such, DNA

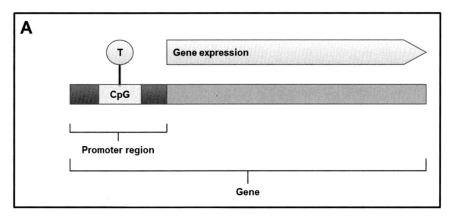

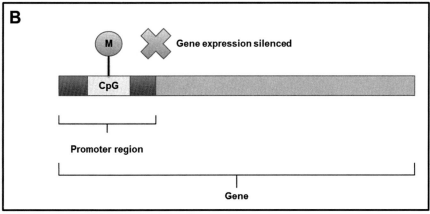

Fig. 16.1 DNA methylation and gene silencing at promoter region

methylation is of particular concern, as it holds the potential to alter gene expression of proteins which have implications even for behavioral development (Griffiths & Hunter, 2014; Murgatroyd, Wu, Bockmühl, & Spengler, 2010).

Epigenetic Modifications by Environmental Conditions in Animal Model

DNA methylation of the promoter region of stress-related genes has been investigated in animal models and humans. Seminal studies in rats have revealed that suboptimal caregiving environment associates with heightened methylation of the gene (i.e., *NR3C1*) encoding for corticosteroid receptors (Meaney & Szyf, 2005). Glucocorticoids (i.e., cortisol in humans) bind to glucocorticoid receptors (GRs) which mediate their cellular effects. Under stressful condition GRs regulate cortisol secretion and attenuate the activation of the hypothalamic-pituitary-adrenal (HPA) axis by a negative feedback action (Tsigos & Chrousos, 2002). An increased methylation of *NR3C1* leads to decreased expression of GRs in the brain, and a low density of GRs is associated with higher stress reactivity. Rats exposed to low quality of maternal caregiving behavior exhibited higher methylation of the *NR3C1*, lower expression of GRs in brain tissues, and heightened susceptibility to stress later in life, compared to rats reared by mothers characterized by high quality of caregiving behavior (Champagne & Curley, 2009). In sum, stressful environmental conditions (i.e., variations in maternal care during the neonatal period) affect the offspring through stable epigenetic variations of the chromatin structure (i.e., DNA methylation). Notably, a reverse protective effect was also observed in a cross fostered condition; pups born from mothers with low quality of care, but reared by high quality-of-care mothers, showed low *NR3C1* methylation and high GR brain expression and HPA axis stress reactivity pattern comparable to pups born and reared by high quality-of-care mothers (Szyf, 2009). This suggests that the effect of early adverse conditions on gene expression might be moderated by caring interventions.

Epigenetic Modifications by Environmental Conditions in Humans

Human behavioral epigenetic studies have suggested that early adverse conditions, including prenatal stress, are associated with epigenetic modifications (Lester et al., 2011). For example, infants born to mothers who had a high number of depressive symptoms during the third trimester of pregnancy had increased *NR3C1* methylation compared to peers which were not exposed to maternal prenatal depression (Oberlander et al., 2008). Similar findings have been reported by other research groups (Braithwaite, Kundakovic, Ramchandani, Murphy, & Champagne, 2015; Caspi et al., 2003; Conradt, Lester, Appleton, Armstrong, & Marsit, 2013) suggesting that early exposure to stress might lead to epigenetic modifications of HPA axis functioning, through alterations at the level of the promoter region of the *NR3C1* gene. For example, newborn infants with high *NR3C1* methylation have been found to have more asymmetrical reflexes measured through the NICU Network Neurobehavioral Scales (Lester et al., 2015). Furthermore, in full-term infants, placental DNA methylation of *NR3C1* was related to greater cortisol reactivity and infant self-regulation in response to social stress (i.e., the still-face procedure; Tronick, Als, Adamson, Wise, & Brazelton, 1978) at 4 months (Conradt et al., 2015). Importantly, epigenetic processes are sensitive to maternal responsiveness, even in presence of maternal depressive symptoms. Conradt et al. (2016) have documented that mothers with depressive symptomology who were more responsive during a face-to-face interaction had infants with less DNA methylation of *NR3C1* compared to mothers with depressive symptoms who were also less responsive.

It has been suggested that the serotonin transporter gene (i.e., *SLC6A4*) is another key epigenetic regulator of the impact of early adverse experiences on subsequent development in human infants and children. The serotoninergic system is one of the major systems associated with stress regulation and is affected by exposures to early life adversities (Lesch, 2011). The serotonin transporter is a key regulator of serotonergic signaling in the brain, and its expression is regulated by genetic and epigenetic factors. In particular, higher methylation of specific CpG sites within the *SLC6A4* promoter region has been linked with reduced serotonin transporter expression (Philibert et al., 2007, 2008; Provenzi, Giorda, Beri, & Montirosso, 2016). Early adverse experiences, such as abuse during childhood (Beach, Brody, Todorov, Gunter, & Philibert, 2010; Vijayendran, Beach, Plume, Brody, & Philibert, 2012) and the exposure to maternal depression during pregnancy (Devlin, Brain, Austin, & Oberlander, 2010), have been associated with patterns of altered methylation at the level of different CpG sites within the *SLC6A4* promoter region. This altered epigenetic pattern at the level of the serotonergic system associates with negative outcomes in adults. Booij and colleagues (2015) documented that greater childhood abuse correlated with higher overall *SLC6A4* methylation, which in turn was associated with smaller hippocampal volume.

Overall, these findings corroborate that exposure to pre- and postnatal adverse environmental conditions have an impact on the epigenome in human subjects, altering the methylation status and the transcriptional capability of specific stress-related genes.

Application of Epigenetic Study to Preterm Infants and NICU Stay

A Model for PBE Research

The application of behavioral epigenetics to the field of prematurity and NICU stay is far more recent. Recently, a theoretical model has been proposed (see Fig. 16.2) and grounded in clinical and research evidence about the role of both prenatal and postnatal environmental encounters in contributing to the emerging phenotype of preterm infants (Montirosso & Provenzi, 2015). The model highlights three main areas of interest.

First, prenatal environment might contribute to preterm birth and to risk status of preterm infants by epigenetic mechanisms. On the one hand, adverse prenatal conditions (e.g., maternal stress in pregnancy) have also been associated with heightened risk of preterm birth, potentially via inflammations or infections of the placenta (Wadhwa, Entringer, Buss, & Lu, 2011). Indeed, epigenetic biomarker of increased methylation at an imprinted gene related to fetal growth (i.e., *PLAGL1*)

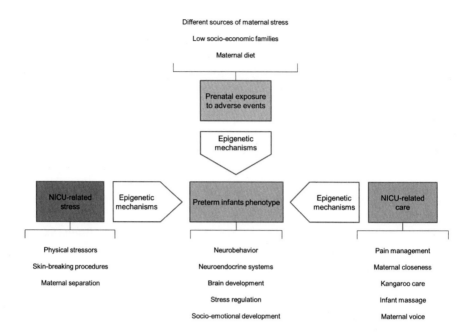

Fig. 16.2 Prospective model for preterm behavioral epigenetics research

has been reported in the case of preterm birth associated with placental infections (i.e., chorioamnionitis and funisitis; Liu et al., 2013). As such, it is plausible to hypothesize that suboptimal conditions of gestation and fetal growth might lead to epigenetic modifications which might increase in some way the risk of preterm delivery (Moog et al., 2016).

Second, the NICU-related stress (e.g., painful stimulation) might be associated with altered methylation of stress-related genes and further contribute to the preterm infants' phenotype. Recent research provides evidence for the existence of environmental-driven epigenetic modifications at genes involved in pain processing (Denk & McMahon, 2012). Human twins discordant for pain sensitivity have been shown to have differentially methylated genes related to pain response (Bell et al., 2014). Importantly, recent emerging findings suggest an association between pain-related stress exposure and epigenetic variations in very preterm infants (see below).

Third, we speculate that early alterations of DNA methylation patterns due to stressful stimulations might be reversed through the exposure to caring and protective environmental conditions. Previous authors have suggested that NICU practices of parental involvement and family-centered interventions might serve such a protective and reversal effect of DNA methylation (Maddalena, 2013; Provenzi & Barello, 2015; Samra, McGrath, Wehbe, & Clapper, 2012). Unfortunately, there is still a paucity of studies documenting epigenetic correlates of caring interventions in humans, with no research in prematurity. In the next sections, insights for future research on potential applicability for understanding how the DC practices can have impact on gene expression by epigenetic mechanisms are discussed.

Emerging Evidence from PBE Research

During recent years, evidence is emerging regarding the epigenetic vestiges of preterm birth and early adverse exposures during NICU stay. Research published in this field has been focused on two specific stress-related genes, namely, the *NR3C1* and the *SLC6A4*. Kantake and colleagues (Kantake, Yoshitake, Ishikawa, Araki, & Shimizu, 2014) reported on *NR3C1* methylation at birth and at 4 days of age in very preterm (VPT) infants and in a counterpart of full-term controls. The *NR3C1* promoter region methylation was assessed in cord blood at birth and in peripheral blood at 4 days. Results highlighted that methylation rates increased from birth to discharge at several CpG sites in very preterm infants, but it remained stable in full-term infants. At day 4, the *NR3C1* methylation was significantly higher in preterm infants compared to full-term counterpart. Moreover, the level of *NR3C1* methylation at day 4 was a predictor of later medical complications during the neonatal period.

A retrospective investigation focused on the epigenetic consequences of pain-related stress exposure in NICU on the *SLC6A4* gene at school age (Chau et al., 2014). The findings suggest that 7-year-old very preterm children had higher *SLC6A4* methylation at specific CpG sites compared to full-term infants, suggesting an association between the number of skin-breaking procedures (i.e., pain-related stress) during NICU stay and *SLC6A4* methylation. Notably, in very preterm children, but not in the full-term children, the altered methylation observed during school age was associated with behavioral problems rated by the mothers through questionnaire (i.e., CBCL scales). More recently, a prospective micro-longitudinal project has assessed *SLC6A4* methylation status at birth and at NICU discharge in very preterm infants and only at birth in full-term infants (Provenzi et al., 2015). There is no difference in CpG-specific *SLC6A4* methylation at birth between VPT and full-term infants, suggesting that birth status does not affect epigenetic regulation of the serotonin transporter gene. However, in very preterm infants, *SLC6A4* methylation significantly increased from birth to discharge at specific CpG sites. The increase was significantly predicted by the number of skin-breaking procedures to which very preterm infants were exposed during the NICU stay. It should be noted that the length of NICU stay and neonatal confounders (e.g., gestational age, birth weight, Apgar score) were not associated with discharge methylation at the *SLC6A4* gene. Interestingly, the methylation level of these specific CpG sites was associated with temperamental difficulties at 3 months (Montirosso et al., 2016a). Higher methylation at discharge was predictive of lower duration of orienting and approach at 3 months (corrected age for prematurity). Finally, when infants were exposed to the stressful maternal still face, very preterm infants reported higher negative emotionality compared to full-term controls. The extent of negative emotionality display was significantly predicted by the *SLC6A4* methylation increase observed at NICU discharge (Montirosso et al., 2016b).

Overall, these findings confirm that in preterm infants early stress exposure is associated with epigenetic variations, which in turn can affect stress response and neurodevelopment outcomes.

Can Early Caring Interventions in NICU Reverse Stress-Related Methylation Changes?

During early life, DNA methylation could be susceptible to positive experiences and environmental manipulations. As abovementioned, animal studies have not only showed that low caregiving quality associated with increased methylation of stress-related genes and with poorer cognitive and socio-emotional development outcomes (Meaney & Szyf, 2005). When rats born from mothers characterized by low quality of caregiving are cross fostered by mothers characterized by high quality of care, they show levels of methylation of the *NR3C1* gene which are similar to those of rats born and reared by high quality-of-care mothers (Cervoni et al., 2004). Moreover, positive experiences for rats, such as being sensitively touched during the early postnatal period, have been shown to decrease the production of glucocorticoids during the first day of life (Jutapakdeegul, Casalotti, Govitrapong, & Kotchabhakdi, 2003). Interestingly, this change was associated with an increased expression of the gene encoding for the hippocampal GRs. In sum, the occurrence of protective environmental factors, even after the exposure to early adverse rearing conditions, appeared to be able to reverse the pattern of altered DNA methylation, thus leading to more favorable outcomes in later life.

In the light of this evidence, one could wonder if stress-related modifications of DNA methylation might be reversed by subsequent exposures to protective or caring environments – such as DC practices in NICU (Samra et al., 2012) – even in human infants. Notwithstanding, whether these findings could be applied directly to human subjects – and infants, specifically – is questionable. Several issues are unresolved, and the behavioral epigenetic research in animals and humans is not at the same scientific stage (Lester et al., 2011). Nevertheless, it is noteworthy that first evidence of DNA methylation reversal in association with caring intervention and protective environmental conditions is starting to emerge. In a study assessing the association between caring interventions and DNA methylation alterations in human subjects, the level of methylation of the serotonin transporter gene (*SLC6A4*) promoter region was measured before and after a cognitive behavior therapy in 116 children with anxiety disorders (Roberts et al., 2014). Change in DNA methylation from pre- to post-intervention paralleled outcomes in children who respond well to the psychotherapeutic intervention. Specifically, while responder children showed increased methylation of a specific CpG site of the *SLC6A4* gene, nonresponders showed a decrease. These findings suggest that different patterns of methylation increase or decrease might be associated with different responses to psychotherapy in children. Similarly, Perroud and colleagues (Perroud et al., 2013) reported that human subjects diagnosed with borderline personality disorder and treated with an intensive behavior therapy showed differential patterns of methylation of the brain-derived neurotropic factor (*BDNF*) gene, in relation to treatment outcomes. Responder subjects exhibited a decrease over time in *BDNF* methylation, whereas nonresponders showed an opposite increasing pattern. Finally, Unternaehrer et al. (2015) asked to a group of adults to retrospectively assess the quality of care received from their mothers by questionnaire (i.e., the Parental Bonding Instrument). DNA methylation of genes coding for the *BDNF* and oxytocin (OXTR) from peripheral blood samples was assayed. Low maternal care in childhood was significantly associated with greater methylation of both these stress-related genes. Despite it was a cross-sectional and retrospective study, the work by Unternaehrer et al. (2015) is the first documenting epigenetic correlates of maternal care variations similar to those highlighted by Meaney and colleagues (Meaney & Szyf, 2005) in animal model.

Important Questions and Future Research Directions for Preterm Behavioral Epigenetics

Summing up, one might reasonably hypothesize that DNA methylation might be modified "for good" through caring interventions and protective environments in humans. Thus, although further research is needed, these findings appear to support the hypothesis that an environment characterized by high quality of care might have epigenetic effects on stress-related genes in human subjects. This scenario might have potential implications for DC practices and early parental interventions in the NICU (Provenzi & Barello, 2015). From this perspective, the application of the epigenetic lens to the context of prematurity is intriguing and warrants future attention within the PBE agenda. Here we would like to highlight some areas of investigations which encompass different aspects of early intervention and prevention for the prematurely born infant (Altimier, Kenner, & Damus, 2015), with the aim of bridging the gap between psychobiological research and clinical practice in NICUs (Samra et al., 2012).

First, as reported in previous chapters, DC interventions such as holding, kangaroo care, parental involvement in pain management, and maternal voice have shown to exert long-term beneficial and protective effects for preterm infants' development. Nonetheless, there is relative inconsistency in literature about the specific applications and effects of different DC practices (Montirosso et al., 2012; Coughlin, Gibbins, & Hoath, 2009). The light side of PBE might be regarded as conveying a biologically grounded evidence-based proxy to inform the parental involvement interventions. Epigenetic correlates of different activities and practices of caregiver engagement should be investigated. As shown in a longitudinal study on the protective role of DC, different features of DC associate with diverse behavioral outcomes for the preterm infant (see: Montirosso et al., 2017). As such, one might expect that not all the modalities of caregiver engagement exert similar, if any, epigenetic effect on the developing biology of prematurely born infants.

Moreover, the PBE research should investigate which genes are better candidates for bearing the epigenetic marker of protective DC practices in NICU. Epigenetic changes at different stress-related genes result in alterations of diverse physiologic systems of stress response. Early life changes in the HPA axis functioning or the serotoninergic system have different implications for socio-emotional development and for health conditions later in life. A specific gene of interest for parental interventions in the NICU could be the oxytocin gene (*OXTR*). Indeed, oxytocin is associated with affiliative behaviors (Weisman, Zagoory-Sharon, & Feldman, 2012) that are threatened and challenged by maternal separation in NICU (Flacking et al., 2012). Intriguingly, variations in the methylation of this gene have been found to associate with early exposure to stressful environments in human newborns (Unternaehrer et al., 2016) and with maternal care quality in adult humans (Unternaehrer et al., 2015).

One of the most critical point is to inquire if stress-related and care-related epigenetic variations are actually working at the same epigenetic substrate or within the same genetic regions. In other words, it should be relevant to study if the reversal effect documented for rats is also at work in human infants. As such, future studies should not be limited only to the investigation of the relationship between DC practices and gene-related methylation. Rather, in order to account for the effects on the epigenome and on the subsequent neurobehavioral and socio-emotional development, it seems important to investigate together the epigenetic correlates of NICU-related stress and DC practices.

It should also be noted that the stability of methylation is not given for granted and there is still need of longitudinal and prospective studies, especially in humans. While the majority of previous behavioral epigenetic studies in humans have revealed stress-related (Beach et al., 2010) and care-related methylation (Unternaehrer et al., 2015) changes in specific genes, they were for the most part retrospective in their nature. This is mainly due to the type of early adversity that was investigated (e.g., abuse and maltreatment) which is of course unpredictable in infants and children development. On the contrary, we can reliably forecast that prematurely born infants will be separated from the mother and that they will be exposed to numerous sources of stress during the relative long hospitalization in the NICU. As such, the PBE research field holds the potential of providing reliable and prospective information about the associations between early life encounters and DNA methylation, for better or for worse (Provenzi, Borgatti, & Montirosso, 2017).

Finally, future studies are warranted to address the epigenetic correlates of neuroprotective DC practices at different time points across preterm infant, children, and adult development. On the one hand, short-term outcomes would be relevant to understand the immediate impact of parental interventions on the developmental biology of preterm infants. This would be of great importance to improve our knowledge of the more suitable time window to promote physical contact, massage, and skin-to-skin holding in a biologically sustainable and effective way for the infant. For example, it is well known that early epigenetic regulation of the HPA axis and of the serotonergic system might set a heightened disease risk later in life (Maccari, Krugers, Morley-Fletcher, Szyf, & Brunton, 2014). On the other hand, long-term neuroprotective effects of NICU DC practices need to be addressed with longitudinal studies. This research will be of great value to build a grounded and time-scaled meter of the biological and neuroprotective effects of NICU quality of care in a life-span healthcare perspective.

Given the topic of this book, one might expected that even maternal voice might exert epigenetic effect on the developing biology of prematurely born infants. As suggested in previous chapters, maternal vocal stimulation (i.e., speaking or singing) has significant effects on infant developing. Nonetheless, to date, no study has inquired the link between maternal voice and epigenetic mechanisms. That said, there could be a rationale to anticipate some speculations. Maternal voice represents a species-specific experience, and infants show a strong orientation to human-made sounds and music (Panksepp & Trevarthen, 2009). Indeed, infants prefer melodic phrases and pleasant sounding rather than dissonant and mechanical sounds (Trehub, 2001). Importantly, infants' listening is attuned with maternal vocal patterns, including time, pitch range, and rhythms which convey the emotional dimensions of early dyadic communications (Jaffe, Beebe, Feldstein, Crown, & Jasnow, 2001). Thus, vocal behavior of mothers, which is characterized by an inherent communicative musicality, contributes to the quality of interactions with infant and supports self-regulation (Papousek, 1981). Likely due to its emotional power, the musicality of maternal voice could affect infant stress regulation. This view is supported by adult research which has emphasized the relationship between music and stress modulation (Theorell, 2014). Studies show that music can alleviate feelings of stress and acute and chronic pain (Bernatzky, Presch, Anderson, & Panksepp, 2011; Cepeda, Carr, Lau, & Alvarez, 2006; Chlan, Engeland, Anthony, & Guttormson, 2007). Moreover, research evidence suggests that early exposure to maternal voice promotes the physiological stability (i.e., decrease in heart rates, higher oxygen saturation rates, lower sign of stress) and capacity of self-regulation (Filippa, Devouche, Arioni, Imberty, & Gratier, 2013; Picciolini et al., 2014). Thus, like other caregiving behaviors, maternal voice might influence behavioral and endocrine stress regulation (i.e., HPA axis) in young infants. We suggest that future studies should be aimed at investigating whether the effects of maternal voice on infants' developmental outcomes might be at least partially mediated by the same epigenetic processes involved in the relationship between maternal quality of care and stress regulation in animal models (Szyf, 2009) and humans (Unternaehrer et al., 2015).

Conclusion

Evidence from animal and human research documents the effects of a variety of early environmental adversities on the behavioral and neuroendocrine development of the offspring. These studies highlight that these effects are relatively stable and involve alterations in gene expression associated with altered patterns of DNA methylation and alteration of the stress response. Interestingly, caregiving behaviors and early care emerge as critical regulators of the epigenome in the offspring. As such, early caring interventions and protective practices should be targeted by future epigenetic studies, especially in the context of at-risk prematurely born infants. From this perspective, the PBE research field has the potentials to improve our understanding of both the effects of NICU-related stress and the protective and buffering role of DC practices (Provenzi & Montirosso, 2015)

Key Messages

- Behavioral epigenetics refer to functional modifications of the DNA transcriptional activity, which are highly susceptible to environmental adversities and protective stimulations.
- Preterm infants are long-lasting hospitalized and cared for in neonatal intensive care units (NICUs), in which they are exposed both to stressful and protective stimulations.
- The application of behavioral epigenetics to the field of prematurity and NICU stay is revealing epigenetic pathways through which early adversity is embedded in neurobehavioral development of preterm infants.
- Future research is warranted to target the epigenetic correlates of protective care interventions in the NICU, including specific strategies to enhance mother-infant closeness and bonding such as maternal voice.

Please, consider to use Fig. 16.2 *as figure supporting these take-home messages.*

References

Aita, M., Johnston, C., Goulet, C., Oberlander, T. F., & Snider, L. (2013). Intervention minimizing preterm infants' exposure to NICU light and noise. *Clinical Nursing Research, 22*, 337–358. doi:10.1177/1054773812469223

Altimier, L., Kenner, C., & Damus, K. (2015). The Wee Care Neuroprotective NICU Program (Wee Care): The effect of a comprehensive developmental care training program on seven neuroprotective core measures for family-centered developmental care of premature neonates. *Newborn and Infant Nursing Reviews, 15*(1), 6–16. doi:10.1053/j.nainr.2015.01.006

Beach, S. R. H., Brody, G. H., Todorov, A. A., Gunter, T. D., & Philibert, R. A. (2010). Methylation at SLC6A4 is linked to family history of child abuse: An examination of the Iowa Adoptee sample. *American Journal of Medical genetics. Part B, Neuropsychiatric Genetics : The Official Publication of the International Society of Psychiatric Genetics, 153B*(2), 710–713. doi:10.1002/ajmg.b.31028

Bell, J. T., Loomis, A. K., Butcher, L. M., Gao, F., Zhang, B., Hyde, C. L., ... Spector, T. D. (2014). Differential methylation of the TRPA1 promoter in pain sensitivity. *Nature Communications, 5*. doi:10.1038/ncomms3978

Bernatzky, G., Presch, M., Anderson, M., & Panksepp, J. (2011). Emotional foundations of music as a non-pharmacological pain management tool in modern medicine. *Neuroscience and Biobehavioral Reviews, 35*(9), 1989–1999. doi:10.1016/j.neubiorev.2011.06.005

Booij, L., Szyf, M., Carballedo, A., Frey, E.-M., Morris, D., Dymov, S., ... Frodl, T. (2015). DNA Methylation of the serotonin transporter gene in peripheral cells and stress-related changes in Hippocampal volume: A study in depressed patients and healthy controls. *PLoS One, 10*(3), e0119061. doi:10.1371/journal.pone.0119061

Braithwaite, E., Kundakovic, M., Ramchandani, P., Murphy, S., & Champagne, F. A. (2015). Maternal prenatal depressive symptoms predict infant NR3C1 1F and BDNF IV DNA methylation. *Epigenetics, 10*(5), 408–417.

Brummelte, S., Grunau, R. E., Chau, V., Poskitt, K. J., Brant, R., Vinall, J., ... Miller, S. P. (2012). Procedural pain and brain development in premature newborns. *Annals of Neurology, 71*(3), 385–396. doi:10.1002/ana.22267

Caspi, A., Sugden, K., Moffitt, T. E., Taylor, A., Craig, I. W., Harrington, H., ... Poulton, R. (2003). Influence of life stress on depression: Moderation by a polymorphism in the 5-HTT gene. *Science, 301*(5631), 386–389. doi:10.1126/science.1083968

Cepeda, M. S., Carr, D. B., Lau, J., & Alvarez, H. (2006). Music for pain relief. *Cochrane Database System, 19*, CD004843.

Champagne, F. A., & Curley, J. P. (2009). Epigenetic mechanisms mediating the long-term effects of maternal care on development. *Neuroscience and Biobehavioral Reviews, 33*(4), 593–600. doi:10.1016/j.neubiorev.2007.10.009

Chau, C. M. Y., Ranger, M., Sulistyoningrum, D., Devlin, A. M., Oberlander, T. F., & Grunau, R. E. (2014). Neonatal pain and COMT Val158Met genotype in relation to serotonin transporter (SLC6A4) promoter methylation in very preterm children at school age. *Frontiers in Behavioral Neuroscience, 8*, 1–12. doi:10.3389/fnbeh.2014.00409

Chlan, L. L., Engeland, W. C., Anthony, A., & Guttormson, J. (2007). Influence of music on the stress response in patients receiving mechanical ventilatory support: A pilot study. *American Journal of Critical Care, 16*(2), 141–145.

Conradt, E., Fei, M., LaGasse, L., Tronick, E., Guerin, D., Gorman, D., ... Lester, B. M. (2015). Prenatal predictors of infant self-regulation: The contributions of placental DNA methylation of NR3C1 and neuroendocrine activity. *Frontiers in Behavioral Neuroscience, 9*, 130. doi:10.3389/fnbeh.2015.00130

Conradt, E., Hawes, K., Guerin, D., Armstrong, D. A., Marsit, C. J., Tronick, E., & Lester, B. M. (2016). The contributions of maternal sensitivity and maternal depressive symptoms to epigenetic processes and neuroendocrine functioning. *Child Development, 87*(1), 73–85. doi:10.1111/cdev.12483

Conradt, E., Lester, B. M., Appleton, A. A., Armstrong, D. A., & Marsit, C. J. (2013). The roles of DNA methylation of NR3C1 and 11beta-HSD2 and exposure to maternal mood disorder in utero on newborn neurobehavior. *Epigenetics : Official Journal of the DNA Methylation Society, 8*(12), 1321–1329. doi:10.4161/epi.26634

Coughlin, M., Gibbins, S., & Hoath, S. (2009). Core measures for developmentally supportive care in neonatal intensive care units: Theory, precedence and practice. *Journal of Advanced Nursing, 65*(10), 2239–2248. doi:10.1111/j.1365-2648.2009.05052.x

Denk, F., & McMahon, S. B. B. (2012). Chronic pain: Emerging evidence for the involvement of epigenetics. *Neuron, 73*(3), 435–444. doi:10.1016/j.neuron.2012.01.012

Devlin, A. M., Brain, U., Austin, J., & Oberlander, T. F. (2010). Prenatal exposure to maternal depressed mood and the MTHFR C677T variant affect SLC6A4 methylation in infants at birth. *PLoS One, 5*(8), e12201. doi:10.1371/journal.pone.0012201

Filippa, M., Devouche, E., Arioni, C., Imberty, M., & Gratier, M. (2013). Live maternal speech and singing have beneficial effects on hospitalized preterm infants. *Acta Paediatrica*, *102*(10), 1017–1020. doi:10.1111/apa.12356

Flacking, R., Lehtonen, L., Thomson, G., Axelin, A., Ahlqvist, S., Moran, V. H., … SCENE Group, SCENE Group. (2012). Closeness and separation in neonatal intensive care. *Acta Paediatrica*, *101*(10), 1032–1037. doi:10.1111/j.1651-2227.2012.02787.x

Gray, L., Watt, L., & Blass, E. M. (2000). Skin-to-skin contact is analgesic in healthy newborns. *Pediatrics*, *105*(1), e14.

Griffiths, B. B., & Hunter, R. G. (2014). Neuroepigenetics of stress. *Neuroscience*, *275*, 420–435. doi:10.1016/j.neuroscience.2014.06.041

Grunau, R. E. (2013). Neonatal pain in very preterm infants: Long-term effects on brain, neurodevelopment and pain reactivity. *Rambam Maimonides Medical Journal*, *4*(4), e0025. doi:10.5041/RMMJ.10132

Hyman, S. E. (2009). How adversity gets under the skin. *Nature Neuroscience*, *12*(3), 241–243. doi:10.1038/nn0309-241

Jaffe, J., Beebe, B., Feldstein, S., Crown, C. L., & Jasnow, M. D. (2001). Rhythms of dialogue in infancy: Coordinated timing in development. *Monographs of the Society for Research in Child Development*, *66*(2), 1–132.

Jutapakdeegul, N., Casalotti, S. O., Govitrapong, P., & Kotchabhakdi, N. (2003). Postnatal touch stimulation acutely alters corticosterone levels and glucocorticoid receptor gene expression in the neonatal rat. *Developmental Neuroscience*, *25*, 26–33. doi:10.1159/000071465

Kantake, M., Yoshitake, H., Ishikawa, H., Araki, Y., & Shimizu, T. (2014). Postnatal epigenetic modification of glucocorticoid receptor gene in preterm infants: A prospective cohort study. *BMJ Open*, *4*(7). doi:10.1136/bmjopen-2014-005318

Lesch, K. P. (2011). When the serotonin transporter gene meets adversity: The contribution of animal models to understanding epigenetic mechanisms in affective disorders and resilience. *Current Topics in Behavioral Neurosciences*, *7*, 251–280. doi:10.1007/7854_2010_109

Lester, B. M., Marsit, C. J., Giarraputo, J., Hawes, K., LaGasse, L. L., & Padbury, J. F. (2015). Neurobehavior related to epigenetic differences in preterm infants. *Epigenomics*, *7*(7), 1123–1136. doi:10.2217/epi.15.63

Lester, B. M., Tronick, E., Nestler, E., Abel, T., Kosofsky, B., Kuzawa, C. W., … Wood, M. A. (2011). Behavioral epigenetics. *Annals of the New York Academy of Sciences*, *1226*, 14–33. doi:10.1111/j.1749-6632.2011.06037.x

Liu, Y., Hoyo, C., Murphy, S., Huang, Z., Overcash, F., Thompson, J., … Murtha, A. P. (2013). DNA methylation at imprint regulatory regions in preterm birth and infection. *American Journal of Obstetrics and Gynecology*, *208*(5), 395.e1–395.e7. doi:10.1016/j.ajog.2013.02.006

Maccari, S., Krugers, H. J., Morley-Fletcher, S., Szyf, M., & Brunton, P. J. (2014). The consequences of early-life adversity: Neurobiological, behavioural and epigenetic adaptations. *Journal of Neuroendocrinology*, *26*(10), 707–723. doi:10.1111/jne.12175

Maddalena, P. (2013). Long term outcomes of preterm birth: The role of epigenetics. *Newborn and Infant Nursing Reviews*, *13*(3), 137–139. doi:10.1053/j.nainr.2013.06.010

Meaney, M. J., & Szyf, M. (2005). Maternal care as a model for experience-dependent chromatin plasticity? *Trends in Neurosciences*, *28*(9), 456–463. doi:S0166-2236(05)00189-X

Montirosso, R., Del Prete, A., Bellu, R., Tronick, E., Borgatti, R., & NEO-ACQUA Study Group. (2012). Level of NICU quality of developmental care and neurobehavioral performance in very preterm infants. *Pediatrics*, *129*(5), e1129–e1137. doi:10.1542/peds.2011-0813

Montirosso, R., & Provenzi, L. (2015). Implications of epigenetics and stress regulation on research and developmental care of preterm infants. *Journal of Obstetric, Gynecologic, and Neonatal Nursing*, *44*(2), 174–182. doi:10.1111/1552-6909.12559

Montirosso, R., Provenzi, L., Fumagalli, M., Sirgiovanni, I., Giorda, R., Pozzoli, U., … Borgatti, R. (2016a). Serotonin transporter gene (SLC6A4) methylation associates with neonatal intensive care unit stay and 3-monthold temperament in preterm infants. *Child Development*, *87*(1), 38–48. doi:10.1111/cdev.12492

Montirosso, R., Provenzi, L., Giorda, R., Fumagalli, M., Morandi, F., Sirgiovanni, I., ... Borgatti, R. (2016b). SLC6A4 promoter region methylation and socio-emotional stress response in very preterm and full-term infants. *Epigenomics, 8*(7), 895–907. doi:10.2217/epi-2016-0010

Montirosso, R., Tronick, E., & Borgatti, R. (2017). Promoting neuroprotective care in neonatal intensive care units and preterm infant development: Insights from the neonatal adequate care for quality of life study. *Child Development Perspectives, 11*(1), 9–15.

Moog, N. K., Buss, C., Entringer, S., Shahbaba, B., Gillen, D. L., Hobel, C. J., & Wadhwa, P. D. (2016). Maternal exposure to childhood trauma is associated during pregnancy with placental-fetal stress physiology. *Biological Psychiatry, 79*(10), 831–839. doi:10.1016/j.biopsych.2015.08.032

Murgatroyd, C., Wu, Y., Bockmühl, Y., & Spengler, D. (2010). Genes learn from stress: How infantile trauma programs us for depression. *Epigenetics, 5*(3), 194–199. doi:10.4161/epi.5.3.11375

Oberlander, T. F., Grunau, R., Mayes, L., Riggs, W., Rurak, D., Papsdorf, M., ... Weinberg, J. (2008). Hypothalamic-pituitary-adrenal (HPA) axis function in 3-month old infants with prenatal selective serotonin reuptake inhibitor (SSRI) antidepressant exposure. *Early Human Development, 84*, 689–697. doi:10.1016/j.earlhumdev.2008.06.008

Panksepp, J., & Trevarthen, C. (2009). The neuroscience of emotion in music. In S. Malloch & C. Trevarthen (Eds.), *Communicative musicality: Exploring the basis of human companionship*. Oxford, UK: Oxford University Press.

Papousek, H. (1981). The common in the uncommon child: Comments on the child's integrative capacities and on parenting. In M. Lewis & L. A. Rosenblum (Eds.), *The uncommon child*. New York, NY: Plenum.

Perroud, N., Salzmann, A., Prada, P., Nicastro, R., Hoeppli, M. E., Furrer, S., ... Malafosse, A. (2013). Response to psychotherapy in borderline personality disorder and methylation status of the BDNF gene. *Translational Psychiatry, 3*, e207. doi:10.1038/tp.2012.140

Philibert, R., Madan, A., Andersen, A., Cadoret, R., Packer, H., & Sandhu, H. (2007). Serotonin transporter mRNA levels are associated with the methylation of an upstream CpG island. *American Journal of Medical Genetics, Part B: Neuropsychiatric Genetics, 144B*(1), 101–105. doi:10.1002/ajmg.b.30414

Philibert, R. A., Sandhu, H., Hollenbeck, N., Gunter, T., Adams, W., & Madan, A. (2008). The relationship of 5HTT (SLC6A4) methylation and genotype on mRNA expression and liability to major depression and alcohol dependence in subjects from the Iowa adoption studies. *American Journal of Medical Genetics. Part B, Neuropsychiatric Genetics, 147B*(5), 543–549. doi:10.1002/ajmg.b.30657

Picciolini, O., Porro, M., Meazza, A., Giannì, M. L., Rivoli, C., Lucco, G., ... Mosca, F. (2014). Early exposure to maternal voice: Effects on preterm infants development. *Early Human Development, 90*(6), 287–292. doi:10.1016/j.earlhumdev.2014.03.003

Provenzi, L., & Barello, S. (2015). Behavioral epigenetics of family-centered care in the neonatal intensive care unit. *JAMA Pediatrics, 169*(7), 697. doi:10.1001/jamapediatrics.2015.0367

Provenzi, L., Borgatti, R., & Montirosso, R. (2016). The light side of preterm behavioral epigenetics: An epigenetic perspective on caregiver engagement. In: Graffigna, G. (Ed.), *Promoting patient engagement and participation for effective healthcare reform*. IGI Global.

Provenzi, L., Borgatti, R., & Montirosso, R. (2017). Why are prospective longitudinal studies needed in preterm behavioral epigenetic research? *JAMA Pediatrics, 171*(1), 92–92.

Provenzi, L., Fumagalli, M., Sirgiovanni, I., Giorda, R., Pozzoli, U., Morandi, F., ... Montirosso, R. (2015). Pain-related stress during the Neonatal Intensive Care Unit stay and SLC6A4 methylation in very preterm infants. *Frontiers in Behavioral Neuroscience, 9*, 99. doi:10.3389/fnbeh.2015.00099

Provenzi, L., Giorda, R., Beri, S., & Montirosso, R. (2016a). SLC6A4 methylation as an epigenetic marker of life adversity exposures in humans: A systematic review of literature. *Neuroscience and Biobehavioral Reviews, 71*, 7–20. doi:10.1016/j.neubiorev.2016.08.021

Provenzi, L., & Montirosso, R. (2015). "Epigenethics" in the Neonatal Intensive Care Unit: Conveying complexity in health care for preterm children. *JAMA Pediatrics, 169*(7), 617–618. doi:10.1001/jamapediatrics.2015.43

Ranger, M., Chau, C. M., Garg, A., Woodward, T. S., Beg, M. F., Bjornson, B., ... Grunau, R. E. (2013). Neonatal pain-related stress predicts cortical thickness at age 7 years in children born very preterm. *PLoS One, 8*(10), e76702. doi:10.1371/journal.pone.0076702

Roberts, S., Lester, K. J., Hudson, J. L., Rapee, R. M., Creswell, C., Cooper, P. J., ... Eley, T. C. (2014). Serotonin transporter methylation and response to cognitive behaviour therapy in children with anxiety disorders. *Translational Psychiatry, 4*(9), e444–e445. doi:10.1038/tp.2014.83

Samra, H. A., McGrath, J. M., Wehbe, M., & Clapper, J. (2012). Epigenetics and family-centered developmental care for the preterm infant. *Advances in Neonatal Care: Official Journal of the National Association of Neonatal Nurses, 12*(Suppl 5), S2–S9. doi:10.1097/ANC.0b013e318265b4bd

Smith, G. C., Gutovich, J., Smyser, C., Pineda, R., Newnham, C., Tjoeng, T. H., ... Inder, T. (2011). Neonatal intensive care unit stress is associated with brain development in preterm infants. *Annals of Neurology, 70*(4), 541–549. doi:10.1002/ana.22545

Szyf, M. (2009). The early life environment and the epigenome. *Biochimica et Biophysica Acta - General Subjects, 1790*(9), 878–885. doi:10.1016/j.bbagen.2009.01.009

Theorell, T. (2014). Stress and music. In: Theorel, T. (Ed.) *Psychological health effects of musical experiences: Theories, studies and reflections in music health science.* Dordrecht, the Netherlands: Springer.

Trehub, S. E. (2001). Musical predispositions in infancy. *Annals of the New York Academy of Sciences, 930*, 1–16. doi:10.1111/j.1749-6632.2001.tb05721.x

Tronick, E., Als, H., Adamson, L., Wise, S., & Brazelton, T. B. (1978). The infant's response to entrapment between contradictory messages in face-to-face interaction. *Journal of the American Academy of Child Psychiatry, 17*(1), 1–13. doi:10.1016/S0002-7138(09)62273-1

Tsigos, C., & Chrousos, G. P. (2002). Hypothalamic-pituitary-adrenal axis, neuroendocrine factors and stress. *Journal of Psychosomatic Research, 53*(4), 865–871. doi:10.1016/S0022-3999(02)00429-4

Unternaehrer, E., Bolten, M., Nast, I., Staehli, S., Meyer, A. H., Dempster, E., ... Meinlschmidt, G. (2016). Maternal adversities during pregnancy and cord blood oxytocin receptor (OXTR) DNA methylation. *Social Cognitive and Affective Neuroscience, 11*(9), 1460–1470. doi:10.1093/scan/nsw051

Unternaehrer, E., Meyer, A. H., Burkhardt, S. C. A., Dempster, E., Staehli, S., Theill, N., ... Meinlschmidt, G. (2015). Childhood maternal care is associated with DNA methylation of the genes for brain-derived neurotrophic factor (BDNF) and oxytocin receptor (OXTR) in peripheral blood cells in adult men and women. *Stress, 18*(4), 451–461. doi:10.3109/10253890.2015.1038992

Vijayendran, M., Beach, S. R., Plume, J. M., Brody, G. H., & Philibert, R. A. (2012). Effects of genotype and child abuse on DNA methylation and gene expression at the serotonin transporter. *Frontiers in Psychiatry, 3*, 55. doi:10.3389/fpsyt.2012.00055

Wadhwa, P. D., Entringer, S., Buss, C., & Lu, M. C. (2011). The contribution of maternal stress to preterm birth: Issues and considerations. *Clinics in Perinatology, 38*(3), 351–384. doi:10.1016/j.clp.2011.06.007

Weaver, I. C. G., Cervoni, N., Champagne, F. A., D'Alessio, A. C., Sharma, S., Seckl, J. R., ... Meaney, M. J. (2004). Epigenetic programming by maternal behavior. *Nature Neuroscience, 7*(8), 847–854. doi:10.1038/nn1276

Weisman, O., Zagoory-Sharon, O., & Feldman, R. (2012). Oxytocin administration to parent enhances infant physiological and behavioral readiness for social engagement. *Biological Psychiatry, 72*, 982–989. doi:10.1016/j.biopsych.2012.06.011

Chapter 17
Family-Based Interventions and Developmental Care Programmes: Rationale, Difficulties and Effectiveness

Jean-Michel Roué, Stéphane Rioualen, and Jacques Sizun

Abstract Family-based interventions and developmental care programmes are becoming more widespread in neonatal units and after discharge. These early family-centred, developmentally oriented interventions are based on theoretical framework that supports the rationale for early intervention, including the following: (a) bonding and attachment processes theory, (b) brain development and synaptogenesis and (c) a family-centred philosophical approach. These interventions are time-consuming and costly, so their impact must be rigorously evaluated. Randomised controlled trials are the gold standard for clinical research but are not always suitable for investigating all aspects of an intervention. Other research methods might be useful, including animal research, qualitative research, observational studies using large cohorts and benchmarking. It is also important to evaluate the implementation of complex interventions. Early interventions can be administered during the neonatal intensive care unit and/or after discharge. Here we evaluate the following programmes: the Newborn Individualized Developmental Care and Assessment Program, Creating Opportunities for Parent Empowerment, Family Nurture Intervention, the Infant Behavioral Assessment and Intervention Program, the Mother-Infant Transaction Program, the Infant Health and Development Program, and the Victorian Infant Brain Studies intervention. The theoretical framework, nature and aims of these early interventions differ, but developmental support for the child, parenting education and parental psychosocial support are common elements. Most of the interventions are "cue-based" rather than "protocol-based" approaches that are designed to support the "sensitive parenting" development process. No programme focuses specifically on the mother's voice, but all support the mother–child relationship in general, including promoting sensitive communication using vocal, visual and behavioural channels.

J.-M. Roué • S. Rioualen • J. Sizun (✉)
Université de Brest, LIEN (EA 4685), Brest, France; CHRU Brest,
Pôle de la Femme de la Mère et de l'Enfant, Brest, France
e-mail: jacques.sizun@chu-brest.fr

© Springer International Publishing AG 2017
M. Filippa et al. (eds.), *Early Vocal Contact and Preterm Infant Brain Development*, DOI 10.1007/978-3-319-65077-7_17

Important improvements in prenatal and neonatal medicine have decreased the mortality rates of preterm populations (Ancel et al., 2015; Costeloe, Hennessy, Haider, et al., 2012; Express Group, 2009), thereby allowing neonatologists to focus more on functional outcomes. Concerns remain regarding possible delays in neurodevelopmental outcomes when the children are older. The long-term adverse outcomes after extreme prematurity include intellectual disability, cerebral palsy, blindness and deafness (Jarjour, 2015). Milder disabilities involving cognition, behaviour and learning are increasingly recognised among older preterm children and young adults. Late preterm children also have an increased risk of lower general cognitive ability (Chan, Leong, Malouf, & Quigley, 2016).

These developmental delays could be due to or associated with medical illnesses such as periventricular leukomalacia, intraventricular haemorrhage, sepsis and/or necrotising enterocolitis (NEC) (Linsell, Malouf, Morris, Kurinczuk, & Marlow, 2015, 2016). Research shows that outcomes may also be associated with non-medical factors like sex, ethnicity, family socioeconomic and educational level, nutrition and breastfeeding (Rozé, Darmaun, Boquien, et al., 2012) and NICU environment (Montirosso et al., 2016). Moreover, preterm infant outcomes are strongly correlated with parental mental well-being (Huhtala et al., 2014). In older children, the influence of parental education is important as well (Linsell et al., 2016).

Improving the outcomes of preterm infants is a public health goal. The first steps are to reduce the burden of preterm birth and to disseminate evidence-based medical strategies that could reduce the rates of NEC and HIV and other risk factors (Zeitlin, Manktelow, Piedvache, et al., 2016). The child's early environment, both physical and emotional, should be modified if necessary to support optimal brain development.

Early interventions in the NICU or after discharge, which are also called "developmental care" or "brain care" interventions, aim to modify environmental sources of stress (environmental approaches), to promote neurobehavioural organisation using specific techniques such as nonnutritive sucking or swaddling (behavioural approaches) and to promote parental understanding of infant behaviours (educational approaches) (Browne & White, 2011). There are multiple early interventions that are based on different theoretical frameworks with various degrees of evidence of efficacy.

Rationale

Early family-centred and developmentally oriented interventions are based mainly on the following, which support the rationale for early intervention:

Bonding and Attachment Process Theory

Bonding and attachment, which occur in the context of close and early relationships, form the basis of human development. "Bonding" refers to the very early development of emotional feelings of a mother towards her infant. Mothers experience negative feelings (sadness or anxiety) when they are separated from their children or when their ability to protect and comfort their children is blocked. Good quality bonding has a positive impact on future parenting behaviour and child development (George & Salomon, 2008). Conversely, failure to establish this early bond can have negative effects on the mother–child relationship and negatively affect the child's development.

From the perspective of the newborn, attachment stems from the baby's natural instinct to seek comfort, protection and nurture. Infants gradually develop attachments to the caregivers who respond to their physical and emotional needs. This attachment is essential to a child's stable psychosocial development and functioning (Benoit, 2004; Branchi & Cirulli, 2014; Bucci, Roberts, Danquah, & Berry, 2015).

Physical and emotional closeness that is established through sensory interactions is essential for establishing this parent–infant relationship. Further, obstacles to the initiation of the mother–child bond in case of hospitalisation may have long-term effects on the newborn's behavioural and mental development. Elective caesarean section, intrapartum hormonal manipulation, preterm delivery and bottle-feeding could alter the physiological neuroendocrine mechanisms involved in attachment and bonding (Olza-Fernández, Marín Gabriel, Gil-Sanchez, Garcia-Segura, & Arevalo, 2014).

Understanding the behavioural cues of the newborn is essential for providing responses that are adapted to his or her specific needs. Parents and NICU staff members may have difficulty understanding the behaviour of premature newborns. Skin-to-skin contact and breastfeeding represent important opportunities that support the bonding and attachment processes for hospitalised newborns in the NICU (Flacking, Lehtonen, Thomson, et al., 2012).

Brain Development and Synaptogenesis (Bourgeois, 2010)

The perinatal period and infancy are marked by major brain development, which is influenced by genetic factors, cellular interactions, innate activity and environmental stimulation (Lagercrantz & Ringstedt, 2001). Synaptogenesis is an important part of brain development that is characterised by the rapid overproduction of synapses, followed by a phase of synapse elimination (National Research Council and Institute of Medicine, 2000). The most appropriate circuits persist, depending on environmental factors. Thus, early experience could play an important role in shaping the future brain of the infant (Kolb, Mychasiuk, & Gibb, 2014). For healthy development, both "experience-expectant" experiences (specific stimulations that occur at the right time) and "experience-dependant" mechanisms (synaptic contact formation that is related to individual experience) are important (Bourgeois, 2010).

Deprivation or disorganisation of these essential environmental stimulations can permanently compromise future behavioural functioning. It is possible that the early NICU environment, including factors like hyperstimulation (such as excess sound and light), hypostimulation (e.g. a lack of vestibular stimulation) and a disorganised agenda (e.g. no difference between day and night), could negatively impact the synaptogenesis process and thus the neurofunctional outcome of hospitalised high-risk infants (Perlman, 2001).

The Family-Centred Care (FCC) Philosophy

According to the American Academy of Pediatrics, "family-*centered* care is an approach to the planning, delivery, and evaluation of health care that is grounded in a mutually beneficial partnership among patients, families, and providers that recognizes the importance of the family in the patient's life" (Institute & Family-Centered, 2012). This philosophy includes the parents as the primary caregivers in decision-making processes and in the delivery of health care. Parents are not considered to be visitors in the NICU but rather to be actors and partners of the medical and nursing staff. Their expertise is recognised, supported and valued (Institute for Patient and Family-centered Care, 2016). In contrast, with the more limited family-*focused* model of care, a professional provides care "from the position of an expert, assessing the patient and family, recommending a treatment or intervention and creating a plan for the family to follow" without clear participation of the parents in the decision-making process (Institute for Patient and Family-centered Care, 2016).

In the past, NICU practices and culture have focused exclusively on emergency and technical tasks. NICU professionals have been encouraged to suppress their emotional involvement in all clinical situations (Anand & Hall, 2008). This explains why implementing effective FCC approaches in the NICU requires major changes in practices, education and culture (Karazivan, Dumez, Flora, et al., 2015). As the parents also experience stress during the newborn's stay in the NICU, it is important to consider approaches that will best support them in their role.

According to this theoretical framework, the following could be considered necessary for improving the neurodevelopmental outcomes of high-risk newborns:

- The need for appropriate sensory input to enhance brain development in the NICU
- Close mother–child physical and emotional proximity, even when the newborn is hospitalised
- Support for the parents both during the hospitalisation and the transition to home in order to help them cope with stress and to improve their mental well-being

Evaluation

The effects of these early interventions must be rigorously evaluated to understand the underlying mechanisms, to analyse the efficacy of the components, to minimise the human and financial costs and to develop research in unproven domains (Sizun & Westrup, 2004). However, scientific evaluation of family-centred interventions raises specific methodological issues.

Evaluation Issues

Randomised control trials (RCTs) are the gold standard for clinical research and the basis of evidence-based medicine. Unfortunately, it is more difficult to design RCTs for non-pharmacological interventions, and the designs are subject to specific biases (Jadad & Enkin, 2007).

- Some intervention programmes need preliminary staff training before the trial begins, and the care team may have difficulties in using the previous approach.
- The intervention may extend over several weeks or months and be implemented to varying degrees over time, making it difficult to investigate the causality between the intervention and the outcome.
- Recruitment of the control population can be difficult, as parents may be reluctant to accept the inclusion of their child in the control group.
- "Contamination" between control and treatment groups needs to be carefully avoided. That is, individuals allocated to a control group may inadvertently receive some aspects of the intervention if they are in physical proximity to the treated group. Conversely, it is important to check whether patients in the experimental group receive the full intervention (quality and amount).
- The RCT may not always be ethically feasible in the context of family-based interventions, as for breastfeeding studies.
- Blinding (for the patient, parents and/or professionals) is difficult, or even impossible, for non-pharmacological interventions.
- The control group may receive the current standard of care, but the definition of the current standard of care changes over time.
- Choosing the main outcome is difficult. Many trials are based on the evaluation of a composite outcome, such as death and development (e.g. the Bayley scale) at 2 years of age. As suggested by Marlow (2015), the robustness of this outcome and the direct causal pathway from the intervention to death and disability must be questioned.
- The RCT could fail to reflect the more complex reality of the babies, parents and staff experiences in the NICU. RCT design is not always suited to explore all aspects of an intervention. For example, measures of the quality of the mother–child bonding experience over time, parental and infant quality of life parameters, parental skills in interacting with the premature infant and nursing staff

motivation to use early interventions are not easily understood using standardised RCT designs (Pierrat, Goubet, Peifer, & Sizun, 2007).

- The detailed descriptions of non-pharmacological interventions are often insufficient (Glasziou, Meats, Heneghan, & Shepperd, 2008). Lack of sufficient information to replicate intervention protocols is a methodological concern. A checklist, such as the Template for Intervention Description and Replication (TIDieR), could be used to help trial replication and to allow identification of common elements across different interventions (Hoffmann, Glasziou, Boutron, et al., 2014).

Alternative Research Strategies

Alternative research strategies could be helpful for evaluating interventions.

To avoid contamination bias, it has been suggested that cluster randomisation be used rather than individual randomisation. Unfortunately, a cluster trial needs a much larger patient sample than a RCT and can be susceptible to recruitment bias (Torgerson, 2001). Participant-informed consent is also challenging (Giraudeau, Caille, Le Gouge, & Ravaud, 2012). It has been suggested that a cluster randomised trial is only more efficient than individual randomisation when contamination exceeds 30% (Torgerson, 2001).

- When it could be unethical or impractical to do random allocation, non-randomised studies could be used to evaluate the impact of an intervention. A careful design is needed to limit the bias and to control for confounders, exposure measurement, completeness of follow-up and blinded outcome assessment (Deeks, Dinnes, D'Amico, et al., 2003). For instance, observational studies have been designed to measure the impact of mother's milk or developmental care on newborns (Pierrat, Coquelin, Cuttini, et al., 2016; Rozé et al., 2012).
- Qualitative research methods can be used to study the knowledge and behaviour of parents and staff members, their compliance with developmental practices and facilitators and barriers to the implementation of evidence-based techniques (Pope & May, 2006). Qualitative methods locate the observer or researcher within the natural environment and consist of interpretations and representations that are not easily measured using quantitative methods. These methods have been used, for example, to study issues related to breastfeeding for preterm newborns (Alves et al., 2013) and the experiences of parents in the NICU (Provenzi & Santoro, 2015).
- Benchmarking is a strategy by which the practices of the best-performing units are identified, analysed, adopted and adapted in order to improve the performance of other units (Walsh, 2003). One example of benchmarking in developmental care is the Neonatal Intensive Care Quality Improvement Collaborative Year 2000 (NIC/Q 2000) supported by the Vermont Oxford Network. Several themes were explored in this study, including the prevention of cerebral lesions

in very low birth weight newborns (Carteaux et al., 2003). Developmental care was among the ten selected "potentially best practices". The authors reported that despite a scarcity of empirical evidence, this strategy was found at each of the four sites chosen for the quality of their results.

– Animal studies are necessary for medical research when it is impractical or unethical to use humans (American Physiological Society, 2016). For instance, the negative impact of early mother–child separation in the neonatal period has been demonstrated in rodents (Meaney & Szyf, 2005) and mammals (Henry, Richard-Yris, Tordjman, et al., 2009).

Impact of Family-Centred Early Intervention

Early interventions can be administered during the NICU stay and/or after discharge. Various programmes have been evaluated. The theoretical framework, nature and agenda of the interventions differ in different studies.

– The *Newborn Individualized Developmental Care and Assessment Program* (NIDCAP) is an individualised developmental approach to support and care that is based on reading each preterm infant's behavioural cues and then formulating a care plan. This plan enhances and builds upon the strengths of the infant and family and involves the parents as the primary caregivers of the baby. Based on the synactive theory of development as its theoretical framework, NIDCAP uses behavioural observation as a tool to understand the needs of the baby and his or her current developmental goals (Als & McAnulty, 2011). Within each subsystem (autonomic, motoric, state, interaction), the behaviours are interpreted as approach (stable/engagement) or as self-regulation or stress (unstable/disengagement) behaviours. NIDCAP implementation requires a 2-year training for health professionals plus active involvement of the medical, nursing and administrative hospital leaders in order to change some aspects of the NICU and hospital system. Clinical trials have suggested that NIDCAP has a positive impact on the brain at term age as measured by behavioural, functional and anatomic parameters (Als, Duffy, McAnulty, et al., 2004). A meta-analysis concluded that NIDCAP had a positive impact on the length of hospitalisation and on development at 9–12 months of age and no measured impact on the composite primary outcomes of death or major sensorineural disability at 18 months (corrected age) (Ohlsson & Jacobs, 2013). The use of this composite outcome in a meta-analysis of 32–34-week preterm infants has been criticised (Haumont, Amiel-Tison, Casper, et al., 2013), but small groups have reported some positive impact on medium- or long-term outcomes (Kleberg, Westrup, & Stjernqvist, 2000, McAnulty, Duffy, Kosta, et al., 2012). Access to the training is possible through the NIDCAP federation international (NFI), which offers training in America and Europe in different languages (www.nidcap.org).

- The *Creating Opportunities for Parent Empowerment* (COPE) programme, which is based on self-regulation and control theories, is designed to help parents learn about the NICU environment, to understand how their premature baby may react to the environment and to identify ways in which they can support their baby's development (Melnyk, Feinstein, Alpert-Gillis, et al., 2006). The educational process is based on specific materials, including a CD, a book with developmental information and magnets that list developmental milestones. The content in the booklet addresses what the NICU may look or sound like, acknowledges that it is a distressing time for parents and encourages parents to engage in activities such as recording developmental milestones, writing about their baby and taking pictures to document growth. A single RCT that involved 260 26–34-week gestational age newborns from two NICUs suggested that the use of COPE resulted in a 3.8-day shorter length of stay in the NICU, less stress in the NICU and less depression and anxiety at 2 months corrected infant age.
- The *Family Nurture Intervention (FNI)* is designed to establish and support the mother–infant emotional connection (Welch & Myers, 2016). The FNI is based on a "calming process" between the mother and infant. Interactions between the mother and infant are facilitated and include odour-cloth exchange, sustained touch, vocal soothing and eye contact. When the infant is medically stable, the interactions include holding and calming sessions. A single-centre RCT involving 115 families with 150 preterm infants at 26–34 weeks postmenstrual age demonstrated that the mothers had better maternal sensitivity during caregiving in the NICU and when the infant was 4 months old as well as decreased symptoms of anxiety and depression. The infants showed advanced maturation in frontal brain activity at term age. At 18 months, FNI infants showed improved cognitive and language scores as measured by the Bailey III score and a decreased risk for autism (M-CHAT) (Welch & Myers, 2016).
- *The Infant Behavioral Assessment and Intervention Program* (IBAIP), like the NIDCAP, is based on the synactive theory of development. The IBAIP is designed to support infants with developmental risks at their homes from term to approximately 8 months of age. By focusing on environmental, behavioural and early developmental factors, this programme aims to support the infant's self-regulatory competence as well as the infant's multiple developmental functions in an integrative way via responsive and positive parent–infant interactions. An RCT at 7 Dutch NICUs involving 176 preterm newborns <32 weeks postmenstrual age or birth weight < 1500 g demonstrated significant and clinically relevant intervention effects on cognitive development at 6 months and at 5.5 years of corrected age and on motor development at 6, 12 and 24 months and 5.5 years of corrected age. Subgroup analyses indicated improved developmental outcomes in the most vulnerable (very preterm and very low birth weight infants) such as infants with bronchopulmonary dysplasia (Van Hus, Jeukens-Visser, Koldewijn, et al., 2016).
- The *Mother-Infant Transaction Program* (MITP) is based on the "transactional model of development" and is influenced by the conceptual design of the

Neonatal Behavioral Assessment Scale by Brazelton (Ravn, Smith, Lindemann, et al., 2011). The MITP trains mothers to recognize and support the needs of the individual infant and to initiate positive stimulation based on the mother's learned appreciation of her infant's sensory regulation and stimulation needs. Seven 1-h sessions take place in the hospital during the last week before discharge, and four sessions take place during the first 3 months at home, with the infant, mother and father present. A 1-h debriefing session has been added to the modified version of the programme (MITP-M). Different RCTs have been conducted to test the efficacy of the MITP and the MITP-M. One trial involving 106 preterm newborns born between 30 and 36 weeks suggested that the MITP reduced postpartum depression but did not find any positive effects on self-reported maternal stress or perceived infant communication (Ravn et al., 2011). Another trial in Norway that involved 146 newborns with birth weights <2000 g reported a higher score of maternal sensitivity/responsiveness at 1 year, fewer behavioural problems reported by parents at 5 years (Nordhov, Rønning, Ulvund, et al., 2012) and fewer attention problems and better adaptation to school at ages 7 and 9 years in the intervention group (Landsem et al., 2015).

–   The *Infant Health and Development Program* (IHDP) is an educational intervention based on the biosocial model of early development. The intervention consisted of home visits every week for the first year of life and every other week in the second and third years, daily centre-based education beginning at 12 months (corrected for the duration of gestation) continuing until 36 months of age and parent support groups. A large multisite RCT included nearly 1000 newborns with a gestational age of less than 37 weeks, 377 in the intervention group versus 608 in the control group, stratified into two low birth weight groups (lighter, ≤2000 g, versus heavier, 2001–2500 g). Infants in the intervention group had higher IQ scores and fewer behavioural problems than those in the control group at age 3 years. At 8 years, there were no significant differences between the intervention and control groups for full-scale IQ or for the verbal or performance IQ subscales. A significant difference in full-scale IQ was demonstrated only for the heavier low birth weight intervention group (McCarton, Brooks-Gunn, Wallace, et al., 1997). There were no statistically significant differences in the risk for special education, remedial reading, remedial math or speech therapy (Litt, Glymour, Hauser-Cram, et al., 2015).

–   The *Victorian Infant Brain Studies* intervention (VIBeS Plus) consisted of nine 1.5- to 2-h home visits during the first year of life that were conducted by a psychologist and a physiotherapist. The intervention aimed to educate the parents "about infant self-regulation and techniques for improving postural stability, coordination, and strength and to support the parents' mental health and parent-infant relationship throughout the first year". One site RCT included 120 very preterm infants (<30 weeks). There were no statistically significant differences between the treatment and the control groups at 2 or 4 years of age in terms of cognitive, language or motor composite scores (Spencer-Smith, Spittle, Doyle, et al., 2012; Spittle, Anderson, Lee, et al., 2010). However, children in the intervention group were reported by their primary caregivers to exhibit fewer externalising and dysregulated behaviours and showed increased competence compared to control subjects. Caregivers in the intervention group had fewer anxiety symptoms than caretakers in the control group (Spencer-Smith et al., 2012).

Systematic Review of Early Interventions in Preterm Newborns

There are several recent systematic reviews of the effects of early interventions in preterm newborns. They differ according to their objectives, research questions and criteria for selecting studies (Table 17.1). The usual limitations of these studies are discussed, including small sample sizes; clinical, methodological and statistical heterogeneity among the studies; lack of homogeneity in the samples in terms of sociodemographic data; changes to the intended delivery mode of the intervention; unequal distribution of neurological impairment between groups; interventions conducted only in Western cultures (USA, Australia, Norway); and randomisation bias (Benzies et al., 2013; Evans et al., 2014; Frolek Clark & Schlabach, 2013; Herd et al., 2014; Spittle et al., 2015; Vanderveen et al., 2009; van Wassenaer-Leemhuis et al., 2016).

Role of the Mother's Voice in Early Intervention Programmes

The common elements in these early interventions include developmental support for the child, parenting education and parental psychosocial support (Benzies et al., 2013). None of these programmes focus specifically on the mother's voice, but all support the mother–child relationship in general, including promoting sensitive communication using vocal, visual and behavioural channels. Most of the interventions are "cue-based" rather than "protocol-based" approaches that are designed to support the "sensitive parenting" development process.

Implementation

Family-centred programmes can be described as complex. An intervention is complex when it is composed of multiple interacting components, when changes in behaviours are required in those who deliver or receive the intervention and when a degree of flexibility is accepted (Craig, Dieppe, Macintyre, et al., 2008). The absence of a measured positive impact of the intervention can be due to incorrect or incomplete implementation. There are important differences in evidence-based family-centred practices between countries in Northern vs Southern Europe

Table 17.1 Systematic reviews of randomised controlled trials (RCTs) of early interventions for preterm newborns

Reference	Research domain	Included studies	Findings	Limitations as reported by the authors of the review
Vanderveen, Bassler, Robertson, and Kirpalani (2009)	Interventions that involve parents and aimed to improve neurodevelopment at 12 months corrected age or older	25 RCTs	At 12 months, the intervention group had significantly higher mental and physical performance scores. At 24 months, the mental performance scores improved more in the intervention group, but the physical performance scores were not statistically significantly different. The improvement in neurodevelopmental outcome was not sustained at 36 months or 5 years	Clinical, methodological and sometimes statistical heterogeneity among the studies
Frolek Clark and Schlabach (2013)	Interventions used by occupational therapists that aimed to improve cognitive development in children from birth to age 5	13 RCTs	The intervention group showed greater improvement in early cognitive development in infancy and at preschool age with inconclusive evidence for school-age children. Educating parents of preterm infants to be more sensitive to their child's needs and more responsive in interactions increased cognitive outcomes and joint attention	

(continued)

Table 17.1 (continued)

Reference	Research domain	Included studies	Findings	Limitations as reported by the authors of the review
Benzies, Magill-Evans, Hayden, and Ballantyne (2013)	Categorisation of the key components of early intervention programs: psychosocial support for the parents, parenting education and developmental support for the child Determination of the effects of the components on parents and preterm infants	18 RCTs (only 11 for parent outcome)	Focusing only on parent education or parent education plus child developmental support had no effect on parental stress Studies with positive effects on anxiety or depressive symptoms showed positive effects on child development over the short term and up to 24 months Studies that showed positive effects on maternal sensitivity/responsiveness were associated with positive infant mood at 12 months	Lack of sociodemographically homogeneous samples Only English studies Significant heterogeneity among the studies
Herd, Whittingham, Sanders, et al. (2014)	Preventative parenting interventions conducted starting at birth that aimed to improve the child's internalising and externalising behaviour	12 RCTs 3 pooled for the meta-analysis	Small but significant effect on child behaviour The MITP-M and the VIBeS Plus programme achieved more lasting behavioural outcomes using a shorter intervention and lower dosage than the other preterm parenting interventions	Only data from 3 of 12 RCTs could be pooled for the meta-analysis Interventions conducted only in Western cultures (USA, Australia, Norway)

Evans, Whittingham, Sanders, et al. (2014)	Parenting interventions that aimed to improve the relationship outcomes between mothers and their preterm infants	11 RCTs and 6 quasi-RCTs	Seven of the interventions found improvements in the quality of the mother–infant relationship for mothers Four of the interventions found improvement in the quality of the mother–infant relationship for infants, with effect sizes ranging from small to large	Heterogeneity of the interventions and of the assessment measures
Spittle, Orton, Anderson, et al. (2015)	Early interventions (posthospital discharge) that aimed to prevent motor or cognitive impairment	12 RCTs with appropriate allocation concealment	Cognitive outcomes improved at infancy and at preschool age, but the effect was not sustained at school age The interventions had a significant effect on motor outcome Interventions had no effect on the rate of cerebral palsy among survivors	Significant heterogeneity among studies for cognitive outcomes at infancy and at school age
van Wassenaer-Leemhuis, Jeukens-Visser, van Hus, et al. (2016)	Early preventive and home-based (family-centred) interventions (posthospital discharge) that aimed to improve cognitive development at age two (narrative review)	6 RCTs extracted from the meta-analysis by Spittle et al. (2015)	Four of the six programs led to improved child cognitive and/or motor development Two programs (MITP and IBAIP), which were focused on responsive parenting, improved cognitive outcome until 5 years of age Only IBAIP improved both motor and cognitive outcomes until 5 years of age The programs that also focused on maternal anxiety remediation led to improved maternal mental well-being	

IBAIP Infant Behavioral Assessment and Intervention Program, *MITP* Mother–Infant Transaction Program, *VIBeS* Victorian Infant Brain Studies

(Greisen, Mirante, Haumont, et al., 2009). Thus, it could be important to analyse cultural or organisational factors that affect the implementation of these early interventions (Chaudoir, Dugan, & Barr, 2013).

Conclusion

Evidence supports the use of early intervention programmes in the NICU or after discharge for preterm newborns. Interventions that are cue based and family centred appear the most efficacious. The specific role of the mother's voice in these early interventions is complex and difficult to evaluate. Additional research is needed to evaluate the cost–benefit balance, the impact at school age, the most adapted implementation strategies and the feasibility of large-scale training and dissemination.

> **Key Messages**
> - Evidence supports the use of early intervention programmes in the NICU or after discharge for preterm newborns.
> - None of the early intervention programmes focus specifically on the mother's voice, but all support the mother–child relationship in general, including promoting sensitive communication using vocal, visual and behavioural channels.
> - Additional research is needed to evaluate the cost–benefit balance, the impact at school age, the most adapted implementation strategies and the feasibility of large-scale training and dissemination.

References

Als, H., Duffy, F. H., McAnulty, G. B., et al. (2004). Early experience alters brain function and structure. *Pediatrics, 113*(4), 846–855.

Als, H., & McAnulty, G. B. (2011). The Newborn Individualized Developmental Care and Assessment Program (NIDCAP) with Kangaroo Mother Care (KMC): Comprehensive care for preterm infants. *Current Women's Health Reviews, 7*(3), 288–301.

Alves, E., Rodrigues, C., Fraga, S., Barros, H., & Silva, S. (2013). Parents' views on factors that help or hinder breast milk supply in neonatal care units: systematic review. *Archives of Disease in Childhood-Fetal and Neonatal Edition, Fetalneonatal-2013, 98*(6), F511–F517.

American Physiological Society. *Why do scientists use animals in research?* http://www.the-aps.org/mm/sciencepolicy/animalresearch/publications/animals/quest1.html. Accessed October 5, 2016.

Anand, K. J., & Hall, R. W. (2008). Love, pain, and intensive care. *Pediatrics, 121*(4), 825–827.

Ancel, P.Y., Goffinet, F., EPIPAGE-2 Writing Group, et al. (2015). Survival and morbidity of preterm children born at 22 through 34 weeks' gestation in France in 2011: Results of the EPIPAGE-2 cohort study. *JAMA Pediatrics, 169*(3), 230–238.

Benoit, D. (2004). Infant-parent attachment: Definition, types, antecedents, measurement and outcome. *Paediatrics & Child Health, 9*(8), 541–545.

Benzies, K. M., Magill-Evans, J. E., Hayden, K. A., & Ballantyne, M. (2013). Key components of early intervention programs for preterm infants and their parents: A systematic review and meta-analysis. *BMC Pregnancy and Childbirth, 13 Suppl 1*, S10.

Bourgeois, J. P. (2010). Reflections on the origin of the human brain. In H. Lagercrantz, M. Hanson, L. R. Ment, & D. M. Peebles (Eds.), *The newborn brain: neuroscience and clinical applications.* Cambridge, UK: Cambridge University Press.

Branchi, I., & Cirulli, F. (2014). Early experiences: Building up the tools to face the challenges of adult life. *Developmental Psychobiology, 56*(8), 1661–1674.

Browne, J. V., & White, R. D. (2011). Foundations of developmental care. *Clinics in Perinatology, 38*(4), xv–xvii.

Bucci, S., Roberts, N. H., Danquah, A. N., & Berry, K. (2015). Using attachment theory to inform the design and delivery of mental health services: A systematic review of the literature. *Psychology and Psychotherapy, 88*, 1–20.

Carteaux, P., Cohen, H., Check, J., George, J., McKinley, P., Lewis, W., et al. (2003). Evaluation and development of potentially better practices for the prevention of brain hemorrhage and ischemic brain injury in very low birth weight infants. *Pediatrics, 111*, e489–e496.

Chan, E., Leong, P., Malouf, R., & Quigley, M. A. (2016). Long-term cognitive and school outcomes of late-preterm and early-term births: A systematic review. *Child: Care, Health and Development, 42*, 297–312.

Chaudoir, S. R., Dugan, A. G., & Barr, C. H. (2013). Measuring factors affecting implementation of health innovations: A systematic review of structural, organizational, provider, patient, and innovation level measures. *Implementation Science, 17*(8), 22.

Costeloe, K. L., Hennessy, E. M., Haider, S., et al. (2012). Short term outcomes after extreme preterm birth in England: Comparison of two birth cohorts in 1995 and 2006 (the EPICure studies). *BMJ, 345*, e7976.

Craig, P., Dieppe, P., Macintyre, S., et al. (2008). Developing and evaluating complex interventions: The new Medical Research Council guidance. *BMJ, 337*, 979–983.

Deeks, J. J., Dinnes, J., D'Amico, R., et al. (2003). Evaluating non-randomised intervention studies. *Health Technology Assessment, 7*(27), 1–173.

Evans, T., Whittingham, K., Sanders, M., et al. (2014). Are parenting interventions effective in improving the relationship between mothers and their preterm infants? *Infant Behavior & Development, 37*(2), 131–154.

EXPRESS Group, Fellman, V., Hellström-Westas, L., Norman, M., et al. (2009). One-year survival of extremely preterm infants after active perinatal care in Sweden. *JAMA, 301*(21), 2225–2233.

Flacking, R., Lehtonen, L., Thomson, G., et al. (2012). Separation and Closeness Experiences in the Neonatal Environment (SCENE) group. Closeness and separation in neonatal intensive care. *Acta Paediatrica, 101*, 1032–1037.

Frolek Clark, G. J., & Schlabach, T. L. (2013). Systematic review of occupational therapy interventions to improve cognitive development in children ages birth-5 years. *The American Journal of Occupational Therapy, 67*(4), 425–430.

George, C., & Salomon, J. (2008). The caregiving system: A behavioral systems approach to parenting. In J. Cassidy & P. R. Shaver (Eds.), *Handbook of attachment: Theory, research and clinical applications* (pp. 833–856). New York, NY: The Guilford Press.

Giraudeau, B., Caille, A., Le Gouge, A., & Ravaud, P. (2012). Participant informed consent in cluster randomized trials: Review. *PLoS One, 7*(7), e40436.

Glasziou, P., Meats, E., Heneghan, C., & Shepperd, S. (2008). What is missing from descriptions of treatment in trials and reviews? *BMJ, 336*, 1472–1474.

Greisen, G., Mirante, N., Haumont, D. et al. ESF Network. (2009). Parents, siblings and grandparents in the neonatal intensive care unit. A survey of policies in eight European countries. *Acta Paediatrica, 98*, 1744–1750.

Haumont, D., Amiel-Tison, C., Casper, C., et al. (2013). NIDCAP and developmental care: a European perspective. *Pediatrics, 132*(2), e551–e552.

Henry, S., Richard-Yris, M. A., Tordjman, S., et al. (2009). Neonatal handling affects durably bonding and social development. *PLoS One, 4*(4), e5216.

Herd, M., Whittingham, K., Sanders, M., et al. (2014). Efficacy of preventative parenting interventions for parents of preterm infants on later child behavior: A systematic review and meta-analysis. *Infant Mental Health Journal, 35*, 630–641.

Hoffmann, T., Glasziou, P., Boutron, I., et al. (2014). Better reporting of interventions: Template for intervention description and replication (TIDieR) checklist and guide. *BMJ, 348*, g1687.

Huhtala M., Korja R., Lehtonen L. et al.; PIPARI Study Group. (2014). Associations between parental psychological well-being and socio-emotional development in 5-year-old preterm children. *Early Human Development, 90*(3), 119–124.

Institute, F. P., & Family-Centered, C. A. R. E. (2012). Patient-and family-centered care and the pediatrician's role. *Pediatrics, 129*(2), 394.

Institute for Patient and Family-Centered Care (2016). *Is there a difference between family-centered care and family-focused care?* http://www.ipfcc.org/faq.html. Accessed October 5, 2016.

Jadad, A. R., & Enkin, M. (2007). Bias in randomized controlled trials. In A. R. Jadad & M. Enkin (Eds.), *Randomized controlled trials: questions, answers, and musings* (pp. 29–47). Malden, MA: Blackwell Publishing.

Jarjour, I. T. (2015). Neurodevelopmental outcome after extreme prematurity: A review of the literature. *Pediatric Neurology, 52*(2), 143–152.

Karazivan, P., Dumez, V., Flora, L., et al. (2015). The patient-as-partner approach in health care: A conceptual framework for a necessary transition. *Academic Medicine, 90*(4), 437–441.

Kleberg, A., Westrup, B., & Stjernqvist, K. (2000). Developmental outcome, child behaviour and mother-child interaction at 3 years of age following Newborn Individualized Developmental Care and Intervention Program (NIDCAP) intervention. *Early Human Development, 60*(2), 123–135.

Kolb, B., Mychasiuk, R., & Gibb, R. (2014). Brain development, experience, and behavior. *Pediatric Blood & Cancer, 61*(10), 1720–1723.

Lagercrantz, H., & Ringstedt, T. (2001). Organization of the neuronal circuits in the central nervous system during development. *Acta Paediatrica, 90*(7), 707–715.

Landsem, I. P., Handegård, B. H., Ulvund, S. E., Tunby, J., Kaaresen, P. I., & Rønning, J. A. (2015). Does an early intervention influence behavioral development until age 9 in children born prematurely? *Child Development, 86*(4), 1063–1079.

Linsell, L., Malouf, R., Morris, J., Kurinczuk, J. J., & Marlow, N. (2015). Prognostic factors for poor cognitive development in children born very preterm or with very low birth weight: A systematic review. *JAMA Pediatrics, 169*(12), 1162–1172.

Linsell, L., Malouf, R., Morris, J., Kurinczuk, J. J., & Marlow, N. (2016). Prognostic factors for cerebral palsy and motor impairment in children born very preterm or very low birthweight: A systematic review. *Developmental Medicine and Child Neurology, 58*(6), 554–569.

Litt, J. S., Glymour, M., Hauser-Cram, P., et al. (2015). The effect of the Infant Health and Development Program on special education use at school age. *The Journal of Pediatrics, 166*, 457–462.

Marlow, N. (2015). Is survival and neurodevelopmental impairment at 2 years of age the gold standard outcome for neonatal studies? *Archives of Disease in Childhood. Fetal and Neonatal Edition, 100*(1), F82–F84.

McAnulty, G., Duffy, F. H., Kosta, S., et al. (2012). School age effects of the newborn individualized developmental care and assessment program for medically low-risk preterm infants: Preliminary findings. *Journal of Clinical Neonatology, 1*(4), 184–194.

McCarton, C. M., Brooks-Gunn, J., Wallace, I. F., et al. (1997). Results at age 8 years of early intervention for low-birth-weight premature infants. The Infant Health and Development Program. *JAMA, 277*, 126–132.

Meaney, M. J., & Szyf, M. (2005). Maternal care as a model for experience-dependent chromatin plasticity? *Trends in Neurosciences, 28*(9), 456–463.

Melnyk, B. M., Feinstein, N. F., Alpert-Gillis, L., et al. (2006). Reducing premature infants' length of stay and improving parents' mental health outcomes with the Creating Opportunities for Parent Empowerment (COPE) neonatal intensive care unit program: A randomized, controlled trial. *Pediatrics, 118*(5), e1414–e1427.

Mercer, J. (2006). *Understanding attachment: Parenting, child care, and emotional development.* Westport, CT: Praeger Publishers.

Montirosso, R., Giusti, L., Del Prete, A., Zanini, R., Bellù, R., & Borgatti, R. (2016). Does quality of developmental care in NICUs affect health-related quality of life in 5-y-old children born preterm? *Pediatric Research, 80*(6), 824–828..

National Research Council and Institute of Medicine. (2000). From neurons to neighborhoods: The science of early childhood development. Committee on Integrating the Science of Early Childhood Development. In J. P. Shonkoff & D. A. Phillips (Eds.), *Board on Children, Youth, and Families, Commission on Behavioral and Social Sciences and Education.* Washington, D.C.: National Academy Press.

Nordhov, S. M., Rønning, J. A., Ulvund, S. E., et al. (2012). Early intervention improves behavioral outcomes for preterm infants: Randomized controlled trial. *Pediatrics, 129*(1), e9–e16.

Ohlsson, A., & Jacobs, S. E. (2013). NIDCAP: A systematic review and meta-analyses of randomized controlled trials. *Pediatrics, 131*(3), e881–e893.

Olza-Fernández, I., Marín Gabriel, M. A., Gil-Sanchez, A., Garcia-Segura, L. M., & Arevalo, M. A. (2014). Neuroendocrinology of childbirth and mother-child attachment: The basis of an etiopathogenic model of perinatal neurobiological disorders. *Frontiers in Neuroendocrinology, 35*(4), 459–472.

Perlman, J. M. (2001). Neurobehavioral deficits in premature graduates of intensive care – Potential medical and neonatal environmental risk factors. *Pediatrics, 108*(6), 1339–1348.

Pierrat V., Coquelin A., Cuttini M. et al. and the EPIPAGE-2 Neurodevelopmental Care Writing Group. (2016). Translating neurodevelopmental care policies into practice: The experience of neonatal ICUs in France-The EPIPAGE-2 Cohort Study. *Pediatric Critical Care Medicine, 17*(10), 957–967.

Pierrat, V., Goubet, N., Peifer, K., & Sizun, J. (2007). How can we evaluate developmental care practices prior to their implementation in a neonatal intensive care unit? *Early Human Development, 83*(7), 415–418.

Pope, C., & Mays, N. (2006). *Qualitative research in health care.* Oxford: Blackwell Publishing.

Provenzi, L., & Santoro, E. (2015). The lived experience of fathers of preterm infants in the neonatal intensive care unit: A systematic review of qualitative studies. *Journal of Clinical Nursing, 24*(13–14), 1784–1794.

Ravn, I. H., Smith, L., Lindemann, R., et al. (2011). Effect of early intervention on social interaction between mothers and preterm infants at 12 months of age: A randomized controlled trial. *Infant Behavior & Development, 34*(2), 215–225.

Rozé, J. C., Darmaun, D., Boquien, C. Y., et al. (2012). The apparent breastfeeding paradox in very preterm infants: Relationship between breast feeding, early weight gain and neurodevelopment based on results from two cohorts, EPIPAGE and LIFT. *BMJ Open, 2*(2), e000834.

Sizun, J., & Westrup, B. (2004). Early developmental care for preterm neonates: A call for more research. *Archives of Disease in Childhood. Fetal and Neonatal Edition, 89*(5), F384–F388.

Spencer-Smith, M. M., Spittle, A. J., Doyle, L. W., et al. (2012). Long-term benefits of home-based preventive care for preterm infants: A randomized trial. *Pediatrics, 130*, 1094–1101.

Spittle, A., Orton, J., Anderson, P. J., et al. (2015). Early developmental intervention programmes provided post hospital discharge to prevent motor and cognitive impairment in preterm infants. *Cochrane Database of Systematic Reviews, 11*, CD005495.

Spittle, A. J., Anderson, P. J., Lee, K. J., et al. (2010). Preventive care at home for very preterm infants improves infant and caregiver outcomes at 2 years. *Pediatrics, 126*, e171–e178.

Torgerson, D. J. (2001). Contamination in trials: Is cluster randomisation the answer? *BMJ, 322*(7282), 355–357.

Van Hus, J., Jeukens-Visser, M., Koldewijn, K., et al. (2016). Early intervention leads to long-term developmental improvements in very preterm infants, especially infants with bronchopulmonary dysplasia. *Acta Paediatrica, 105*(7), 773–781.

van Wassenaer-Leemhuis, A. G., Jeukens-Visser, M., van Hus, J. W., et al. (2016). Rethinking preventive post-discharge intervention programmes for very preterm infants and their parents. *Developmental Medicine and Child Neurology, 58*(Suppl 4), 67–73.

Vanderveen, J. A., Bassler, D., Robertson, C. M. T., & Kirpalani, H. (2009). Early interventions involving parents to improve neurodevelopmental outcomes of premature infants: A meta-analysis. *Journal of Perinatology, 29*, 343–351.

Walsh, M. C. (2003). Benchmarking: Techniques to improve neonatal care: Uses and abuses. *Clinics in Perinatology, 30*, 343–350.

Welch, M. G., & Myers, M. M. (2016). Advances in family-based interventions in the neonatal ICU. *Current Opinion in Pediatrics, 28*(2), 163–169.

Zeitlin, J., Manktelow, B.N., Piedvache, A. et al.; EPICE Research Group. (2016). Use of evidence based practices to improve survival without severe morbidity for very preterm infants: Results from the EPICE population based cohort. *BMJ, 54*, i2976.

Index

© Springer International Publishing AG 2017   329
M. Filippa et al. (eds.), *Early Vocal Contact and Preterm Infant Brain
Development*, DOI 10.1007/978-3-319-65077-7